The Yoga of Power

The YOGA *of* POWER

Yoga as Political Thought and Practice in India

SUNILA S. KALÉ AND
CHRISTIAN LEE NOVETZKE

COLUMBIA UNIVERSITY PRESS *NEW YORK*

Columbia University Press
Publishers Since 1893
New York   Chichester, West Sussex

Library of Congress Cataloging-in-Publication Data
Names: Kalé, Sunila S., 1973– author. | Novetzke, Christian Lee, 1969– author.
Title: The yoga of power : political thought and practice in India /
Sunila S. Kalé and Christian Lee Novetzke.
Description: New York : Columbia University Press, [2025] |
Includes bibliographical references and index.
Identifiers: LCCN 2024022791 (print) | LCCN 2024022792 (ebook) |
ISBN 9780231179249 (hardback) | ISBN 9780231220019 (trade paperback) |
ISBN 9780231549462 (ebook)
Subjects: LCSH: Yoga—History. | India—Politics and government.
Classification: LCC BL1238.52 .K353 2025 (print) | LCC BL1238.52 (ebook) |
DDC 320.55—dc23/eng/20240627

Cover design: Julia Kushnirsky
Cover image: The Picture Art Collection / Alamy Stock Photo

We dedicate this book to the memory of

आई

Pushpa Vitthal Paranjape

1926–2023

Contents

CONTENTS

Preface

IN 2014–2015, yoga and politics were in the air. Three events around this time prompted us to think about the interconnections between yoga and the political world. The first took place in the domain of U.S. legal politics. A dispute between parents of elementary schoolchildren and a local public school in Encinitas, California, reached the state's appeals court for a final judgment in 2015. Since 2011, the public school had been offering yoga instruction to its students, supported by a grant from the Pattabhi Jois Foundation, a private yoga organization. The objecting parents argued that yoga instruction contravened the Establishment Clause of the U.S. Constitution's First Amendment, which is understood to mean that government institutions cannot "establish" or support any specific religion. They further argued that yoga was a Hindu practice and that performing yoga poses was akin to reciting prayers or, as one expert witness called it, a kind of "camouflage" for the real purpose of proselyting Hinduism. In its defense, the school system argued that yoga, as it was being taught in its curriculum, was a form of meditative exercise with no relationship to any religion or ideology.[1] The judge ruled, paradoxically, that yoga is both religious and not religious, and that the public school's yoga instruction fell into the nonreligious category; therefore, it did not violate First Amendment protections.

A second intersection in 2015 occurred in the field of cultural politics, where there was a surge of public debate and discussion in North America about whether yoga, as it was taught and practiced outside India, was a form of cultural appropriation. In November 2015, a free yoga course at the University of Ottawa was abruptly cancelled. The leaders of the Student Federation that made the decision to terminate the course argued that yoga was part of "sacred spiritual practices" that were being decontextualized and stripped from their rightful cultural owners, who were oppressed groups marginalized by "colonialism and western supremacy."[2] A year after the course's cancellation, it was reinstated, but this time with a person of Indian-Canadian origin as the instructor.

A third intersection of yoga and politics unfolded in the world of international relations in the wake of India's 2014 parliamentary elections, which brought to power the Bharatiya Janata Party as India's governing party and Narendra Modi as prime minister. Modi addressed the United Nations General Assembly for the first time in late 2014 in a speech in which yoga appeared prominently. He suggested that yoga could offer a solution to the world's most pressing challenges, like global climate change, and called for the UN to recognize yoga's global importance, a motion that was adopted in the General Assembly by 177 of 193 member states. Since 2015, International Day of Yoga has been celebrated in many parts of the world every June 21. Some at the time considered Modi's invocation of yoga to be an inappropriate mingling of yoga and politics, two worlds that many practitioners and observers alike believed should not mix.

One of us is a scholar of politics and development in India (Kalé) and the other a scholar of Indian religion, culture, and history (Novetzke). These three events made us wonder if the abundant intersecting of yoga and politics was more normalcy than anomaly. We began to sort what we were observing into two related but distinct grooves: yoga *and* politics, and yoga *as* politics. We knew that yoga had long mixed with the political world in India's past—think of the Mughal king Akbar's fascination with yogis and their battles with one another or the medieval warrior ascetics of the Mughal period in India. All three of the events in 2014–2015 share a similar quality, one in which yoga as psychophysical practice and philosophy becomes entangled with political institutions and political actors, instances of yoga *and* politics. Reading more widely in yoga studies literature to understand these events made us wonder if a deeper vein of political thought and action might be contained within the concept of yoga, something beyond the mere mixing or meeting of psychophysical yoga practice and the political world.

Could yoga name a form of political action and thought itself? Should yoga also be understood *as* a form of politics?

These questions inaugurated several years of research and writing. We wrote essays that addressed the three events mentioned above, and we published a few pieces of public scholarship that delved into these issues. Our research in India took us into several worlds. We drank chai in government offices in New Delhi while waiting to interview bureaucrats seated behind stacks of bound files. We visited venerable institutions of India's modern scientific study of yoga and interviewed key leaders who viewed yoga as a mode of rational inquiry into the body, mind, self, and social world. We spent time in the former Princely State of Aundh, viewing the large collections of yoga materials and art in the Raja's library and museum, and exploring India's first open prison, established in that tiny Princely State more than eighty years ago. We met with the Raja's descendants in Pune, and the descendants of others who had grown up in Aundh. We spoke to former supreme court judges about yoga and secularism in India and had conversations about yoga as political thought with anyone who would take the time to talk to us. We also dipped into the vast sea of Sanskrit texts, supplementing our own cursory ability to read Sanskrit with the extraordinary work of many translators and text editors. We read primary documents from India's remarkable anticolonial thinkers, in English as well as in Marathi and Hindi. In many of these texts, the word yoga conveys a broad conceptual world unmatched in English sources. The result is this book, in which we argue that yoga as a term names a long history of political thought and practice that intersects with but is also distinct from the more common understandings of yoga as philosophy and psychophysical practice.

A Note on Diacritics, Sources, and Citations

WE USE STANDARD DIACRITICAL MARKS to transliterate Sanskrit, Marathi, and Hindi. For all non-English words and titles of works, we use italics and diacritical marks. We do not use diacritical marks for people's titles and proper names, place names, or words of non-English origin now common in English, such as "yoga." Wherever possible, we write non-English words and titles as the original authors rendered them. For example, the *Bhagavad Gītā* may be rendered as "the Gita" or "the *Gītā*" or "The Bhagwat Geeta," in works by others in English.

We divide our bibliography between primary and secondary sources. Primary sources list original text editions, any English translations that we adopt as our primary source for a non-English work, memoirs, government documents, archives, newspapers, periodicals, films, and plays. Secondary sources include scholarly works, consulted translations, consulted original text editions, and anything else we cite but do not treat as a primary document.

Original edition sources in Sanskrit, Marathi, Hindi, and English are given in primary sources. For key texts, like the *Ṛg Veda*, *Mahābhārata*, *Bhagavad Gītā*, and the *Arthaśāstra*, we provide a citation to the textual edition we use within "primary sources" listed under both the title of the work and the name of the first editor. For example, the reader will find information about the Sanskrit source text we use for citations regarding the *Mahābhārata* under both "*Mahābhārata*" and under "Sukthankar et al. 1966."

We do not use the name of the purported author of many of these texts because authorship is uncertain. Therefore, the reader should search for these works under the work's title.

When we adopt an English translation as our primary source for translation, we note this and include it in the bibliography under primary sources. For example, our primary source for translations of the *Arthaśāstra* is Olivelle 2013. If we do not accept a single translation of a text or use multiple translations for a text, these are given in secondary sources. Unless otherwise noted, all other translations from Sanskrit, Marathi, or Hindi are our own.

We list the names of all newspapers, periodicals, annual series, and archival materials in our bibliography. We give specific citational information in the relevant note, but do not list separately each newspaper article or issue from an annual series in the bibliography. The exception is for news stories that we consider to be primary documents, for which we give full citations in the primary sources section of the bibliography. For interviews, we provide location information in notes and identify government officials by their institutional affiliation in our notes but do not provide specific names or dates in order to protect the anonymity of our interlocutors.

The Yoga of Power

Introduction

THIS IS A BOOK ABOUT YOGA, but it is not about *that* yoga. Our book does not center what you'll find in a modern yoga studio, the yoga of *prāṇāyāma*, *āsana*, *mantra*, or *namaste*. It is not the yoga philosophy of Patanjali or the psychophysical yoga of the *Haṭhapradīpikā*, although these forms of yoga do appear in this book and in the intellectual history we chart.

Instead, the yoga of this book is the yoga of poets and kings, warriors and heroes, princes and revolutionaries; it is the yoga of leaders finding ways to govern and of insurgents rising up from under the weight of colonialism. The yoga that we study here echoes from the ancient past in a way that resonates forcefully in the political present. This is a book about the yoga that names what people do to hold sway over other people, things, concepts, and political structures. This is a book about the yoga of power.

Our subject is a strand of yoga that runs from the ancient and classical periods to the present; it is woven through some of the oldest textual sources of India's past and integrated into key moments in the history of modern India. Yet this kind of yoga is rarely highlighted in history or textual sources, has no established place in existing scholarship, and does not receive attention as "yoga" in most scholarly studies. This is because the modern study of yoga and its practice focuses primarily on two spheres of yoga commonly identified as the "psychophysical" and the "philosophical."[1] Within these two spheres scholars do trace lines of politics, society, economy, and power, but they do not trace a distinct genealogy for understanding yoga as political thought and practice. Psychophysical yoga is epitomized by the traditions of *haṭha* yoga that proliferate body positions (*āsana*), breathing techniques (*prāṇāyāma*), and other physical means to achieve psychospiritual well-being or empowerment. This sphere includes modern postural yoga forms like Ashtanga Yoga, Power Yoga, Iyengar Yoga, Vinyasa Yoga, and hundreds of other modern innovations. The second sphere of yoga, philosophical yoga, is typified by ancient texts like the *Yoga Sūtras*[2] and their modern reinterpretations, such as Vivekananda's *Raja Yoga*. The most well-known of the ancient texts of yoga philosophy is attributed to Patanjali, who presents methods of concentration (*dhāraṇā*), meditation (*dhyāna*), and transcendence (*samādhi*). These two spheres of yoga have been made famous in India over millennia. And over the last 150 years, charismatic individuals like Vivekananda in the late nineteenth century and Iyengar, Pattabhi Jois, and Indra Devi in the twentieth century have brought these kinds of yoga global renown.

In this book, we identify a third sphere of yoga, as old or older than the other two, and running through them and with them from the past into the present. This sphere of yoga names ideas, practices, and theories of action that can be traced to India's oldest text, the *Ṛg Veda* (ca. 1400 BCE–1000 BCE);[3] some of India's most famous texts, such as the *Mahābhārata* (ca. 400 BCE–400 CE)[4] and within it, the *Bhagavad Gītā*;[5] and texts central to ancient Indian political thought, such as the *Arthaśāstra* (ca. 250 CE).[6] Through these textual traditions, we trace a concept of yoga as a means of controlling one's antagonists (enemies, opponents, others) as well as the conditions that antagonize (hostile neighbors, unstable political or economic conditions, uncontrolled information or misinformation). Yoga as a political concept resurfaces in the modern period, used by key figures of resistance to colonial rule, such as B. G. Tilak and M. K. Gandhi, where it names a mode of political action under the yoke of foreign rule. This line of yoga as political thought and practice is entwined with the twentieth-century popularization of one of the quintessential forms of modern postural yoga, the Surya Namaskar, itself situated amid the kind of subdued resistance to colonial rule undertaken within some Indian Princely States. Our book traces yoga as political thought and practice through these textual sources, cultural forms, and political contexts, set alongside and overlapping at points with the spheres of yoga as psychophysical practice and yoga as philosophy. We illustrate this point in figure Intro.1.

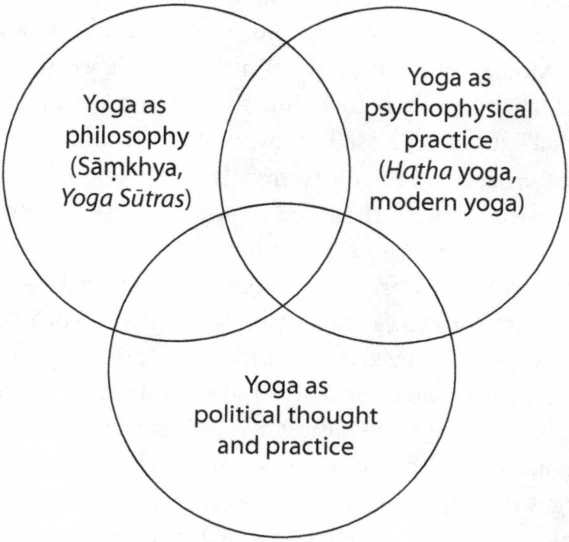

FIGURE INTRO.1 Three spheres of yoga

Throughout the book, we refer to two key terms: yoga and the political. The first is a very common word in Indian languages—like Sanskrit, Hindi, and Marathi—and over the last century or so has become commonplace in English and other European languages as well. But it is a word that means different things in different contexts, even in English, and so it makes sense to clarify our use of this word. We also identify three more specialized characteristics of yoga as political theory and practice that we draw from our analysis of how the word circulates in the texts and events that we study in this book. The other term, the political, is an essential concept with its own branching and bifurcating meaning, especially after the interventions of feminism, Marxism, poststructuralism, postmodernism, and postcolonialism, and so we want to be clear about how we understand this term as well.

Yoga

Yoga is just one of those words. It has multiple meanings even in English over the last two hundred years of its use, and its scope is far wider in Indian languages like Sanskrit, Marathi, and Hindi, where it has existed for many more centuries. For example, in the standard Sanskrit-English dictionary by Monier-Williams, the definition of this word, including compounds in which it appears, takes up five columns over two pages and the word "yoga" alone is glossed by over 106 different English words and phrases.[7] Yoga proved so difficult to translate into English and other European languages that the effort caused a serious academic kerfuffle in early nineteenth-century European scholarship, drawing in the likes of G. W. F. Hegel to declare that the word simply could not be translated at all.[8] And so it seems essential for us to say what we mean by this word across the uses we trace in this book in Sanskrit, Marathi, Hindi, and English.

Ask any good yoga scholar or teacher of yoga what the word yoga means and they might start with the basics: a yoke.[9] In this sense, yoga means to yoke an animal, usually a horse, as we will see in chapter 1. From this idea of yoking emerges meanings for the word around harnessing, fastening, linking, and as such, uniting for some purpose. It is often a person, someone in charge, who is doing the yoking of another thing, like an animal. This is the most literal and probably oldest meaning of this word—going back some thousands of years in languages like Sanskrit and Avestan. The two words—"yoga" and "yoke"—are cognates, which suggests that the concept of the yoke is extremely old and elemental to the Indo-European world, whatever that was or is. The word yoga also has many meanings outside the scope of what a person does—like naming a constellation of stars or a stroke of good timing, the auspicious confluence of events, a coincidence. But in this book, when we refer to yoga, we are specifically talking about a thing a person does with intention to someone or something else in an effort to apply force and thereby control that person or thing.

When people use the word yoga, they usually are not referring to yoking an animal. While the generalized concept of the yoke is perhaps implicit, the word yoga more likely refers to controlling some aspect of life like mind, body, and breath or some cosmic force like death, rebirth, or the liberation of the soul. The word has its broadest sense in all these contexts as "a means of controlling something," and it is this simple definition that we adopt here. One can replace "means" with technique, application, device, apparatus, strategy; one can replace "control" with use, manage, apprehend, and so on; and the "something" at the receiving end of yoga can be anything from animals (especially horses joined to chariots) and facets of the self (breath, body, emotion, desire, mind, limbs, attention) to aspects of the cosmic world (*karma*, rebirth, the nature of reality).

We suggest in this book that the word yoga also has been used over the last several millennia to reference aspects of the political world, like economies, enemies, information, and power itself. In English, the word's usage is restricted to the psychophysical and philosophical, but its range far exceeds this in the other Indian languages we examine in this book, including Sanskrit, Marathi, and Hindi. In these languages, the applications of this word are vast, ranging from prosaic meanings like link, join, method, and way to the usual highly specialized meanings around physical and philosophical forms. Nevertheless, even in these languages, most contemporary invocations of the word yoga refer to philosophy or psychophysical practice. But our point in this book is that these many uses of the word yoga are not the *only* uses of the word as a technical or practical term. As one can imagine, any word or idea that involves techniques of control is likely to find its way into the world of social and political power. Our book expands the concept of yoga to see how the term names a theory, or even strategy, of power. We think that there are additional characteristics that inhere in the concept of yoga as a theory of power—namely, how the field of power is delineated, the nature of relationships within this field, and the purpose or ends of contention among actors within it. We refer to three additional qualities of yoga as a political concept: transitive, intramural, and dialectical.

Yoga Is Transitive

Yoga, like a transitive verb, usually requires a subject (the one doing the yoga) and an object (the thing upon which the yoga is done). When one is "doing yoga" in the psychophysical sense, one is engaged in a process of controlling something—perhaps the turning of thought or inflexible muscles. When your yoga teacher asks you to set an "intention" for your yoga practice, we think they are telling you to identify the "something" you plan to control through yoga, even if it is your insatiable desire for control itself. We believe this is also the case in the political realm, where yoga names a means, strategy, or technique for having power over someone or something, often including oneself in the effort to impose discipline and control over one's own thoughts and behavior as a political actor. This passing through of power and control of an object by a subject is what we call the transitive property of yoga. At other times, yoga can mean the goal or attainment of a state of control, the endpoint of the action of yoga.[10]

One will often find yoga, through the concept of the "yoke," translated as "union."[11] This translation implies some equality between the one yoking and the one yoked, as if they are unified by mutual consent. What we argue in our book, however, is that yoga in the world of politics does not register the concept of a mutual "union" but rather power applied by one thing or person *over* another thing or person, whether or not the object desires to be yoked. In other words, yoga for us is not a kind of amicable or equal union; instead, it is the imposition of power by one over another. As a process, yoga implies an asymmetry of power; as a goal, it implies the resolution of that asymmetry in favor of the one who has undertaken yoga. Throughout this book, we will endeavor to show how yoga is configured as a term that names this transitive, asymmetric nature of control and domination, expressed in the realms of politics and power. Yoga is then the instrumentalization of power. One of the primary modes of psychophysical yoga is *haṭha yoga*, expressed in texts such as the *Haṭhapradīpikā*, where the word *haṭha* means "violence, force." This word is interpreted within psychophysical yoga to mean "forcing the mind to withdraw from external objects."[12] Our idea about yoga as a political concept relates to this quality of *haṭha*. We argue that yoga, extending from its meaning of "yoking" or "harnessing," carries with it a sense of *force*, that is, it requires force and is itself a means of force.

Related to this concept of "force" is our understanding that yoga contains an epistemological force as well, what we render as "to apprehend" at various points in the book. By this we mean that yoga is also a way to apprehend, to know something. In political contexts yoga is sometimes used to name ways to understand or acquire knowledge about something or someone, often against the will of the thing or person. The implication is that by understanding something, one can control it, too. Knowledge is power, even with yoga. Just as the word "apprehend" in English conveys both to understand and to capture physically, we show how yoga is often considered a mode of knowing something, a way to grasp knowledge and also a way to control and make use of it *as force*. This aspect of yoga is particularly prevalent in the *Arthaśāstra*, as we will see. In this sense, yoga also means to circumscribe, restrain, and direct knowledge, especially "intelligence," in the field of politics. When yoga indicates ideas like gathering intelligence or disseminating misinformation, the sense of apprehension conveys a strategic gathering and use of knowledge. Throughout the book, we also attend to how yoga appears as a form of apprehension, a mode of seeing the world in order to act upon and control it.[13]

We define yoga *as a means, method, technique, or strategy by a subject to control an object in a shared field of power*. Our theory of power is drawn from the characteristics of yoga as a thing someone does, as we have articulated here. As Michel Foucault argues, power is a relational force,[14] a way of acting upon another, altering fields of knowledge and structures of order.[15] Yoga is itself power when it describes the control a subject achieves over an object. This unidirectional flow of power in yoga can be further refined as both intramural and dialectical.

Yoga Is Intramural

Yoga operates in an *intramural* system, occurring within a social, religious, political, or cosmic sphere that is shared by both the subject and object of yoga. In our analysis, we do not find that yoga "works" on subjects outside a shared, prescribed field of power. Yoga implies a conjoined system for its application of force.[16] Yoga as political thought and action assumes an emic relationship between subject and object that is defined by internally shared elements. Yoga can be utilized as a strategy of control because the subject and object both operate by the same norms and rules. In all the instances of yoga as political thought and action that we explore, the subject shares the same field of power with the object of its yoga, and a shared concept of yoga creates an intramural sphere.

One way to illustrate what we mean by this intramural sense of yoga is to consider the *Bhagavad Gītā* and the epic in which it is located. The action of the *Bhagavad Gītā* takes place on a battlefield where two armies, the Pandavas and Kauravas, are related not just as enemies in the shared battle to come but also by shared blood as members of a large extended family. They also share the same general rules of war, even if those rules are transgressed. When we write of the intramural nature of yoga, we mean this shared space of contention where adversaries mutually dwell and the rules of which empower or disempower each according to their yoga, their strategy in conflict.

Sometimes the aim of yoga is to alter the parameters of the political and the modalities of politics itself, to apprehend, control, and redefine the entire political field. We can see this perhaps most clearly with an example from the modern era: M. K. Gandhi's corporeal politics. By his yoga, Gandhi ruptured the boundaries between public and private, the body politic and his physical body, and sought to redefine the language of politics through his dress, language, diet, comportment, and his own body.[17] Yoga, as an intramural political force, can mean the effort or strategy by a subject to alter parts of the field or even the whole of a given political order.

Yoga Is Dialectical

We describe yoga as the control of an object by a subject and we express this relationship as a dialectics of power. From Socrates to modern Western philosophy and law, the dialectical process—of resolving two opposed points of view to achieve a more perfect synthesis—is a central feature of how change is understood and defined. This concept underwrites the ideas of G. W. F. Hegel and Karl Marx most famously, but it is an old concept and one that is hardly unique to Europe.[18] We suggest that the dialectics of yoga differs from the teleological and totalizing theories of figures like Hegel and Marx because yoga resolves oppositional or agonistic categories without compelling a particular end point; there is no "end of history" written into yoga.[19] In other words, each individual application of yoga—of force on an object by a subject—has its own unique teleology that does not map onto a universal progression of some kind. If we had to draw a comparison to dialectical theory in European thought, the dialectic of yoga is closer in spirit to Theodor Adorno's "negative dialectics."[20] Writing after the horrors of World War II, Adorno argues that the dialectical process in the modern world would not necessarily achieve a "positive" end. He proposes that one might accept the Hegelian-Marxist dialectical process yet jettison their assumptions about progress, their ideas that the end of history would lead to pure freedom, liberalism, or a communist utopia.

We argue that each dialectical application of yoga between subject and its object of control is idiosyncratic rather than universal. Yoga evinces no universal teleology through its dialectics, it moves toward no set goal in some general way. Instead, it is a dialectical approach to a unique, idiomatic condition specific to the subject that undertakes yoga for some goal related to an object. We do not read yoga within a grand arc of history, providence, or progress.

In yoga, the finale remains unwritten. For example, in its psychophysical and philosophical forms, yoga has long proposed solutions to the mind-body or soul-nature problem that are not universal but rather adapted to each theological, political, or cultural-physical context in which the technique is used. Yoga is at home in dualist and nondualist philosophical and theological schools of thought. Yoga is shared by Hindus seeking the True Self, by Buddhists seeking No-Self, by Muslims seeking Allah, or by atheists seeking to chill. And psychophysical yoga's application to the mind-body problem crosses the barriers of the religious and secular, the premodern and modern, the scientific and spiritual because the core dialectic to which yoga is addressed starts with a subject, usually an individual, set against a world of infinite dialectical possibilities, both physical and metaphysical, theoretical and theological: the Self against the self, but also other selves, the world, the cosmos, even death. In some cases, the dialectic's resolution is ultimately a rejection of the very premises on which the dialectic is first constructed. In many forms of Buddhism, the object—the Self—is revealed as an illusion to be extinguished like a candle's flame. The resolution that yoga proposes is not a "synthesis" in the Hegelian sense. Instead, a subject dominates an object by means of a yoga; the endpoint is that very domination.

Some readers may feel that what we are calling "yoga" in the texts, sources, and contexts we cite throughout this book is a homonym of the "real yoga," which is primarily psychophysical practice and philosophy, embedded in lineages and genealogies, and aimed toward some kind of self-realization. Our subject, one might argue, is related to those kinds of yoga only by the mere accident of sound and spelling. Such arguments have been made to distinguish medieval *haṭha* yoga from modern postural yoga or philosophical yoga, or even forms further afield, like "goat yoga" or "broga" (yoga among "bros"). We feel that the word yoga that knits together all these admittedly very different forms cannot be dismissed as merely homonymic. Generally speaking, Sanskrit does not evince homonyms as one finds in English, although it is true that words in Sanskrit and other Indic languages are often replete with meaning.[21] A scholar of Sanskrit once remarked, "Every word in Sanskrit means itself, its opposite, the name of a god, a word for an elephant."[22] Our aim in this book is not to foreclose the possible contexts in which yoga circulates or to argue about what is or is not "real yoga," but rather we want to draw out from this plurality a clear strand of meaning that names political thought and action over a broad sweep of text and time.

The Political

The Maṇḍala Theory

Our understanding of yoga as a political concept is intertwined with the idea of the *maṇḍala*, or "circle" of friends and enemies. Here we draw on the conceptualization of the political sphere in the *Arthaśāstra*, a classical Sanskrit text of political economy and strategy.[23] One reason we center the *maṇḍala* theory is that the *Arthaśāstra*, as we will see in chapter 2, links it to yoga as a term of political theory and practice.[24] The *maṇḍala* theory envisions a world where a king is surrounded by neighboring forces, both hostile and friendly. A contiguous state is assumed to be a foe, either to be converted into an ally or defeated; a state contiguous to a foe is assumed to be an ally, either actual or potential, and so on (see figure Intro.2).

The *maṇḍala* political theory describes this field of neighboring states vying for power and the *Arthaśāstra* prescribes strategies for its management. As Upinder Singh explains, the *Arthaśāstra*'s ideal "leader should try to stretch himself out as the hub in the circle—that is, become the center of a galaxy of kings. Ultimately, the *vijigīṣu* [the aspiring victor] has to overreach (*atisaṁdhā*) not only the enemies, but all the elements in the circle."[25] In line with our discussion of the intramural above, the king, while seeking supremacy among kings, negotiates with and against others with whom he shares the same political sphere, similar political goals, and the same intentions toward conquest and stability. Perhaps they even share the same instruction manuals such as the *Arthaśāstra*. Other kings and other kingdoms are therefore not wholly "other," to be annihilated; rather, they serve as potential resources. In this conceptualization of the field of power, there are neither permanent friends nor permanent enemies; there is always the possibility of flipping an enemy to a friend, and of a friend turning traitor.

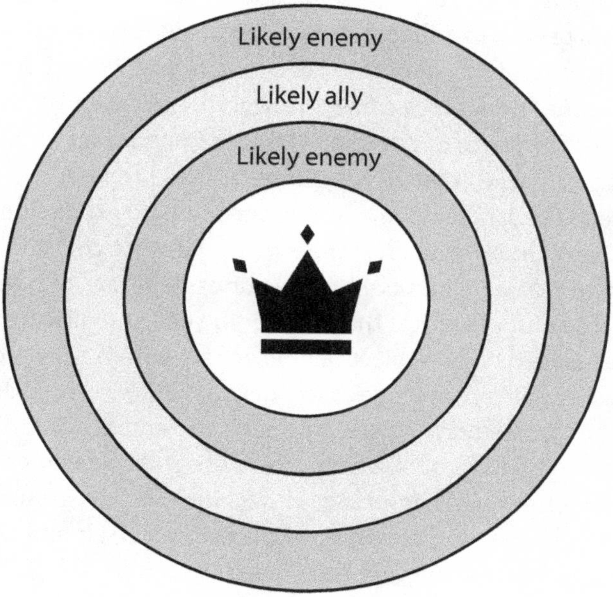

FIGURE INTRO.2 Maṇḍala theory

Agonism

While the kings who are guided by the *maṇḍala* theory share the same political world, they do so in a fashion of constant struggle and conflict. To describe this field of struggle, we adopt the term "agonism" used by the political theorist Chantal Mouffe. Mouffe defines the political as a shared field of agonism, of productive conflict in which political opponents battle for power.[26] In this notion of the political, there is no permanent equilibrium, only constant flux. In the texts and events we analyze to uncover yoga as a political concept, these twin ideas of the *maṇḍala* and agonism define the political.

The earliest meanings of "agonism" in English name "the victor's prize . . . in strenuous struggle," especially in combat or competition.[27] Above, we describe yoga as operating within an intramural or emic system where yoga is the means of control of something (opponents, resources, militaries, information, the self, etc.) in contention with others who also seek power in this field. Yoga here is the art, perhaps sometimes a martial art, of managing agonism for one's benefit in a shared arena. This conceptualization of the political and power is reminiscent of the French sociologist Pierre Bourdieu's field theory where the "rules of the game" are shared, and power is a force marked and distributed by forms of capital.[28] This is in opposition to other concepts of the political, such as that of Carl Schmitt, who proposes the primacy of the friend/enemy distinction and war, as the ultimate expression of politics, means the "existential negation of the enemy,"[29] a horrifying and dismal idea of the political that we have not found in our explorations of yoga.

The concept of the political that inheres in yoga as political thought and practice assumes that the subject and object act within a shared, intramural, and flexibly dialectical space as the field of contest rather than with an absolute enmity, as among agents who seek the annihilation of the other. Indeed, the annihilation of all enemies would mean the end of all politics, and the end therefore of the world that yoga inhabits as a means of empowerment. It would spell the cessation of the *maṇḍala* itself and thus the end of political opportunity, the very thing yoga seeks to leverage for benefit.

By "politics," then, we do not mean the messy, often venal, frequently corrupt world of electoral politics, either in the United States, India, or anywhere else. Rather, by "politics" and "the political" we mean an orientation to the world and a conception of the world as a place where power is constantly at play. Yoga, in this sense, does not entail any particular or partisan ideology or theology. Other scholars have shown how yoga as psychophysical or philosophical practice has been used to aid liberalism, neoliberalism,[30] and capitalism,[31] as well as fascism and democracy.[32] The political ends of yoga are vast and unrestricted, and there are many great studies of how yoga enters such modern political worlds. Our position is not that any one of these is inherent within the sense of yoga as political, psychophysical, or philosophical practice. Yoga is in this way agnostic to political ends; if this were not the case, its cooption by so many divergent political agendas would not be possible. Our chapters are organized and titled to underscore a handful of these multiple possible ends of yoga: war and peace, political strategy, revolutionary nationalism, and sovereignty under colonial rule. We do not pretend to exhaust all such possibilities. Rather our aim is to offer a conceptualization of yoga as political theory and practice, drawing on our understanding of how the term has circulated in a handful of important texts and episodes of history.

Disciplines and Fields

Our collaboration sits at the crossroads of several fields of scholarship: South Asia studies, religious studies, political theory, and yoga studies. We are both scholars of South Asia, dedicated to understanding a region of the world through a deep engagement with its language, culture, and history. One effect of this commitment is that our book is grounded in reading texts in Indian languages and Indian contexts, visiting places, and talking with people, even about the ancient past. While English is one of those Indian languages, we also draw on sources in Sanskrit, Marathi, and Hindi. The use of Sanskrit is common in the study of yoga as a subject, but the exploration of yoga through other Indian languages is less common, even for the modern period, when some of the founding figures of modern physical yoga, like Tirumalai Krishnamacharya, wrote their key works in languages other than English or Sanskrit.[33] Sanskrit sources make up the bulk of chapters 1 and 2 of this book; in chapters 3 and 4, Marathi, Hindi, and English sources sit alongside Sanskrit texts. Our commitment to the study of South Asia also means that we have sought opportunities to ground our analysis through fieldwork, which we have undertaken in India several times since 2016. This is most evident in our work on the modern period in chapter 4 and in the conclusion when we discuss the afterlives of yoga in the postcolonial state. We hope our book has the mark of an area studies orientation through a rooted approach to language, culture, place, and an analysis of power.

We engage two additional fields of study that intersect in this book: religious studies and political theory. One way that we see the productive collaboration of our disciplinary backgrounds and the interplay of the primary subjects of these disciplines—religion and politics—is through the concept of political theology.[34] Our view of political theology is inspired by the broad sweep of this concept in Western thought, from Hegel, Marx, Friedrich Nietzsche, Immanuel Kant, Max Weber, and others.[35] Many of these thinkers did not use the term but nonetheless observed that political concepts at the heart of Western modernity were Christian in their origin or rooted in other theological concepts. This insight was not limited to European intellectual history; the idea that concepts and practices shift back and forth between the spaces of the religious/theological and the mundane/secular is found worldwide.

We do not call political theologies "secularized concepts," which presupposes that the concept in question has been evacuated of its religious or theological content.[36] That is no truer of the ideas emerging from India that we discuss than it is of Kant's categorical imperatives drawn from Christian moralism or Hegel's Weltgeist in history. Political theologies can be the very opposite of secularized concepts. These ideas are not necessarily or even usually shorn of their religious natures just because they take on political force. For us, the term is useful as a way to name the constant flow of ideas between and among the political and the religious, which is another way to say what so many have said, that the worlds of politics and religion are not and have never been separated. We situate yoga in this intermedial space by challenging the idea that yoga is fundamentally religious or spiritual and so its political forms are secondary or aberrant. At the same time, we show how yoga as a political theory and practice is expressed in the language of "religion" as well. Our use of the term "political theology" is an effort to bypass these artificial distinctions.

A curious fact about yoga, from the point of view of political theology, is that it appears to invert the Western paradigm of political theology in which an idea moves from the religious to the secular-political. Yoga, as we trace it, is not grounded in theology but rather in the mundane world. Yoga is an idea forged in relation to war and violence as a feature of political life, but it is set in a ritualized poetic field. As we discuss in chapter 1, the first uses of the term yoga, set around 3,500 years ago in the *Ṛg Veda*, are within martial and political worlds where war itself is sacred ritual undertaken by humans and gods in concert. Like the evocative image of the *maṇḍala* as concentric rings of power, yoga is unrestricted by either the categories of the sacred or mundane, but deployed within and between them to serve the ends of those who use yoga to empower themselves. We use "political theology" to capture with a term of English critical theory this intermediate idea. Our aim is to contribute to a new history of the political, as Prathama Banerjee suggests, that may not be derived solely from Euro-Western models.[37] We write in the vein of Foucault's claim that we are at "the end of the era of Western philosophy . . . [and] . . . if a philosophy of the future exists, it must be born outside of Europe or it must be born of encounters and reverberations between Europe and non-Europe."[38] This book is a contribution to this "philosophy of the future" rooted in an Indic past and present woven around the idea of yoga.

The general idea of political theology requires a concept to be neither religious nor political in its totality, but always somewhere in between.

Many a modern state still begs for divine favor, and heaven remains full of holes.[39] The distinctions between politics and religion are historical contingencies overwritten time and again. Yoga, in all its forms, seems to exist in this liminal space, as we have discussed in other work.[40] In some cases, one will read religion replete in our text—as perhaps in chapters 1 and 3, both of which engage the Hindu *Bhagavad Gītā*. In others, religion may appear more like an aesthetic in the background of political strategy—as in chapter 2 on the *Arthaśāstra* or chapter 4 on the modern liberal secular efforts of the Raja of Aundh.

In addition to South Asia studies, religious studies, and political theory, we have only recently entered a fourth area of scholarship: yoga studies. Since 2016, we have published three articles and several pieces of public scholarship about yoga in political worlds.[41] Thus, we are new entrants to this growing, dynamic field that crosses an array of disciplines and approaches, including philology, literary studies, religious studies, theology, history, sociology, anthropology, political science, law, medicine, and contemplative studies, where questions of race, sex, gender, sexuality, caste, class, and religion proliferate. Our book may take a novel approach by exploring yoga as a political concept, but we travel a road that has been paved by extraordinary work on the texts, histories, and contemporary ideas of yoga. Other scholars have studied yoga's long textual history as well as its historical practices and artistic representations.[42] Some of these studies examine the intersection of yoga and organized groups of yogis engaging in political fields, particularly within the premodern Indian world.[43] Studies of the development of modern yoga have engaged moments when the physical practices of yoga touched on the world of politics, from the precolonial and colonial eras to the present.[44] Recent work has likewise noticed yoga's political valence when studying how yoga philosophy and practice intersect with U.S. popular cultures,[45] its cultures of race,[46] capitalism and neoliberalism,[47] and its impulses toward discipline.[48] Some scholarship has also analyzed yoga's connections to contemporary Hindu right politics.[49] Although most of these studies deal with politics in one way or another, none foregrounds the conceptualization of yoga as political thought and practice as their thematic core.

By looking deliberately at those points where yoga, religion, and politics intersect, we contend with texts and contexts that have often been overlooked by these fields individually. For example, neither religious studies nor yoga studies extensively takes up the term yoga when it appears in texts and contexts like the *Ṛg Veda*, *Arthaśāstra*, or the concept of *karma-yoga* in anticolonial nationalist thought. These are all places in which the word yoga names practices that are very different from how the field of yoga studies has defined the term as either philosophy or psychophysical practice and sometimes configured as religious practice and spirituality. Studies of politics, history, and political theory also tend to overlook yoga's place in the political philosophies of important figures because the term is assumed to reference aspects of their theology, philosophy, or spirituality rather than constituting a central axis of their political ideas.[50]

In much of political science and political theory, yoga is not intelligible as a theory of politics.[51] In proposing that yoga constitutes a distinct political theory and mode of political action, we share Prathama Banerjee's aim to "move on from the moment of (postcolonial/decolonial) critique and undertake the positive and experimental task of reassembling diverse philosophies and experiences of struggle from across the world."[52] Doing so means "converting political actors into political thinkers," as Shruti Kapila puts it.[53] In this book we take seriously the political thought of influential political figures, as Kapila suggests, but we also mine for their political meaning texts and practices that sometimes have been miscoded as solely religious or spiritual. As Adom Getachew and Karuna Mantena put it, to diversify political theory requires not only critiquing Eurocentric thought but also shifting "the terrain of theorizing to better attend to politics in 'most of the world.' "[54] We believe that the concept of yoga provides fertile ground to consider how political thought and practice have been conceptualized both in India's ancient textual past as well as its modern period. Our notion of yoga is certainly related to political concepts in other parts of the world, as we hope our discussion in this introduction conveys, but we believe it also deserves to be understood on its own terms. Whether defined as war (as in the *Ṛg Veda*) or as action unattached to its ends (as in the nationalist era's *karma-yoga*), yoga has proven to be a durable resource for political actors and thinkers over millennia within South Asia. It is an outline of this history that we trace here.

This is a book that draws heavily from a social force of gender and caste that has dominated most literary and political production in India over the course of its long history, and that is Brahmanical patriarchy. Most of the figures we study in this book are Brahman or "elite caste" (*dvija*, "twice-born") men. The major texts of both the ancient and modern periods that we discuss likely were written by such men and for such men. Any study of the intersection of politics, kingship, and Sanskrit (or Marathi or Hindi) literary worlds will rely disproportionately on this gender-caste demographic and the work produced from within it. Too often this world defined by caste patriarchy comes to stand in for "Indian" in some normative sense, and for "Hindu," too.[55]

In our other work, we have written on non-Brahman fields of art, literature, politics, and practice; paid attention to social inequality, especially around caste and gender; and focused on the politics of social equity around caste, religion, and gender,[56] including in the field of yoga practice.[57] In this book, when the possibilities arise, we likewise attend to issues of gender, caste, and social order. But a history of gender and caste within the political formation of yoga is beyond the scope of this book as we have articulated it for the moment. This does not mean that the male authors and agents of the material we study all shared the same points of view or the same views on power, or that our focus suggests a normative boundary for the subjects we study. But it does mean authors of our sources and texts mostly shared the same social ontology within the long-standing network of Brahmanical patriarchy that underwrites most literary production in the Sanskrit, Marathi, English, and Hindi materials we cover. Insofar as we acknowledge this fundamental lacuna in our present work, we also hope for future scholarship to fill this critical space.

Plan of the Book

The rest of this book is divided into two parts. The two chapters that make up part I provide a selective survey of ancient and classical texts that we believe are foundational to the conceptualization of yoga as political thought and practice in an Indic and primarily Hindu vein of thought. The two chapters that make up part II on the modern period examine how the genealogy for yoga charted in part I surfaces as political idiom and practice in the twentieth century. The reader will note that a great deal of time transpires between the historical periods of part I (ca. 1400 BCE to 200 CE) and part II (late nineteenth and early twentieth centuries). Between the two parts, we offer a brief "interlude" that we hope will convince our readers of the historical continuities in yoga as political thought and practice that link the two eras.

Another way to make sense of the book's organization is to consider that its two halves are separated not only by time but also by our research aims, methods, and sources. Part I consists of textual and philological analyses of Sanskrit materials. Our aim is like that of James Mallinson and Mark Singleton in their *Roots of Yoga*; we, too, seek to chart "[t]he yoga whose roots . . . prevailed in India on the eve of colonialism."[58] Their interest is psychophysical yoga, whereas ours is yoga as political thought and practice. Our goal in part II is to understand how yoga served as a resource for political activists and princely rulers in the late nineteenth and twentieth centuries. We use English, Marathi, and Hindi materials such as records of speeches, court cases, state archives, newspapers, autobiographies, periodicals, plays, and films. We also draw on fieldwork conducted between 2016 and 2023 when we visited government ministries, institutions, and bureaucracies, as well as private institutions, all of which deal with yoga. Many of these are discussed in the conclusion.[59] We hope to show that these numerous contemporary engagements with yoga draw from a deep historical reservoir in which the word properly belonged to the world of the political.

Chapter 1 focuses on two texts, the oldest literary work from India, the *Ṛg Veda*, and the largest single composition from India or from anywhere in the world, the epic *Mahābhārata*, and within it, India's most famous classical text, the *Bhagavad Gītā*. In the *Ṛg Veda*, we show that yoga indicates various concepts of war and mastery over powerful forces but never names any form of psychophysical or philosophical practice. We extend this discussion to see how yoga as a political concept shapes both the narrative of the war told in the *Mahābhārata* as well as the peace that follows war. In the epic, the spheres of psychophysical and philosophical yoga intersect with the political. Across these texts, we trace yoga as a key concept within an evolving discourse around governance and political power. We argue that the early meaning of yoga in *Ṛg Veda* as mastery in war, a way of controlling something powerful, underwrites many of the word's meanings in the *Mahābhārata* and the *Bhagavad Gītā* within it.

In chapter 2, we trace the meaning of yoga within classical India's preeminent text of political theory and practice, the *Arthaśāstra* (ca. 200 CE).

We examine yoga as a term for various kinds of political, informational, and military strategies, noting how the meanings of the word within the political field explored in chapter 1 find a new formalization within the *Arthaśāstra*. At key moments in the text, yoga is central to conceptualizations of how a king should govern himself, his kingdom, and his relations with other polities. Yoga as political strategy in the *Arthaśāstra*, while coterminous with the full emergence of yoga as psychophysical and philosophical practice, remains distinct from these streams. At this crucial stage of Indic Sanskritic thought in the first centuries of the common era, yoga retained a set of highly technical meanings around political strategy, thought, and practice. We particularly attend to the word *yoga-kṣema*, introduced in chapter 1 but fully expanded in the *Arthaśāstra*. We argue this term represents a political theory and practice that is neither fully war nor peace but rather a realpolitik perspective that peaceful governance is maintained through martial force.

In the interlude, we briefly suggest how some of the ideas in part I of the book move through time to meet the subjects of part II. We rely on a range of scholarship about ideas, texts, and forces from the fourth century CE to the early nineteenth century CE to demonstrate important lines of continuity between the textual origins of yoga we present in part I and its circulation as a term of politics in the modern period. Aware of the chasm this interlude thinly bridges, we offer this section not as a substantive historical or textual engagement but rather as an invitation to further exploration of how yoga as political thought and practice endures from the classical to modern periods.

Chapter 3 is the first of two chapters on the modern colonial period. We track how key figures of India's revolutionary resistance to colonial rule used the concept of yoga, and particularly *karma-yoga*, as a political philosophy of action. We note the overlap of two spheres of yoga, where political thought and practice meets philosophy in modern interpretations of the *Bhagavad Gītā*. We look at the writings of Lala Lajpat Rai, Aurobindo Ghose, B. G. Tilak, M. K. Gandhi, and B. R. Ambedkar and the role of *karma-yoga* in the contexts of their politics. In declaring that yoga requires an active engagement with the contested quotidian world—the world of politics and even violence and warfare if necessary—India's political revolutionaries saw themselves as *karma-yogis*. Yoga was understood in two distinct registers: as a spiritual philosophy and active, sometimes violent, resistance. While many understood these two registers to be contradictory, nationalist advocates of *karma-yoga*, as we show, asserted that they were one and the same.

In chapter 4, we look at the emergence of the Surya Namaskar as a mode of politics in the unique location of India's Princely States and in particular the small state of Aundh in western India. The last Raja of Aundh, Bhawanrao Shriniwasrao Pant Pratinidhi, popularized the Surya Namaskar, perhaps the most common sequence of movements in modern postural yoga. We argue that the Raja's notion of sovereignty demonstrates the overlap and interconnection of yoga as psychophysical practice and yoga as a theory of political action by tying together bodily self-control and political autonomy. His tiny principality embarked on an ambitious program of modernization through self-governance. Rooted in the spread of the Surya Namaskar practice, these changes extended outward throughout Aundh's educational, political, economic, and carceral domains. The Raja's varied efforts actualized the idea that yoking the self was the first step in political sovereignty, a theory and practice epitomized in his use of the Surya Namaskar.

In our conclusion, we address a question left only partially answered by contemporary yoga studies: How has the postcolonial Indian state utilized psychophysical and philosophical yoga for its political purposes? There are many books and articles that address this question in the post-2014 period, but there is much less attention to the prior decades from independence in 1947 to 2014. We chart how the Indian bureaucratic state instrumentalized psychophysical and philosophical yoga from the 1950s onward. Our aim is to contextualize the current entanglements of yoga and the state within a much longer history in which yoga has been used to achieve varied political ends. It may seem that this marks a shift from our previous chapters' focus on yoga *as* politics back to the formulation of yoga *and* politics. What we see happening in this period, however, is a convergence of the two—the harnessing and controlling of psychophysical yoga itself by the state, the yoking of yoga, the control of something enduring and powerful.

PART I

Ancient and Classical Periods

ONE

Yoga as War and Peace in the *Ṛg Veda* and the *Mahābhārata*

TAKE A YOGA TEACHER TRAINING COURSE anywhere in the world and you will likely find yourself contemplating the pithy aphorisms of Patanjali's *Yoga Sūtras* or trying to imagine the feats—mundane to marvelous—described in the *Haṭhapradīpikā*. Many of the largest modern systems of psychophysical yoga attempt to trace their lineages and techniques to these canonical roots.[1] Text is vital for such a concept of "tradition," and these works, among others, make up a vision of the yoga tradition as it is commonly received, taught, and cited. Modern yoga practitioners use such texts to determine the correct Sanskrit pronunciation of different *āsana*s and the proper chanting of *mantras*. They refer to these texts for key ideas such as "yoga is the cessation of the turning of the mind" (*yogaś citta-vṛtti-nirodhaḥ*), the most famous quote from Patanjali. The premodern classical canon of yoga remains an essential component of how yoga is practiced today, even as science and the concerns of modern life become the new subjects of this classical practice.

But is there such a canon for the third sphere of yoga that we are endeavoring to examine, a canon for yoga as political thought and practice? This chapter and the next form our effort to provide such a textual and intellectual genealogy by looking to well-known Sanskrit sources. We approach the question of what a classical canon of yoga as political thought and practice might look like. What are the layers of text and meaning that position yoga as a mode of political thought and action? The second half of the book takes up how the ideas from this textual genealogy inform the field of the political in modern India.

Because there is no existing scholarly route to explore such a classical genealogy of yoga as political thought, one has a blue vista of texts through which to find a path. We have chosen two in this chapter, and one in the next. The first is the oldest literary text of ancient India, the *Ṛg Veda* (ca. 1400 BCE to 1000 BCE). The second is the largest text of India (and perhaps worldwide), the *Mahābhārata* (ca. 400 BCE to 400 CE); contained within this epic is perhaps the most famous text of India, the *Bhagavad Gītā*. These works are foundational texts for Indic thought. In the next chapter, we examine a third text, the preeminent work of political thought and practice in classical India, the *Arthaśāstra*. We have selected these texts for several reasons. They are each of general importance in Indic textual history; they each speak to yoga as political thought and practice; and they are texts that, though ancient, resonate in political worlds in the modern period. One could choose other texts, of course, such as sources from Buddhism, Jainism, Islam, and Sikhism, and our selection does not endorse any political or religious position in which these texts circulate.[2] We offer this selective textual genealogy as an entry point into a conceptual history of yoga as political thought and practice.

The *Ṛg Veda* is highly influential in the development of many strains of Indic thought. While it is foundational for some forms of normative high-caste Hinduism and ritualism, its rejection is essential to Jainism, Sikhism, and Buddhism, and many *bhakti* or devotional traditions.[3] We use the *Ṛg Veda* because, in the historical archive of texts in India, it evinces the oldest use of the word yoga. When yoga appears in the *Ṛg Veda*, it bears no explicit relationship to psychophysical or philosophical yoga.[4] We agree with James Mallinson and Mark Singleton when they write that "it would be wrong to read . . . backwards" into the Vedic texts the presence of the psychophysical and philosophical spheres of yoga.[5] However, we do find in the *Ṛg Veda* evidence of what we identify as the third sphere of yoga, that of political thought and practice. As we will see, yoga in the *Ṛg Veda* takes on a set of meanings related to war, horses, chariots, and the mastery of some object. Rather than contemplation, it is a word situated in a world of action, conflict, and contention, a world of political agonism.

The second text on which we focus in this chapter is the massive epic, the *Mahābhārata*, and within it the *Bhagavad Gītā*, in which yoga in multiple forms appears prominently. Yoga is a concept seeded throughout, and more especially toward its end, after the conclusion of the tragic battle that forms the core of the story. We follow the trail of yoga from the *Ṛg Veda* as it passes through and is reconstructed in this epic, and we situate the *Bhagavad Gītā*'s engagement with yoga in the context of the larger epic of which it is a part.

Many texts of the ancient world—and perhaps many texts of the modern world too—are not singular objects but accumulations of many voices over time, of many editors and critics, of many versions knit together with the concerns of a given era and place. This is true of all the texts of the classical yoga studies canon, and it is true of the texts we study in this chapter and the next. This means we are making sense of fragments just as the texts themselves make sense of fragments.

Preparing for War in the *Ṛg Veda*

The *Ṛg Veda* is the oldest text that we have related to culture on the Indian subcontinent.[6] Its ten books were all composed at different points in time, from approximately 1400 BCE to 1000 BCE. There are many ways to describe this extraordinary text. It is a highly stylized and specialized work of art and ritual, embedded within a religious-cosmological world where humans can entreat deities to their aid through the Vedic sacrifice. It was composed by and for a very small community of people (mostly men it seems) invested in a highly elite sacrificial system, out of which a vast social, cosmological, and ritualistic world was spun. It is a massive work of poetry, composed in a verse called *sūkta*, or "well-said," that largely centers around the performance of ritual sacrifice and praise of deities, natural powers, and other supernatural forces that one hopes to control or entreat. It is not a work of history or sociology, subjects that the text makes no claim to represent in any case.[7] Instead, as a work of poetry about systems of ritual and language, it is a prime example of a "world-building" text, a work of poiesis.

The world that the poets conjure and describe in the *Ṛg Veda* is a martial world.[8] Its key subject is a god of war, Indra, and several of the most important sacrificial rituals described are integrated into cultures of war.[9] For example, the sacrificial act illustrated most frequently in the *Ṛg Veda* is the Soma sacrifice, when the potent elixir, *soma*, is consumed by Indra before battle and, by extension, is ritually consumed through sacrifice by human warriors and priests.[10] One of the essential Vedic rituals of Hindu kingly enthronement is the *aśvamedha*, the horse sacrifice, that enacts and delineates the realm of sovereignty for a king. Performance of this sacrifice is recorded as late as the eighteenth century.[11] Even the poets, called *ṛṣis*, may themselves have been warriors.[12] As with so many texts of religious traditions, the *Ṛg Veda* is not confined to any one purpose or meaning. However, its martial aspect, so essential to understanding the text, is often muted when the *Ṛg Veda* is simply described as a set of religious "hymns." The text is about power: it is for and about people who existed in a martial culture and used the Vedic ritual and invocation of its deities in contest with one another, whether in actual battle or in the rituals of conflict and sacrifice. As we move through the discursive uses of the word yoga in the *Ṛg Veda*, we keep in mind that when the poet-priest-warrior invokes the metaphors of war, he may be drawing from his own deep familiarity with martial culture as a practitioner himself, as a warrior *and* a poet-ritualist.[13]

We chart three tiers of meaning for the word yoga in the *Ṛg Veda*: literal, metonymic, and metaphorical. The literal meaning of yoga is to yoke or harness a horse to a chariot in preparation for war. The metonymic meaning of yoga is then war itself: just as the sword is a common metonym for war, in the *Ṛg Veda* a horse harnessed to a chariot is a metonym for war. The metaphorical meanings stem from these literal and metonymic meanings and come to indicate exercising power or control over something else, usually something powerful. We see this metaphorical meaning especially in relationship to thoughts (*dhī*, *mata*); art, truth, right, rite (*ṛta*); and poetic verse (*veda*).[14]

Making War

Here is an exemplary verse from Book Four (*sūkta* 24) that speaks to some of these many meanings. In these lines, beautifully translated by Stephanie W. Jamison and Joel P. Brereton, Indra is being summoned and *soma* prepared on the eve of war between two Aryan clans in the Vedic world's imagination. We set in bold and brackets the use of the word yoga here:

> Just to him do men separately call at the encounter.[15] Having given up
> Their bodies, they make him [Indra] their preserver,

when the men of both camps, on opposite sides, have come to abandon
(their bodies) in the winning of offspring and descendants.
The settled peoples show their resolve at the **hitching up (for battle) [yoga]**, o
powerful one, while they are gasping on opposite sides in the winning
of the flood.
When the battling clans have rolled together, just then do those on the
one side seek Indra at the moment of confrontation.
Just then do those on the other side perform sacrifice to his Indrian
Strength . . .
The man with fully focused mind who never loses the track—just him
does he [Indra] make his comrade in battles . . .
. . . Through our insightful thought may we be charioteers who always win.[16]

In this text "hitching up (for battle)" is how Jamison and Brereton translate the word yoga. It specifically refers to hitching up horses to chariots in a process of "yoking," which is to say, yoga. This is one of the chronologically oldest references to yoga in the *Ṛg Veda* and indicates the act of readying for battle. In short, yoga metonymically means here and elsewhere "preparing for war."[17] The act of fully focusing the mind may be part of the process of "hitching up for battle," a part of yoga, but it is not explicitly so—the text instead clearly links yoga to war preparation rather than to any philosophical position or psychophysical process. As we discuss in our introduction, one of the several ideas of yoga as a political concept that we propose is that yoga conceives of power as an intramural field in which each side aims to control the other. Yoga, we conjecture, works as any competitive game works: both players play on the same field, on the same board, as in the war game of chess that may have originated in India. Yoga here assumes that the rules are shared among contestants as is the hoped for victory; controlling the other, the agonist, is the means to this end. This verse situates the Vedic sacrifice, and the Vedic hymns themselves, within just such a shared economy of power, to which both sides of the battle adhere, each appealing to Indra for victory, each speaking the same language of ritual, poetry, and contest that the other speaks. Both sides of this battle worship Indra; both sides perform the same rituals; and both sides speak the same language, share the same worldview, exist as recognizable partners in conflict within the same Vedic Aryan frame. The side that is most skillful in these arts (of worship, ritual, poetry, violence) will emerge victorious because the arts themselves are shared. The poets too insert themselves into this economy of power, portraying themselves as warriors, or more specifically as "charioteers" (*rathya*) who win against each other, against rival poet-warrior-priests. The verse suggests that the association of war, horses, chariots, language, poetry, and power is essential for understanding the word yoga in the *Ṛg Veda*. This most elemental use of yoga here, as "hitching up" the horses to chariots for battle, is the seed of all the later meanings we trace within the political field, and perhaps beyond.

As Marianna Ferrara points out, the word yoga appears around twenty-one times in the *Ṛg Veda*.[18] Of these, in seven instances the word simply means harnessing a horse to a chariot, such as those ridden by the Aśvins, or "horsemen";[19] by Indra;[20] and by Agni, the deity of fire.[21] These references occur both in chronologically older books of the *Ṛg Veda* (Two, Five, and Seven) and younger ones (One, Eight, and Ten). Notably, only horses—no other kinds of animals—are associated with the word yoga in the *Ṛg Veda*, and where the word appears metaphorically, as we will see below, the metaphor builds on this literal meaning of harnessing horses as if for war.[22] This association between yoga, war, and horses suggests the transitive sense of yoga as the exertion of force by a subject (one who harnesses), through an action of control (harnessing to a war chariot), upon an object (horses).

This power relationship between intention and object of action, what we have called in our introduction the transitive property of yoga, is important for the development of the idea of yoga as political theory and practice. Many future metaphorical meanings of yoga in a specialized sense rely on this metonymy, on the valence of "yoking a horse to a chariot as if for war," and this is perhaps applicable not only to the word's political uses but also perhaps to its philosophical and psychophysical ones—yoga as the control of something (body, mind, spirit, others).[23] Yoga as a term and concept here suggests the instrumental use of power in conflict. This metonymic meaning emerges from the idea of controlling a horse and its power, diverting its energy away from the animal's own concerns to those of humans: fighting, winning, acquiring something through conflict with other humans. A horse is yoked to a chariot to use its power to the charioteer's advantage in battle, a vehicle of war, controlled by men for their aims and gain. While yoga may appear relatively infrequently in this text, its meaning and use coheres around a sense of controlling something, having power over something.

Rather than a general term for "joining" or "union" of some kind, it is here a technical term embedded in the details of equine warfare technology and extended from this basis to other uses.

In the remaining fourteen instances, yoga's metonymic valence reinforces the idea of yoga as a metaphor for conflict, especially war, as well as intentional control over an object harnessed for the benefit of the person who does the harnessing. We have already seen this in the passage cited at length above. Similar passages situate a poet entreating Indra to join the poet's patrons in battle against a rival clan:

> Will he [Indra] be here for us at our **hitching up (for war) [yoga]**, he for wealth, he in plenty? Will he come to us with prizes of victory?[24]

And later in the same book:

> At every **hitching up (for battle) [yoga]**, at every prize-contest we call to the more powerful one—as his comrades (we call) to Indra for help.[25]

The poet's entreaty forms a contest within a contest: Indra is summoned to support one group over another in battle, and the poets who composed the text see themselves as "charioteers" who are competing with the poets-priests-warriors of the opposing clans, themselves trying to summon Indra. So the battle for Indra's boon is nested within the martial contest for which Indra is invoked; there are two battles, the rhetorical one to persuade Indra and the physical one, for which the invocation is a prelude. The poet harnesses verse like the warrior harnesses the horse to the chariot—both "saddle up" for battle. This metaphorical use of yoga to show a poet's mastery over something is almost as common as the more direct metonymic meaning of "war," even while the idea of hitching up for battle remains at the core of the metaphor's resonance. For example, we read of poets yoking verse itself, that is, the Vedas:

> Who is the wise one who knows the **yoking [yoga]** of the meters [*veda*]? Who has undertaken the holy speech?
>
> What champion do they call the eighth of the priests? Who indeed has discerned the two fallow bays of Indra?[26]

The one who can use poetic speech and ritual to command the gods to attend the Vedic sacrifice is described as a champion; a *śūra*; a valiant, strong hero in battle. The poets (who may also have been warriors) see themselves through the metonym of yoga, of hitching up for war, because they are also in battle with one another. We want to emphasize the repeated martial associations that the skillful ritualist poet, by using the word yoga, accomplishes through both the "yoking" of hard-to-tame poetic meters and the imagery of the poet as a victor in combat and winner of the battle's spoils.[27]

Beyond the taming of meters, the poets also seek to yoke implements of the Vedic ritual[28] as well as highly abstract concepts, such as art, truth, right, rite (*ṛta*) and thought (*dhī*, *mata*):

> Without whom the sacrifice even of one attentive to poetic inspiration
> does not succeed,
> He drives **the team [yoga]** of insightful thoughts.[29]

Later in the same chapter:

> And our **horse-yoked [yoga]** thoughts lick him like cows their tender young
> Our songs approach him, the sweetest smelling of men, like
> wedded wives.[30]
> Agni, guiding (his horses) and crossing the waters—at **the harnessing [yoga]** of
> the truth, the eager
> inspired ones kindle him with the prizes of victory.[31]

And in this instance from the last chapter of the text:

> Impel our ceremony by a sacrifice to the gods; impel our sacred
> formulation to gain the spoils.
> At the **yoking [yoga]** of truth unloosen your udder. Grant us attentive hearing,
> o waters.[32]

The harnessing of thought and truth (*ṛta*) points toward the many future uses of yoga as the "discipline" of something that will follow in all three spheres of yoga we have identified, particularly in relationship to knowledge, action, and devotion in the *Bhagavad Gītā*.[33] The word *ṛta* is a precursor to the word *dharma*, "holding together," and *dharma* will come to absorb most or all of the meanings of *ṛta* in future texts, such as the *Bhagavad Gītā*, the epics, and the *dharmaśāstra* (discipline or practice of law/custom) literature.[34] As we will see, yoga continues to serve as the word for discipline and mastery in all these contexts, and in the *Bhagavad Gītā* and the epics, where war is the context for this discipline to emerge. Here, as elsewhere, the language of these *sūktas* is filled with the boons of martial victory or *vāja*, the "prize of a battle."[35] Just as a warrior yoked to *ṛta* (art, truth, right, rite) is victorious, so too are the Vedic poet-priests victorious in their sacrificial work. Here, *ṛta* is the correct or true performance of the art of the rite: the poet-priest's ability to control the poiesis of the Vedic world, the "artfulness universe," as William K. Mahony says, the cosmic creation and control contained in the word *ṛta*.[36] One might speak of yoga here as a "martial art," the art of harnessing power in conflict of many kinds. The yoga or harnessing of the poet-priest is the control he exerts over *ṛta* itself. And this control is linked through the word yoga to the martial world metonymically represented by horses and chariots and joined to a form of battle or contest.

We have followed the single word "yoga" as it appears in the *Ṛg Veda* and traced its meanings. While it does not refer to conventional ideas of yoga as psychophysical practice or philosophy, its meanings range from harnessing a horse to a chariot for war to harnessing poetry, art, truth, right, rite, and thoughts in poetic battles between poets and in the performance of the Vedic sacrifice. Connecting all of these is the meaning of yoga as a mode of power over something else, a transitive form of discipline and control, situated within an intramural, shared, or emic realm. In a grand sense, it seems as if agonism itself animates the *Ṛg Veda*, and the text therefore provides a solution to this ongoing conflict over power.[37]

Making Peace After War

Another important way that yoga is used in the *Ṛg Veda* draws on its meanings around war and preparation for war in a compound formation with the word *kṣema*, which means something like "peace" and "settlement."[38] This compound word *yoga-kṣema* will become a standard and essential formation of yoga in the political sphere for the *Mahābhārata*, discussed below, and the *Arthaśāstra*, the subject of the next chapter, as well as for many other ideas about political acquisition, stability, and welfare in the centuries to come and even into the present, as we will see. The compound word *yoga-kṣema* serves to signal two sides of power—acquisition and preservation—forming a link that will convey the political meanings of yoga from the ancient past into the current moment.

In the *Ṛg Veda* these two words appear in different modes in relation to one another. In one of the oldest books of the *Ṛg Veda*, *yoga* and *kṣema* are not joined in a compound but articulated as an antonymic pair:

> That king does not falter, by whom Indra drinks the sharp soma whose comrades are cows.
> He drives (the cows) here with his warriors, he smashes Vṛtra; he dwells peacefully, prospering the settled peoples, bearing the name "Well-portioned."
> He will prosper in **peace [*kṣema*]**, and he will prevail at **the hitching up (for War) [yoga]**; (when) the two opponents are clashing together, he will entirely conquer.[39]

This *sūkta* speaks to a dyadic relationship of "the hitching up (for War)" (*yoga*) and "peace" (*kṣema*), two states of political being—at war and at peace—that are in constant tension with each other. But when conjoined in a compound form, yoga and *kṣema* become something more than antonyms expressing ends of a spectrum; they are interdependent concepts that interact in symbiotic formation. The terms used together may have indicated different calendrical "seasons" linked to different activities or modes of property possession appropriate to each: a season for war and a season for settlement.[40] Other examples throughout the text show the mutual imbrication of these terms as they come to form a single compound concept.[41]

Here are two verses from Book Seven:

> O Lord of the Dwelling Place, might we be accompanied by your capable fellowship, joy-bringing, providing the way.
> Protect us at will in **peace [*kṣema*]** and **war [*yoga*]**.—Do you protect us always with your blessings.[42]

And:

> This praise song is for you, Varuṇa, you who are of independent will: let it be set within your heart.

> Let there be good fortune in **peaceful settlement [*kṣema*]** for us and let there be good fortune in **war [yoga]** for us.—Do you protect us always with your blessings.[43]

And in these two verses from Book Ten:

> Indra is master of heaven and Indra of earth, Indra of the waters and Indra of the mountains,
> Indra of the strong and Indra of the wise; Indra is to be called upon in **Peace [*kṣema*]** and Indra in **war [yoga]**.[44]

And:

> Having taken for myself your **yoking up [war] [yoga]** and your **peace [*kṣema*]**, might
> I become the highest. I have trampled on your head.
> From beneath my feet, lift up your speech to me, like frogs from the water, like frogs from the water.[45]

Marianna Ferrara suggests that the verbal root of *kṣema* (*kṣi*) "develops two meanings" that involve not only "to stay, dwell, reside" but also "to have power over, to rule, to possess," and so to conquer and control.[46] It names a peace won by war, by defeating one's enemies and subduing their resistance. When paired with yoga—a term for hitching up horses to chariots for battle—both meanings abide in this term, a state of dwelling and peace made possible by conquest and power. As Ferrara succinctly puts it, *yoga-kṣema* may be considered "rest after war,"[47] and it may also be the threat of war that establishes a period of rest. We would adapt Ferrara's gloss to provide the less pithy but more political "pacification through control." As we will see, *yoga-kṣema* will resonate over millennia, entering the *Mahābhārata*, the *Bhagavad Gītā*, and the *Arthaśāstra* in significant ways, all related to governance through power. The various uses of this term over time preserve the idea of *yoga-kṣema* as an ideal goal, a hoped-for future of stability, security, and freedom, but always from the perspective of the victor, the government, the king, the one who controls the "yoke."[48]

Boris Oguibénine and Marianna Ferrara arrive at similar conclusions in their rich philological studies of the word yoga in the *Ṛg Veda*. Oguibénine theorizes yoga as indicative of "connective practices" (*pratiques connectives*), a central feature of the discourse of the Vedic sacrifice that linked cosmic, social, and material aspects of the world to the sacrificial rituals at the heart of this text.[49] Oguibénine argues that yoga in the *Ṛg Veda* "did not distinguish between the subject and the object of the action of harnessing . . . the inescapable conclusion is that the harnessing action had to be conceived of as an autonomous act, having its own and rather abstract meaning."[50] Oguibénine argues that the text equates the yoke with the yoked.[51] We build on and emend these insights. As we saw above, yoga is used exclusively in contests of power among people, animals, and concepts that share intrinsic relationships: the domestication of a powerful animal; the defeat of rival Aryan clans; the bettering of others who sacrifice to the same god; the control of shared ideas of thought, speech, and art, truth, right, rite; the defeat of a rival poet of the same language who shares the same worldview. Rather than "connective practices," we describe yoga as transitive, naming a mode of acting upon another to subject or control: yoga is a connection that is *forced*; it is the instrument for the application of force, and the state of being yoked, connected, controlled. Rather than see the yoke and the yoked equated or in "union," we see them as connected but with a differential of power; one seeks the subordination of the other. The yoke is the instrument of subjection, but the one who yokes and the yoked commonly exist within the same discursive sphere and share the same system of power. We have described this in the introduction as the intramural quality of yoga, the way it assumes a shared or emic field of power. The combination of intrinsic and transitive properties suggests that yoga mediates power in agonistic relations, among emic communities who share an investment in maintaining, and gaining power, in shared cultural, economic, social, religious, literary, and political spheres.

As we've traced so far, yoga assumes a differential of power: one masters, disciplines, or yokes another (person, thing, idea) with yoga. This implies a triad of relations: the one who yokes, the thing yoked, and the method of yoking that joins them together. "Yoga" will come to name a system or method that links the one who yokes and the object that is yoked toward some end. We agree with Ferrara, who appears to depart from Oguibénine when she finds that yoga in the *Ṛg Veda* "indicates a concrete action that produces strength and stability in battle" and the ability "to yoke in conformity with one's own task," thus leading to "dominance over the one who is yoked."[52] In the section below and the chapter that follows, we trace this concept of yoga, rooted in war and conflict, as it expands throughout subsequent centuries to emerge as a concept about the mediation of power within an agonistic sphere. Yoga comes to signify a practical tool for this mediation to the benefit of the one who wields it, which is not just the harness or yoke but also the power to harness and yoke, the discipline, tactic, strategy, and skill to apply the technique, whatever it may be. If politics is the contest for power with others, then yoga may stand at its center as a theory and practice of acquiring power and harnessing it for one's benefit.

We started our discussion of the *Ṛg Veda* by noting the three categories into which the use of yoga in the text could be divided: a *literal* meaning, "harnessing," which always occurs in relationship to horses bound to chariots as if to prepare for war; a *metonymic* meaning, rendered as "war" itself; and a *metaphorical* meaning, which is attached to some object (art, truth, right, rite; verse, thought) that indicates the control of that object as if one were disciplining and using a horse by harnessing it for war. All three modes also occur within the context of conflict over power—a horse controlled and reined by a charioteer; one clan defeating and pacifying another; the poet mastering art, truth, right, rite, verse, or thought in ways superior to another. We refer to these instances as the agonistic context of yoga, the field of productive conflict, the victor seeking a prize. Yoga will continue to mediate such fields, addressing conflict, war, methods of achieving victory, and modes of mollifying one's opponents.

Making War to Make Peace in the *Mahābhārata* and the *Bhagavad Gītā*

The *Mahābhārata* may be the world's longest poem. At almost two million words across 200,000 lines of text—around ten times the length of the *Iliad* and *Odyssey* combined—composed over hundreds of years by an untold number of people, the *Mahābhārata* epitomizes the word "epic." Relative to its size, the core story of the *Mahābhārata* is concise. It tells of a civil war within a fractured royal family, divided at the time of succession between one branch, the Kurus, and another, the Pandavas. Out of this central narrative hundreds of other stories proliferate. The story of war at the heart of the text is perhaps based on the actual history of a dynastic war in ancient

India, but the epic also serves as a grand archetype that has been reinvented many times in South Asian cultural forms from literature and art to Bollywood cinema and beyond.

One-third of the way into the eighteen books of the *Mahābhārata* is Book Six, which contains the *Bhagavad Gītā*, a relatively brief Sanskrit poem of seven hundred verses spread over eighteen chapters. It is the record of a dialogue between a Pandava warrior, Arjuna, and his charioteer, Krishna, that takes place just before the start of the great and tragic battle at the heart of the story.[53] In the dialogue, Krishna must convince Arjuna to fight a war that appears to the Pandava prince to be unjust, unnecessary, and cruel, in part because it would be waged against his kinsmen. Arjuna's dilemma has resonated with audiences for centuries. As India's best-known text worldwide, the *Bhagavad Gītā* has been translated into almost one hundred languages since the thirteenth century.[54] It is a text Henry David Thoreau took to Walden Pond, was quoted at the dawn of the nuclear age by Robert Oppenheimer, and was often projected as Hinduism's "bible" in the modern period. Even today, Hindu political leaders around the world use it in lieu of the Christian Bible for their oaths of office.[55] Chapter 3 will focus on the political uses of this text and its concept of yoga amid anticolonial efforts in modern India. Here, we focus on the epic in which the *Bhagavad Gītā* is enfolded in order to explore the traces of the ideas outlined above in the *Ṛg Veda*, the rudiments of what we are calling a genealogy of yoga as political theory and practice.

In the earliest, stable iterations of the *Mahābhārata* and the *Bhagavad Gītā*, the word yoga takes on a broad spectrum of meaning. Just as the Vedic poets had lifted yoga from its martial-equine context and deployed it in relation to their mastery of verse, thought, art, truth, right, rite, by the time of the epic, yoga had come to express philosophical concepts, meditative practices, superhuman powers, and means of salvation from rebirth. Now, rather than primarily indicating "harnessing a horse to a chariot as if for war," the term yoga indicates "mastery" and "discipline" of something in a more general sense.[56] James Fitzgerald notes that the Vedic concept of yoga as "harnessing" led to the idea in the epic that "the person in control harnesses the lower-order being or entity for some purpose, for some enterprise or work,"[57] what we suggest is the transitive property of yoga, or the control and subordination of something or someone by another.

What is truly new in the epic is the emergence and intertwining of the three spheres of yoga we identified in our introduction: yoga as a philosophical system (precursor to Patanjali's yoga and often paired with Sāṃkhya philosophical thought),[58] yoga as a psychophysical activity (e.g., meditation and early expressions of *dhyāna* and *prāṇāyāma*), and yoga as political theory and practice (especially in relation to *yoga-kṣema* and *karma-yoga*). Around this time, key texts of the other two spheres of yoga—philosophy and psychophysical practice—are formed, such as the *Kaṭha Upaniṣad* (ca. 200 BCE), a text resonant with metaphors of chariots and horses that we saw in the *Ṛg Veda*.[59] The yoga of the epics and the *Bhagavad Gītā* inherits the old Vedic sense now applied to modes of mastery far beyond horses and chariots, and into the realm of spirit, cosmos, and reality itself. We argue, however, that the engagement with yoga in this myriad way in the epic and the *Bhagavad Gītā* seems always underwritten by the old concept that we traced in the Vedic text. Especially for what is essentially a story of war, yoga in the epic cannot be shaken free of its moorings in conflict, violence, control, and power—the world of politics.

On the one hand, the field of yoga studies has mostly engaged the epic and the *Bhagavad Gītā* to search for genealogies of yoga as philosophy and/or yoga as psychophysical practice, whereas the genealogy of yoga as political thought has often been overlooked despite the fact that this is a text about a political problem, a war. This is understandable given how important the psychophysical and philosophic contexts are for the meaning of the word yoga over the last two thousand years. On the other hand, studies of ancient Indian kingship and martial practice do not generally focus on yoga, perhaps because it is always assumed to reference philosophy or psychophysical practice, and therefore deemed to be irrelevant as a concept of political thought.[60] When the word yoga appears, it is assumed to be in relation to those more established usages. Here we argue that one can trace the political genealogy of yoga by attending to how and when the word appears in the epic, especially in relationship to its core story of war. We suggest that the frequency and distribution of use of the word yoga outlines its importance to two related but distinct tasks in the epic: the preparation for war and, following the war, the preparation for peace and governance. This latter task also requires that stability be maintained by the threat of violence and techniques of subjugation, negotiation, control, domestication, and apprehension. The frequency and distribution of the word yoga in the eighteen books of the *Mahābhārata* is rendered in figure 1.1.

Yoga appears most often in the second half of Book Six (which contains the *Bhagavad Gītā*), before the war begins, and again, almost twice as many times, around Book Twelve, *after the war is done*.[61] These two crescendos of the word yoga in the epic bear a structural similarity to each other. In both locations, yoga appears primarily in the context of discourses delivered by a man designated as a *māhāyogī*—Krishna and Bhishma, respectively—who must convince a reluctant Pandava hero—Arjuna and Yudhishthira, respectively—to take on a duty (*dharma*) relevant to his warrior-ruler status. And in both cases, each of the many techniques used to persuade these reluctant warriors is called a "yoga." The two episodes bookend the tale of the war, which starts in the second half of Book Six and concludes with Book Eleven, "The Book of Women," when many of the epic's female characters perform funeral rites and lamentations.[62] From the view of plot and structure, and whatever else "yoga" may mean in the text, an engagement with

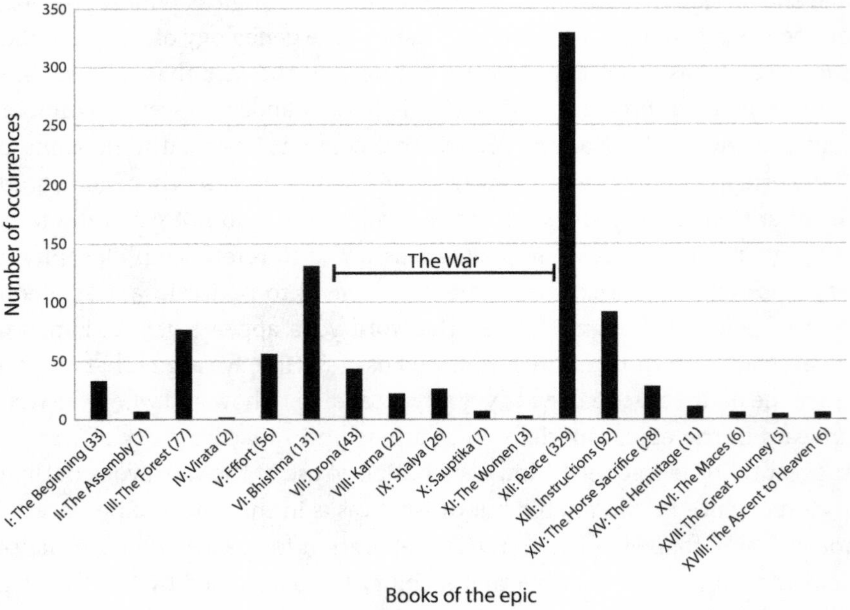

FIGURE 1.1 "Yoga" in the *Mahābhārata*

yoga in all its forms frames the battle at the heart of the epic. This framing suggests that the many meanings of yoga were organized by, linked to, and informed by concepts of war and conflict, that is, politics.

Yoga Before the War

The *Bhagavad Gītā* contains most of the instances of "yoga" in Book Six. As many scholars have noted, the *Bhagavad Gītā* is distinct from the epic's narrative form and structure; it is a kind of poetic and philosophical interlude in a massive prose text that is clearly the result of much refinement and attention over time.[63] This poetic meditation dwells on the many yogas used by Krishna to persuade Arjuna to take up battle because he has literally unyoked himself from his chariot and must be yoked again to fight. At one level, the advice that Krishna gives Arjuna is called "yoga"—disciplines for Arjuna to use to control his own mind, soul, and karmic fate. At another level, the *Bhagavad Gītā* records the yogas used by Krishna to control Arjuna and thus inaugurate the war. All eighteen chapters are also referred to as "yogas"; the text is called a *yogaśāstra* in the commentarial and colophonic traditions that interpret and preserve the *Bhagavad Gītā* for two millennia;[64] and the *Bhagavad Gītā* is revealed by a "lord of yoga" (*yogeśvara*), Krishna, a master of disciplines of control.[65] Just as Arjuna reins himself in with yoga, so too does Krishna rein Arjuna in with yoga. The listener to the divine dialogue is privy to multiple layers of yoga at once, one of the many literary qualities of the text that renders it open to boundless interpretations over the centuries. Many modes of yoga emerge from commentary on the *Bhagavad Gītā*, and three are perhaps best known: the harnessing of knowledge (*jñāna-yoga*), the harnessing of devotion (*bhakti-yoga*), and the harnessing of action (*karma-yoga*).[66] Although these are not strict distinctions in the text itself, much has been written about these three, including which trumps the other and how the three are related. Much also has been written about the presence of other yogas, including Sāmkhya Yoga as well as psychophysical practices, especially of meditation and the control of breath, a particular subject of chapter 6 of the *Bhagavad Gītā*.[67] Yet all these modes of yoga—from the dialogue to each individual discipline, to the structure of the text itself—serve to catalyze not only a war but the end of the war, the way through it to a dubious victory and peace.

The form of yoga from this text that is most enduring from a political point of view is *karma-yoga*, the harnessing of "action" through nonattachment, that is, acting but not being attached to the action or its results or benefits, its "fruits."[68] The ideal yogi is in control when he acts without attachment and by this means does not accrue *karma*.[69] This is the "harnessing" of the potentially damaging repercussions of action (*karma*) on one's soul (*ātman*).[70] Many times Krishna tells Arjuna he must find the means of controlling himself, a term often expressed as *yoga-yukta*, yoked to discipline, to control.[71] This soteriological problem is closely connected with the political problem Arjuna faces because it would be wrong of him—morally wrong—to be attached to the outcome of a war in which he must kill his own family members. But he has to do it; it is his duty, as Krishna reminds him many times. Krishna appears exasperated with Arjuna's recalcitrance and demands that he "cut away his ignorance" and "apply yoga" (*yogam ātiṣṭha*), by which he means "get up" (*uttiṣṭha*) to fight.[72] This exhortation to discipline oneself and then act without attachment is the core concept of *karma-yoga*, an idea that will resonate widely in the modern period's political reinterpretation of this ancient text, a subject of chapter 3. Whatever else the yogas of the *Bhagavad Gītā* may be—and they are a spectrum of extraordinary things, to be sure—they all bear the mark of a story of one warrior trying to convince another to go to war.

The Sanskrit scholar M. A. Mehendale analyzes the three times when Krishna is hailed as a *yogeśvara* or "Lord of Yoga" in the *Bhagavad Gītā*.[73] We find that the three spheres of yoga interweave in these moments in the text. In the first instance, Krishna is called *yogeśvara* when he shows his cosmic form to Arjuna,[74] a moment when his yoga appears to describe his ability to contain and command the eternal cosmos.[75] The second moment occurs in the final book,[76] and here Mehendale argues that Krishna is celebrated as "quite clearly . . . the master of . . . *yogaśāstra*," that is, philosophical and psychophysical yoga.[77] In the very last verse of the *Bhagavad Gītā*, Krishna is called a *yogeśvara* again for a third and final time, at the point when his exhortations have borne fruit and Arjuna finally has been convinced to fight. In this final instance, Mehendale argues, Krishna is celebrated as *yogeśvara*, not because of his divinity or his command of *yogaśāstra* but because he is the "the master of stratagem, master of the expedient means of warfare."[78] Yoga here in this last verse of the *Bhagavad Gītā*, at the precipice of the battle's start, means "strategy in war." This parallels how Krishna's many other martial strategies (sometimes based on deception) will come to form key moments in the war's progression later in the epic.[79] From this point of view, the encompassing "yoga" of the *Bhagavad Gītā* is a set of strategies to control a warrior-prince's reluctance to do his violent duty with the aim to harness his anxiety and thereby start a war. The war is an event in which many other yogas exist, many other strategies for victory, and multiple other kinds of yoga as well. But the point of all yogas, as they are combined and deployed in this text by Krishna, is to get Arjuna to fight.

When Book Six begins, well before we are standing on the battlefield with Arjuna and Krishna listening to their debate about whether or not to go to war, the war's outcome has already been reported by Sanjaya to Dhritarashtra: we know that the great yogi-warrior and leader of the Kaurava army, patriarch of both sides of the battle, Bhishma, is dead, and so we know that the war will turn in favor of the Pandavas eventually.[80] From this epic spoiler the narration proceeds to the *Bhagavad Gītā* followed by a recounting of the first ten days of battle. For the first nine of those days, the Pandavas face an unassailable Bhishma and the tide of war flows against the heroes. On the eve of the tenth day of battle, the Pandavas ask Bhishma to reveal how he can be killed. Bhishma obliges, and the tenth day ends with Bhishma wounded and the Pandavas ascendant in the conflict. The rest of the war is narrated in Books Seven through Eleven, which is titled "The Book of Women," when the last grievances are addressed, funeral rites undertaken, and key female characters of the epic speak their minds about the horrific violence their men have committed. Bhishma keeps himself alive during this time through his powers of psychophysical yoga. The epic war concludes with the bittersweet triumph of the Pandavas, the classic pyrrhic victory, and finally, in Book Twelve, the Book of Peace (*śānti*), Bhishma can teach the *dharmas*, the principles of proper action, that will govern the world after the war.

Yoga After the War

With a hard-won peace, the time has come for Bhishma to provide one last lesson to his former student and grand-nephew, Yudhishthira, who must overcome his desire to renounce the world in disgust (like his brother Arjuna before the battle) and instead focus his mind on ruling the postwar world.

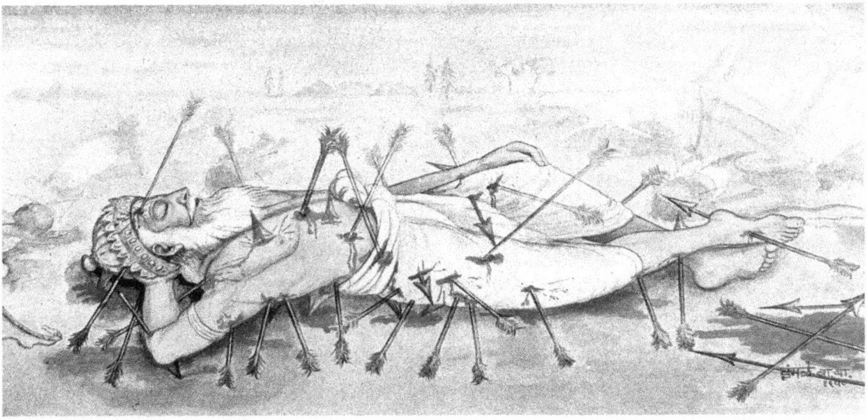

FIGURE 1.2 Bhishma on a bed of arrows
Source: Artist V. B. Imale 1945. Sukthankar 1966, folio. Commissioned by the Raja of Aundh.

Book Twelve records a mortally wounded Bhishma, cushioned upon a bed of spent arrows (figure 1.2), as he endeavors to induce Yudhishthira to do his duty as a warrior-king. The many rationales the old warrior teaches to the new king are called yogas. This might sound familiar. James Fitzgerald has argued that Book Twelve is a kind of prototype of the *Bhagavad Gītā*, which he describes as "a later and improved solution to the same basic problem" of kingship and salvation, making the *Bhagavad Gītā* a "later amelioration" of the teachings of Book Twelve, even though the *Gītā* diegetically precedes it.[81]

Bhishma's instructions (*anuśāsana*) to Yudhishthira take up all of Book Twelve and most of Book Thirteen, the Book of Instruction (*ānuśāsanaparvan*). Together, they cover four main topics: the responsibilities and methods of ruling (*rājadharma*); what to do in times of moral calamity (*āpaddharma*); how to attain release from the phenomenal world, the way of soteriology (*mokṣadharma*), the largest section of Book Twelve; and the teaching on "the obligation of donations" (*dānadharma*), the largest section of Book Thirteen.[82] Yoga as a technical term appears almost 330 times running through all these sections, although the greatest number of references occur in the section on "salvation/freedom" (*mokṣa*), where yoga predominantly names ideas of psychophysical-meditative practices or philosophical concepts, many related to Sāṃkhya, all of which seem to promise the maudlin

Yudhishthira a way out of the trap of human existence that embroiled him in this tragic civil war. Most scholars who study yoga in the epic beyond the *Bhagavad Gītā* turn to this section of the book, where ample material on these two streams of yoga is to be found.[83]

All the yogas of the Book of Peace are aimed toward "pacifying" (*śānti*) Yudhishthira's remorse (*śoka*), what Fitzgerald has called "the persuasion of Yudhiṣṭhira,"[84] a clear parallel to the yoking of Arjuna's "despair" (*arjuna-viṣāda-yoga*) that Krishna must manage. As with the *Bhagavad Gītā*, here too we have a text about politics that presents many strategies for rulership, all proposed as yogas, with most of these possessing the multivalent meaning of salvation from or advantage in the tumultuous world of death and rebirth, self and other that yoga as philosophy and psychophysical practice aim to quell.

Yoga carries multiple meanings throughout the *Rājadharma* and *Āpaddharma* sections,[85] including references to Sāṃkhya[86] and also to *bhakti* as a mode of yoga,[87] but a dominant use of the word in these sections involves governance and power in some way, usually revolving around the idea of yoga as control or mastery of aspects of governance,[88] battle tactics and strategies for gathering information,[89] sowing confusion among the enemy,[90] and running a political system.[91] The word is used in relationship to troop mobilization and movement,[92] the use of force (*bala*) to ensure peace,[93] the creation and discernment of allies,[94] as well as the art of peacemaking.[95] Yoga expresses the need of a king to master and control vital functions of his economy,[96] including judicious taxation.[97] At other times, one reads of *ayoga*, strategically unsound methods of control,[98] including excessive force on a population or just bad policy.[99] Indeed, the text tells us that "all yogas are within *rājadharma*," that is, the question of yoga, whatever the kind, is a question of kings, of proper governance.[100] Although some scholars have understood "yogas" here to mean "kinds of meditation,"[101] these portions of the text are not devoted exclusively or in some cases even primarily to meditation; instead, they engage with proper governance by a king in many realms, as noted above. These are techniques by which a king controls not just his mind or his actions, his *karma*, but the entire political realm. All forms of yoga are appropriate for the king. Put another way: all forms of control are the purview of the sovereign. Yoga as governance here does not preclude the governance of the self, mind, *ātman*, and thought, but it is, we argue, not in any way restricted to these meanings either. In the final passage of the *rājadharma*, as a segue into the *āpaddharma* section, Yudhishthira asks Bhishma what to do in a state of misfortune and calamity (*āpad*)—when ministers are corrupt, one has no allies, one's enemies are strong, and one's state is weak. Bhishma tells Yudhishthira that, in such difficult and uncertain times, he must hold fast to yoga, that is, skill or discipline in political matters:

> Ignorance gives rise to a man's lack of yoga (*ayoga*).
> And although ignorance certainly gives rise to a lack of yoga (*ayoga*),
> Yoga gives rise to prosperity (*bhūti*).[102]

Or put another way:

> Ignorance gives rise to a man's lack of political discipline (*ayoga*).
> And although ignorance certainly gives rise to a lack of political discipline (*ayoga*),
> Political discipline (*yoga*) gives rise to prosperity (*bhūti*).

Recumbent on his bed of arrows, Bhishma imparts this wisdom: a kind of political or royal discipline leads to prosperity, as much for a king as for his kingdom. This has been part of the lesson of the *Bhagavad Gītā*, and it is part of the lesson of the *rājadharma* and *āpaddharma* sections of Book Twelve as well. Everything rests on a well-governed kingdom governed by a self-governed king.

The other primary term we track in the *Ṛg Veda*—*yoga-kṣema*—also appears in the *Mahābhārata* in a way that aligns with the use of the word yoga we have traced above. As before, we visualize the appearance of the term *yoga-kṣema*, or "war and peace," in the *Mahābhārata* in figure 1.3.

Although it appears less frequently than yoga, the word *yoga-kṣema*, like yoga, bookends the story of the war, appearing primarily in Books Five and Six, and Books Twelve and Thirteen. Throughout the epic, the compound word takes on several meanings, all oriented to action, conflict, and resolution of conflict engaged for the sake of securing land, power, wealth, and political stability. The term's meanings range from "war and peace," "acquisition and security," "well-being," and "peace" in general to "secured possessions," "safety/security" itself, and "prosperity" in general.[103] Framing the start of the war, the term *yoga-kṣema* appears six times: four times in Book Five and two times in Book Six, the latter two times within the *Bhagavad Gītā*.[104]

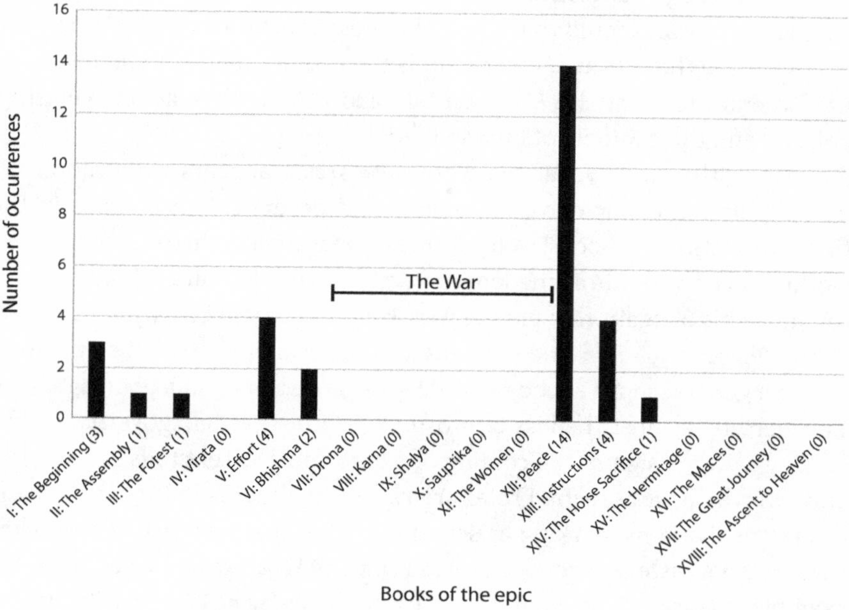

FIGURE 1.3 *Yoga-kṣema* in the *Mahābhārata*

In both places that it appears in the *Bhagavad Gītā*, *yoga-kṣema* conveys the older Vedic meaning of acquiring and securing property through war and the peace that follows, although the engagement with this term might seem contradictory. In the first occurrence of *yoga-kṣema*, Krishna tells Arjuna in chapter 2 that he must be without attachment to *yoga-kṣema*,[105] which is to say, indifferent to the acquisition of property and its security, the entire mission of a good king and the function of a state.[106] Instead, Krishna tells Arjuna he has "the right to action, but not its fruits."[107] The second appearance of *yoga-kṣema* in chapter 9 augments this earlier lesson when Krishna tells Arjuna that to those who worship Krishna, "I bring welfare and security [*yoga-kṣema*]."[108] In the first instance, Arjuna is instructed to renounce attachment and act only in the name of duty, but in the second instance Krishna tells Arjuna that one of the benefits (a fruit?) of devotion or *bhakti* is achieving *yoga-kṣema*. Theological interpretations aside, the lesson to Arjuna appears to be that *yoga-kṣema* is the interest of the warrior-king, whose job is to accumulate and preserve wealth for himself and his kingdom through successful and beneficial negotiations with neighboring kingdoms, or war, should that prove the most fruitful strategy.[109] The word *yoga-kṣema* in the *Bhagavad Gītā* reminds the listener that war and peace are fundamental to what the *Bhagavad Gītā* and the epic are about: kingship, politics, and the conflicts of human life.[110]

As with the word yoga, the word *yoga-kṣema* appears even more frequently after the war ends. The compound occurs thirteen times in the first two sections of Book Twelve as Bhishma instructs the reluctant Yudhishthira on how to rule a kingdom correctly.[111] Yudhishthira initially tries to renounce his obligation to pursue *yoga-kṣema*—a parallel to Arjuna's refusal in the *Bhagavad Gītā*.[112] The meaning of the term appears to be "prosperity" in a general sense as the result of good governance in a good age,[113] or safeguarding against the loss of prosperity because of bad governance in a dark age.[114] One sign of the coming of a dark age, the text tells us, is a situation in which caste (*varṇa*) roles are reversed: Shudras living by alms and Brahmans living by working as servants.[115] The maintenance of orthodox, conservative caste and gender orders is part of *yoga-kṣema* as well here. For example, chapter 13 on "giving" argues that *yoga-kṣema* is primarily won by donations to Brahmans.[116] We also read that *yoga-kṣema* is supported by the king's right to tax his subjects properly,[117] as well as his duty to propitiate deities and ancestors correctly.[118] We are told that *yoga-kṣema* depends on the king,[119] who depends on his priestly advisers (*purohita*), who depend on Brahmans to pacify people's anxieties about religious mysteries (the "unseen" [*adṛṣṭa*]). The king, through force, allays their anxieties about terrestrial threats.[120] The king's and the state's charitable support of the "less fortunate" is also a key aspect of *yoga-kṣema*.[121] A sign of the achievement of *yoga-kṣema* in a kingdom is an educated and thriving aristocracy.[122] In the effort to maintain *yoga-kṣema*, the king must regulate and secure trade and help support (and also tax) the trading community,[123] as well as the cattle-tending economy (which also gets taxed).[124] Indeed, the stability and expansion of these individual livelihoods is itself called *yoga-kṣema* in this text; that is, each economic and social subsystem nested within the larger polity is also described as *yoga-kṣema*, which presents a grand system of interlocking fields that must be maintained, controlled, defended, and allowed to prosper. In short, the term names the stabilization of the social, economic, and political fields, the "harnessing" (*yoga*) of "peaceful settlement" (*kṣema*).

Here *yoga-kṣema* means something like "peace arising from security" or even "a justly secure state," a state that is yoked or harnessed, internally but also externally—ready for war and peace, a land properly governed.[125] As we will see in the next chapter, Indian kingship strategies of this period assume the *maṇḍala* concept, the idea that a ruler is always "encircled" (*maṇḍala*) by potential friends and foes, as discussed in the introduction.[126] This concept of state sovereignty assumes the condition of *yoga-kṣema*, of a stable and secure internal state and economy that feeds a stable and secure external or "foreign" affairs apparatus, which includes an army as well as a network of spies—about which we will say more in the next chapter. This point is reinforced in one section of the *rājadharma* that speaks of the warrior's duties (*kṣatriya-dharma*). Here is Fitzgerald's translation:

> Those familiar with ancient times do not praise the deeds of a kṣatriya who withdraws from battle when his body has not been badly wounded. They say the Law of kṣatriyas is primarily killing. He has no more important duty than the destruction of barbarians . . . the acquisition [*yoga*] of goods, and their preservation [*kṣema*] are enjoined upon him; therefore, the king in particular must make war.[127]

Whatever distance the terms yoga and *yoga-kṣema* have traveled from their simpler, Vedic forms, they remain legible in the epic as terms deployed in contests of political power and its preservation. This is apparent from the meanings of these terms as well as their appearance within the narrative arc of the text.

Conclusion

The *Mahābhārata* and the *Bhagavad Gītā* evince a full integration of the three spheres of yoga that we have identified: the philosophical, the psychophysical, and the political; whereas the *Ṛg Veda* appears to confine the term solely to the political. While yoga as a concept exists only within a political-martial nexus in the *Ṛg Veda*, even there the metonymic and metaphoric uses of yoga to indicate the harnessing (often in conflict or competition) of other things like thought; art, truth, right, rite; and language are already present and may presage the future yogas of meditation, philosophy, and psychophysical practice. From *ṛta-yoga*, harnessing the "artful universe," to *jñāna-yoga*, *bhakti-yoga*, or *karma-yoga* is, linguistically and intellectually speaking, not a great leap. The meanings of these terms all circulate around a strategy, method, or system of control of each object: *ṛta*, *jñāna*, *bhakti*, and *karma*. This may be aspirational—who can really control these lofty powers? And it may be instrumental—as when Krishna employs knowledge, devotion, and action to persuade his reluctant warrior, or the warrior employs these yogas to quell his own doubts and frayed nerves. Indeed, the epic proliferates with yogas organized around the control or strategic use of powerful objects, even one's own self and the turning of one's thoughts. The commonality is that this yoking always furthers one's advantage or advances one toward a goal in the realm of earthly power and control.

We do not argue that this formulation applies to all instances of the word "yoga," although it might. Instead, our aim is to note that the political is the first demonstrable context for the technical use of the term yoga in the *Ṛg Veda*, and this early use echoes in the epic. In the centuries that follow, yoga as psychophysical practice, meditation, and philosophy will grow far beyond the narrow Vedic meaning of "harnessing a horse as if for war," but these subsequent meanings in the realms of philosophy and psychophysical practice will often return to the metaphors of chariots, horses, contests, and heroics, which perhaps implies the way this old Vedic concept is reinvented to apply to new technologies of controlling an object of some kind, new yogas for new eras.

TWO

Yoga as Political Strategy in the *Arthaśāstra*

IN JANUARY 2022, India's finance minister, Nirmala Sitharaman, addressed the Indian parliament to share her vision for India's fiscal future in the annual union budget presentation. The speech lamented the impact of a global pandemic on Indian citizens and their economy, and both noted and promised an increase in public investment as well as an increase in funds allocated to benefit women, farmers, youth, and scheduled castes and tribes. As she reached the middle of her speech, Sitharaman's remarks took a turn: she invoked yoga. But this was not the yoga of breath, mind, body, or spirit. This was the yoga of paying taxes. Sitharaman thanked "the taxpayers of our country who have contributed immensely and strengthened the hands of the government in helping their fellow citizens in this hour of need," then she cited Book Twelve, Bhishma's lesson to Yudhishthira, from the *Mahābhārata*:

> The King must make arrangements for Yogakshema (welfare) of the populace by way of abandoning any laxity and by governing the state in line with Dharma, along with collecting taxes which are in consonance with the Dharma.[1]

In the last chapter, we explored the term *yoga-kṣema* as well as the meaning of the word yoga within this compound. Sitharaman defined this term in her speech as "the welfare of the populace" and the official Government of India publication of the speech glosses the term in the quote above as "welfare." Her implication is that it is the state's *dharma*, its obligation, to levy taxes to ensure the *yoga-kṣema* of the public and the state, its "welfare." As we have already seen, this is a term used in the *Ṛg Veda* and the *Mahābhārata*. The latter is Sitharaman's source for her quote, the same deathbed discourse on yoga by Bhishma that we explored in the last chapter. This is the yoga of statecraft, of controlling a political economy and ensuring stability, in this case, through taxation.

Indian media rippled with surprise and rushed to comment on this "cryptic" reference. Some extended the epic citation, while others complained that invoking an ancient text suggested that India's finance policy was five thousand years out of date.[2] The act of referring to the *Mahābhārata* is certainly nothing new in modern Indian society. A. K. Ramanujan quipped that no Indian "reads the *Mahābhārata* for the first time."[3] The ancient past is layered onto the present in complicated ways, awaiting renewal and fresh fields. Just as the ancient texts and practices of psychophysical yoga have found new life in the modern world, so too do older ideas of yoga as a term with political valence find novel uses in the present. Despite the media surprise, in fact, it is not unusual to find the term *yoga-kṣema* used in contemporary India, especially in relationship to the state and its functions, particularly providing welfare. One prominent example is the government-owned Life Insurance Corporation (LIC) of India, for which the word *yoga-kṣema* serves as part of a slogan within its logo: "*yogakṣemam vahāmyaham*," which the LIC translates as "your welfare is our responsibility"[4] (figure 2.1).

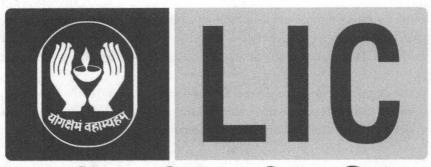

योगक्षेमं वहाम्यहम्

LIC

भारतीय जीवन बीमा निगम

LIFE INSURANCE CORPORATION OF INDIA

FIGURE 2.1 Logo of the Life Insurance Corporation (LIC) of India

The LIC was formed in 1956 after the government nationalized and acquired a host of Indian and foreign-owned insurance companies that had operated in colonial India for many decades but in a fashion deemed unsatisfactory for the needs of a large, poor, and newly independent country. A few years after its formation, a grand new structure was built to serve as the LIC headquarters at Nariman Point in Mumbai and christened "Yogakshema." At the 1963 inauguration of the curving modernist structure, Prime Minister Jawaharlal Nehru said that insurance should be encouraged "in every way" because it provides security to large numbers of people.[5] Security and welfare are the bedrock ideas of the modern state, and in invoking *yoga-kṣema*, modern politicians like Nehru attempted to provide a sense of inevitability for postcolonial India by drawing on an ancient political concept.

Although Sitharaman invoked the *Mahābhārata* to connect taxation and state welfare, the more germane classical text for the idea of *yoga-kṣema* is the *Arthaśāstra* (ca. 200 CE), a treatise on statecraft. In 2010, under the government led by the Indian National Congress (INC) politician, Manmohan Singh, the income tax department commemorated 150 years of taxation by issuing a five-rupee coin stamped with the image of the *Arthaśāstra*'s purported author, Chanakya or Kautilya (figure 2.2).

The *Arthaśāstra* is a classical authoritative study of the theory and practice (*śāstra*) of political economy (*artha*).[6] The *Arthaśāstra*'s subject—*artha*—is

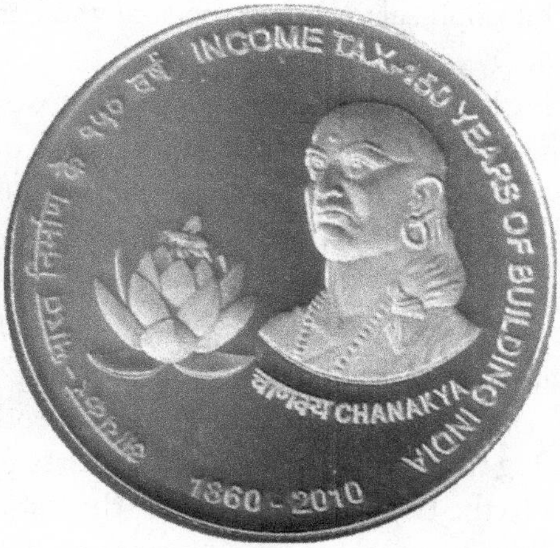

FIGURE 2.2 Five-rupee Chanakya coin, 2010

cognate with the English word "earth," and its meanings range from "wealth," "state," and "power" to "meaning" itself, all grounded in the earthly affairs of human beings. The sense in which it is used in this text is as the field of theory and practice for a king; for the organization of the state, its economic, social, and military affairs; and for success in confronting one's adversaries. *Artha* is one of the "three things" (*trivarga*) of classical Brahmanical *dharmic* thought: *artha*, *kāma*, and *dharma*—wealth, pleasure, and duty. While other authoritative studies exist for the other two things—*kāma* has the famous *Kāmasutra* and *dharma* has the many texts of Dharmaśāstra literature—the *Arthaśāstra* remains the preeminent text of political economy from classical India. Amid other texts within the *arthaśāstra* and *nītiśāstra* genre, it is the exemplar.[7]

Among classical texts, the term *yoga-kṣema* and the idea of yoga as statecraft find perhaps their fullest application in the *Arthaśāstra*. Yoga as a political concept and practice appears throughout the *Arthaśāstra* and forms a core idea in the work, yet it has received very little attention in scholarship on yoga.[8] The reason is perhaps because yoga, in its forms as psychophysical practice or philosophy, is nearly absent from this text, even while its political valences run throughout. Extending from the last chapter, our primary aim in this chapter is to draw from the *Arthaśāstra* its theory of yoga as political thought and practice, both for its own sake, and to establish a set of classical resonances for the chapters on modern India that follow in part II of the book. In this way, we are continuing in line with the broader world of yoga studies that has established a canon on which modern forms of psychophysical and philosophical yoga have been aligned, made divergent, or entirely reinvented.[9]

The *Arthaśāstra* is quite different from the two texts we studied in chapter 1. It has none of the grand history, narrative, or drama of the *Mahābhārata*, nor does it possess the arcane ritual, poetry, or extravagant cosmic imagination of the *Ṛg Veda*. Instead, it is a relatively direct text on the theory and practice of governing a state in India roughly two thousand years ago. As a primary source about the political in this period, the *Arthaśāstra* is an ideal text for our pursuit of a classical genealogy of yoga as political theory and practice.[10] It is also a text that reveals an awareness of both the Vedic corpus and the epic, drawing from and referencing both, thus providing at least a circumstantial link to the two textual studies of the last chapter.[11]

The *Arthaśāstra*, like many texts of the ancient world, including those we studied in chapter 1, was not likely composed in a year or a decade or by a single author. Instead, it was probably assembled over several hundred years.[12] There are a few names given for the author of the text—Vishnugupta, Chanakya, Kautilya—and most scholars who cite this text refer to "Kautilya" as its author. Ours is not a study of the text's authorship, so we leave it to the experts and follow Patrick Olivelle in referring to the author-editor of the final version of the text as Kautilya.[13] It is also interesting to note that there are good reasons to believe the text itself was composed in or around Maharashtra, a key location for chapters 3 and 4.[14]

Most modern commentators on the *Arthaśāstra* describe the ideas contained in this work as either "philosophy" or "realpolitik" because the text makes little use of cosmological or superhuman references and instead grapples with the political exigencies of its day.[15] It is thus a text on the theory and practice of statecraft from the minute levels of courtly interaction among advisers to the vast logics of the movement of troops, the measurement of a state's demographics and economy, and the grand strategy of sustaining one's political power in a world surrounded by potential allies and enemies. The text assumes and serves a male, kingly, powerful audience, and, in the form we have it today, it also reflects the influences and interests of Brahmanical power.[16]

After its "rediscovery" in the early twentieth century, the *Arthaśāstra* was hailed as the preeminent ancient Indian text on a variety of aspects of statecraft, from how to conduct foreign policy and manage the economy to how to ensure the public good within one's political realm.[17] Remarking on the *Arthaśāstra* in the early twentieth century, historian K. V. Ramaswamy Aiyangar said that the text would provide "a corrective to the prevalent belief of our day in the total absorption of the ancient Indian intellect in metaphysical speculation."[18] The work subsequently received important attention from scholars in the Western academy.[19] As the text showed, ancient India was home to complex theories about political economy, grand strategy, and state surveillance. Even someone as seemingly far afield as the American sociologist W. E. B. Du Bois identified in the text a source to chart a non-Western genealogy for the modern welfare state. This occurred not in his social science scholarship but in his foray into the world of science fiction with his 1928 novel, *The Dark Princess*.[20]

After brief fame in the early twentieth century, the *Arthaśāstra* faded somewhat in English-language materials. As Maria Misra argues, the text's dominant note of pragmatism was out of step with the prevailing view that politics should be imbued with a moral purpose, a position shared by the most influential of India's antinationalist and postindependence leaders, especially Nehru and M. K. Gandhi.[21] The text's fortunes would rise again when, from the 1980s onward, Nehru's state-led developmentalism gave way to a neoliberal model of political economy that privileged economic growth, and the end of the Cold War led to the declining importance of the Non-Aligned Movement as a force for organizing foreign policy in the Global South.[22] Both shifts paved the way for the *Arthaśāstra*'s reemergence in the spheres of politics and policy, when it was embraced by centrist market reformers and Hindu nationalist politicians alike.[23]

Mirroring its growing importance for politicians and policymakers, contemporary scholarship has likewise grown apace.[24] Over the last several decades, two main streams of scholarship have emerged. The first and older stream is about the *Arthaśāstra* as a text of political realism in the fields of international relations, intelligence studies, security studies, and foreign policy; the second is focused on the *Arthaśāstra* as a text of management, especially business and wealth management.[25] We focus on the first body of scholarship because it shares our core concerns with the political. Here, the text is often hailed as an important work in a classical genealogy for non-Eurocentric or non-Western theory, along with classical Chinese thought. For example, Philip Davies suggests that what distinguishes the *Arthaśāstra* from the Chinese theorist Sun Tzu (ca. sixth to fifth century BCE) is the *Arthaśāstra*'s insistence that intelligence gathering—its apparatus, logic, and personnel—is central to all facets of governance. The text therefore constitutes one of the few ancient sources of intelligence theory, which is one of the primary conceptual fields designated by "yoga" in the text, as we will see.[26] Roger Boesche (2005) compares the *Arthaśāstra* to a different Chinese author, Han Feizi (ca. third century BCE), whose text is more contemporaneous. The two texts are alike, he argues, in offering pragmatic advice to kings as well as in their take on human nature as fundamentally self-interested. But whereas the Chinese text's guidance is geared toward securing the social status quo, the Indian text is aspirational, advising a ruler on how to maximize the kingdom's wealth.[27]

Among scholars of politics in particular, more common than references to classical Chinese texts, however, are comparisons between Kautilya's *Arthaśāstra* and the Italian diplomat and theorist Niccolo Machiavelli (1469–1527) and his text, *The Prince* (1532).[28] The trend began just a few years after the *Arthaśāstra*'s early twentieth-century translation into English, when Max

Weber describes its logic of kingly advice as having a "radical 'Machiavellianism,'" compared to which even "*The Prince* is harmless."[29] More recently, Stuart Gray compares the entanglements of politics and theology in *The Prince* and the *Arthaśāstra*, arguing that at the core of the latter is a clear political-theological ethic that is lacking in *The Prince*.[30]

What is striking for us regarding scholarship about political theory in ancient India, including work on the *Arthaśāstra*, is the absence of any sustained discussion of yoga as a term of political theory and practice, even though the word, both alone and in various compound forms, appears throughout the text. We can give examples of important work from a range of disciplines—from political science and international relations to political theory, history, and political philosophy. For instance, John Spellman, in his *Political Theory of Ancient India*, does not mention yoga at all. More recently, writing on the *Arthaśāstra*'s relevance for the field of international relations, Medha Bisht defines yoga when it appears in the compound *yoga-kṣema* as "the acquisition of things" and the word yoga alone as one of several schools of Indian philosophy.[31] Upinder Singh, in her *Political Violence in Ancient India*, does cite an important passage in the *Arthaśāstra* that defines *yoga-kṣema*, where she writes: "Peace [*śama*] and activeness [*vyāyāma*] are further described as the source of acquisition and security (or prosperity) (*yogakṣema*) directly in line with the larger goals of the *Arthashastra*."[32] In this context, Singh defines yoga as "acquisition," but she does not elaborate on the meaning of the word in her book beyond this combined definition. Prathama Banerjee draws on a range of premodern sources, including the *Arthaśāstra*, as they form possibilities for the shape of the political in the modern period. She explores the *Arthaśāstra* as an example of "realpolitik" in her analysis, understanding the text to examine the "the science of achieving *artha*" or "efficacy" and tracing its reception and uses in modern India, but again without an explicit discussion of yoga except as a school of philosophy.[33]

To reiterate a point from the introduction, the absence of scholarly attention to *yoga as a political concept* in discussions of ancient Indian texts, history, and political theory is perhaps because of a double omission: on the one hand, those who study yoga (i.e., yoga studies scholars) bypass the political texts and contexts in which yoga as political thought and practice circulates; on the other hand, those who study political theory do not engage the many references to yoga that might have political valence, perhaps assuming that any reference to "yoga" is a reference to its forms as religious thought, spirituality, philosophy, or psychophysical practice.[34] Our work tries to weave a space in between, joining the concerns of these fields but converging on a point often missed in both. For all these reasons, the *Arthaśāstra* is an ideal text to see the place of yoga as a political concept in the ancient worlds of statecraft and strategy.

Yoga as Strategy

As with the uses of the word yoga in contexts studied in chapter 1, the term usually means something very basic in the *Arthaśāstra* such as: to master, control, or harness something; to carry out or undertake some practical activity; and to apply or use something or someone in some way, often with the implication of doing so with successful or skillful completion or control.[35] The *Arthaśāstra* is fundamentally about kingly mastery of the political realm, and so the word yoga is pressed into serving this primary subject by indicating modes of mastery related to various strategies of control. Just as ideas of *jñāna-yoga* as "harnessing knowledge" or *karma-yoga* as "harnessing action" appear in the *Bhagavad Gītā* in the context of war and peace, as we saw in chapter 1, so too one finds many references in the *Arthaśāstra* to harnessing powerful things for some political purpose, especially as a method of subterfuge. For example, we read of various yogas that describe practices of harnessing the ability to confuse, bewilder, or unsettle one's enemy: "harnessing deception" (*māyā-yoga*),[36] "harnessing word-spells" (*mantra-yoga*),[37] "harnessing intoxicating mixtures" (*madana-yoga*),[38] "harnessing vision" or rather visual illusions (*yoga-darśana*),[39] and "harnessing secret doctrines/methods" (*upaniṣad-yoga*).[40]

Scholars of psychophysical and philosophical yoga have noted the intersection of the word yoga and these disciplines of deception, particularly as they are used by ascetics or non-ascetics in the guise of ascetics. For example, David Gordon White refers to the figure of a spy "who puts on the garb of a yogi in order to travel incognito through foreign lands" but also refers to actual yogis who are "spies or agents provocateurs," or to both: "yogi spies, or of spies dressed in the garb of yogis."[41] The *Arthaśāstra* does advise kings on the use of ascetics to gather intelligence and spread misinformation,[42] and it also speaks of spies (who are not ascetics) dressing as ascetics in order to infiltrate enemy domains more easily.[43] This also means, from the point of view of a diligent king, that all people who look like ascetics are potentially enemy spies.[44]

The ascetics of the *Arthaśāstra* are of various kinds (*muṇḍa, siddha, tāpasa*), but it is noteworthy that the *Arthaśāstra* does not use the term "yogi" (e.g., *yogin, yogī, yoginī*) to describe these figures—indeed, the term seems entirely absent from the *Arthaśāstra*.[45] In this literal sense, there are no "yogis" in the *Arthaśāstra*. Although ascetics abound in the text, yoga in its psychophysical or philosophical modes is not used to describe any practice these ascetics undertake or any philosophical position they hold, even among figures who are, in other kinds of texts, described as yogis who practice yoga, such as *tāpasa* (austere ascetics),[46] *muṇḍa* and *muṇḍā* (male and female ascetics with shaved heads), *jaṭila* (ascetics with dreadlocks), *siddhavyañjanā* (learned accomplished ascetics), *parivrājikā* (wandering female ascetics), and *bhikṣukī* (female mendicants who wander and beg for alms).[47] Sometimes such figures possess certain "masteries," certain "yogas," such as *māyā-yoga-vid*, "knowing the harnessing of illusion" or visual deception, but nowhere do we read of their explicit association with psychophysical or philosophical yoga and such abilities are not attributed to psychophysical yogic practice, but to techniques of spycraft and political strategy.[48] One also finds that the activities of secret agents posing as ascetics (*siddhavyañjanarūpa*) are described as yoga, but here this word means skill in deception, with no relationship to psychophysical yoga.[49] Of course, these ascetics may have been practitioners of psychophysical yoga. For example, one reads of secret-agent ascetics "with shaved heads or dreadlocks, living in a secret cave in the mountains, declared to be four hundred years old."[50] Such a description would suit a reclusive yogi well. Our point here is only that no form of the word "yogi" is used to describe these figures in the *Arthaśāstra*, and the text is not prescribing for them or detailing any kind of psychophysical yoga. We may modify White's insights to say that, while there is no explicit reference to "yogis" or anyone practicing psychophysical yoga in the *Arthaśāstra*, there are references to ascetics, who, whether real or in disguise, have a role to play in gathering intelligence, sowing disinformation, and serving as provocateurs for the king. These various disciplines of deception and misinformation are themselves called yoga.

What exactly does the *Arthaśāstra* say about these secret-agent ascetics, and how might this relate to the word yoga in the text? The selection of spies is a key issue for the *Arthaśāstra*, and the word yoga, as well as the figure of the ascetic, are both prominent in this context.[51] For example, the eleventh chapter of the first book of the *Arthaśāstra* is entirely dedicated to the appointment and use of "secret agents" (*gūḍhapuruṣa*).[52] People "presenting" (*vyañjana*) as ascetics of one kind or another are common. The sorts of people who could be recruited to serve as spies include an *udāsthita*, a former actual ascetic who has renounced his vows; a *tīkṣṇa*, a religious zealot; a *tāpasa*, an ascetic who takes on tremendous austerities; and a *bhikṣukī*, a female begging mendicant.[53] The *Arthaśāstra* elaborates whether these several kinds of ascetics are useful for espionage. For example, the *udāsthita* is one who has become disillusioned with the path of asceticism and seeks to pursue wealth and pleasure. He can be enticed by a handsome salary, the *Arthaśāstra* tells us, to put his ascetical garb back on and run an intelligence ring composed of other wandering ascetics.[54] The *Arthaśāstra* expands on this method in relation to traders (*vāṇija*) and farmers (*karṣa*) who have failed in their former professions (*vṛttikṣīṇa*) and so are susceptible to offers to be restored to their former livelihoods in exchange for giving intelligence to the king.[55] This is also the model for recruiting *tāpasa*, who are ascetics who want to return to the worldly pleasures of life (*vṛttikāma*).[56] They can be induced to stay in the guise of an ascetic—appearing with "shaved-heads" (*muṇḍa*) or with "dreadlocks" (*jaṭila*)—to serve both as a spy and as a ringleader of other recruited mendicant spies. In return, they are paid and given food regularly.[57]

The *Arthaśāstra* seems to blur the line between the sincere ascetic and the apostate ascetic in disguise as a sincere ascetic. For example, later in the *Arthaśāstra*, in the fifth chapter of the fourth book, spies take on the guise of ascetics (*siddhavyañjanā*) to sus out plots brewing against the king.[58] Perhaps one could not know, then, if a given ascetic was a real ascetic, a real ascetic who was also a spy, or a spy disguised like a real ascetic. One might say this is the yoga of the ascetic—the ability to shift among worlds to suit a strategy of self-benefit. For this reason, kings are advised both to use ascetics (or former ascetics, or just spies dressed as ascetics) and also to remain suspicious and watchful of all who appear as ascetics.[59] In part, this is because a neighboring king can also be presumed to be following the very same advice on the use of ascetics in the *Arthaśāstra*.

In addition to yoga conveying the meanings and associations of spy craft discussed above, the word in the *Arthaśāstra* has multiple associations with "mastery" of some esoteric art. For example, the text mentions those who have mastered self-mortification (*tapasvin*), know the three Vedas (*vedavid*), can harness illusion (*māyā-yoga-vid*), and have mastery of the *Atharva Veda*.[60] The one who has "mastered illusion" appears also to be able to control the weather, especially rain; to challenge evil spirits; and to help avoid general calamities in the kingdom.[61] These are tangential connections, really vague associations among some ascetics and people who have these supernatural powers of mastery or who enact yoga as a term for their clandestine work. The kinds of superpowers associated with yogis of the psychophysical variety are well known, but here there is no evidence of such figures as practitioners of psychophysical yoga, such as *haṭha*, in this text. Instead, the text gives us examples of how the word yoga indicates mastery, in this case of the sorts of supernatural abilities that are sometimes associated with yoga and yogis in the psychophysical context, but not limited to them.[62] Essentially, the only activity of an ascetic (or apparent ascetic) in this text that is clearly described by the word yoga is some form of espionage work. What then does yoga mean in the *Arthaśāstra* more generally if it does not mean psychophysical practice or philosophy?

We can approach an answer by looking at the two figures in the text whose very identity is described through the term yoga. The first is the "yoga man," or *yoga-puruṣa*. The yoga man appears to be a high-level secret agent, a master of multiple forms of deception and espionage, the James Bond of ancient India. The *yoga-puruṣa* is a recurring figure of the *Arthaśāstra*,[63] described as an agent provocateur who works directly for the king[64] and so is a more elite form of the general "secret agent" or *gūḍhapuruṣa*, noted above.[65] The yoga man seems best equipped to undertake clandestine operations behind enemy lines,[66] especially enacting misinformation campaigns,[67] or employing guerilla tactics,[68] and sometimes operating within the king's own territory as a spy surveilling his own population,[69] such as during dangerous liminal moments of succession within the kingdom.[70] Although mentioned only once, one also reads of the *yoga-strī*, the "yoga woman," who might pose as a wealthy widow to lure one's enemy into compromising situations, especially after infiltrating the enemy's territory, and may carry out assassinations.[71] The *yoga-puruṣa* and *yoga-strī* serve as the direct human instruments of the king's covert strategy; that is, they are the people who carry out the king's yoga, his political vision.

The primary specialized use of the word yoga in the *Arthaśāstra* is as a strategy for action in the field of politics and war. This specialized use combines meanings of utilization and mastery with a particular directive: advantage in conflict with one's opponents. It also often implies secrecy, which is a standard aspect of strategy in general, something one does not divulge to one's enemies. Yoga in these contexts is sometimes described as a "trick," yet this word fails to convey all the senses of yoga here, such as deceptive political tactics; purposeful illusion; campaigns of misinformation, dissimulation, and disguise; the use of secret agents; unconventional or clandestine warfare (*kūṭayuddha*); or a clever countermove in political conflict. Yoga exists here in the field of "intelligence," the strategic gathering and deployment of information to one's political advantage.

Yoga as strategy is often joined in the *Arthaśāstra* with the idea of punishment and the threat of violence, represented by the king's *daṇḍa* or "rod."[72] Yoga in this form takes on several meanings around the general concept of a covert strategy in conflict, politics, and war as opposed to outright attack or physical violence. For example, the term describes strategies for how to reveal the enemy[73] and how to use water for camouflage, called the "strategy of Varuna" (*vāruṇa-yoga*).[74] In such contexts, yoga indicates covert tactics of many kinds that are applied to very specific needs or outcomes.[75] The subject is important enough to the text that the entirety of Book Five of the *Arthaśāstra* deals with *yoga-vṛtta*, "matters of covert strategy." In all these examples, yoga indicates a secret action, especially where overt force would be impractical or impossible. There are also points in the text when yoga does not emphasize deceptive action but simply strategy in a more general sense.[76] The dominant sense of yoga as a political concept in the *Arthaśāstra* is then as a strategy intended to create an advantage over one's adversaries. While the word may not mean "war" in these cases, it certainly involves contention over power, deployed in secret, all in the context of war and peace, settlement and prosperity that are the responsibilities of the king to his polity.

Yoga-kṣema as the Aim of Politics

As in the *Ṛg Veda* and in the *Mahābhārata*, the compound term *yoga-kṣema* appears in the *Arthaśāstra*, and even more prominently than in those texts. Although the word occurs only fourteen times in the *Arthaśāstra*, it figures importantly in the theory and practice of governance expounded in the work.

Most translators of the *Arthaśāstra* render this term in a way that echoes the use of the word in the epic context, especially in Book Twelve, which we surveyed in chapter 1. Olivelle, for instance, translates the term as "enterprise and security,"[77] while R. P. Kangle writes "acquisition and security,"[78] R. Shamasastry renders it "acquisition (of property) and security,"[79] and Upinder Singh defines it as "acquisition and security (or prosperity)."[80] L. N. Rangarajan elaborates on the term as "acquiring new territory and ensuring the security of the state within existing boundaries."[81] In all cases, the term carries the sentiment of governing by virtue of power and the threat and actualization of military power in particular, all set toward accomplishing security, stability, and the conditions for wealth and prosperity.

We are introduced to *yoga-kṣema* at the start of the first book, and almost half of the occurrences of this word appear in this first book alone. The *Arthaśāstra* describes *yoga-kṣema* as one of the essential aspects of governance, or as Mark McClish has noted, it is the very "goal of statecraft" in this text.[82] A state that actualizes *yoga-kṣema* provides stability and security in which certain endeavors can thrive, namely, the pursuit of knowledge (*ānvīkṣikī*), Vedic religion (*trayī*), and economic trade and industry (*vārttā*).[83] In turn, this system of law and order (*nīti*) requires the legitimate use of violence, metonymically represented by the king's staff (*daṇḍa*). And so *yoga-kṣema* is achieved and maintained through governing by "the rule of force" (*daṇḍanīti*), what McClish calls simply "conquest."[84] This mode of state power expressed through *yoga-kṣema*, in Olivelle's translation, "seeks to acquire what has not been acquired, to safeguard what has been acquired, to augment what has been safeguarded, and to bestow what has been augmented on worthy recipients."[85] This fulsome definition of *yoga-kṣema* echoes uses from the *Ṛg Veda* to the epic and into the *Arthaśāstra*. As with violence in the *Bhagavad Gītā*, however, here too violent force (*daṇḍa*) must be rooted in disciplined use (*vinayamūla*) in order to achieve one's ultimate and laudable goal of *yoga-kṣema*; it cannot be the violent and complete domination celebrated in the Vedic texts.[86] Indeed, poverty, greed, and disloyalty arise from the negligent application of *yoga-kṣema*.[87] A king who is perceived as weak might pursue *yoga-kṣema* to show strength;[88] if a king must repair to his fort, he is advised to attribute this defensive move to the desire to maintain *yoga-kṣema* of what remains of his territory, thus preserving the impression of his strength through a tactical retreat;[89] and a king's secret agents who have infiltrated the enemy's government should flatter its ministers with false praise of that kingdom's impressive *yoga-kṣema*.[90] Elsewhere, the *Arthaśāstra* says that *yoga-kṣema* is sustained by other means, such as the need to maintain state secrets;[91] proper lending practices;[92] the selection and support of ministers and chiefs who can extend the king's mission of maintaining *yoga-kṣema*;[93] the proper power-sharing arrangements between a king and his prince at a time of succession;[94] and the king's right and obligation to tax the citizenry,[95] which is reminiscent of the invocation of *yoga-kṣema* by Sitharaman that opened this chapter. The *Arthaśāstra* succinctly tells us that the difference between good policy (*naya*) and bad policy (*apanaya*) is whether the king is properly enacting and maintaining *yoga-kṣema*.[96] The *Arthaśāstra* is in essence a text about how to accomplish *yoga-kṣema*, and many of the disciplined methods used to attain this state are called "yoga."

The concept of *yoga-kṣema* is centrally important for the *Arthaśāstra*, but it is also perhaps a bit archaic; even in the time of the text's composition, the text devotes some space to carefully defining the word's meanings for its audience. A key passage provides a definition of *yoga-kṣema* in the second part of Book Six, which Olivelle has described as the core of the *Arthaśāstra* and as containing the "blueprint" for the structure of the text itself.[97] Here is Olivelle's translation of this passage, with the technical Sanskrit terms supplied in brackets by us:[98]

> Rest [*śama*] and exertion [*vyāyāma*] form the basis of enterprise [*yoga*] and security [*kṣema*].
>
> Exertion [*vyāyāma*] consists of the enterprise [*yoga*] that one furnishes to activities [*karma*] that are being undertaken.
>
> Rest [*śama*] consists of the security [*kṣema*] that one furnishes to the enjoyment of the fruits of one's activities [*karma-phala*].[99]

This passage occurs at the start of Book Six, which is entitled the "Maṇḍala-yoni" or "The Essence of the Circle Theory." This book of the *Arthaśāstra* is dedicated to exploring the political theory of the *maṇḍala*, which we have detailed in the introduction to our book and likened to Chantal Mouffe's idea of the political as a space of agonism. As Stanley Tambiah notes, the idea of the *maṇḍala* permeated the Hindu-Buddhist worlds of South and Southeast Asia and was used to describe not just a king's relations between his adversaries and allies but also a host of social, economic, political, and religious relations, from the mundane to the cosmologically significant.[100] In the *Arthaśāstra*, the *maṇḍala* describes a king's central location in a field of potential allies and enemies. The basic premise noted in the introduction is that any contiguous state poses a threat as an enemy, but this enemy can be turned into an ally through diplomacy, negotiation, shared enmity with another king, or the sheer dominance of superior power. Once an ally, this polity's borders become subject to the rule of the *maṇḍala* as well, and therefore a king assumes his kingdom's contiguous polities are enemies to be defeated or converted into allies. As Upinder Singh puts it, the king should "try to become the center of a galaxy of kings."[101] And so the entire system describes a sphere, a *maṇḍala*, of competing and cooperating power.

Yoga through *yoga-kṣema* is closely linked to the political theory of the *maṇḍala* through the concept of the sixfold strategy (*ṣāḍguṇya*),[102] which is the subject of the following book, Book Seven. Between the two texts, we read that "the basis of *yoga-kṣema* is the sixfold strategy . . . [and] the basis of the sixfold strategy is the *maṇḍala*."[103] As Hartmut Scharfe writes, "This circle [*maṇḍala*] in turn is the basis of the 'aggregate of six strands' [*ṣāḍguṇya*], which again is the basis for 'ease' (*śama*) and 'effort' (*vyāyāma*); these two finally are the basis for acquisition (*yoga*) and rest/security (*kṣema*)."[104] Yoga, through *yoga-kṣema*, is an essential mode of political strategy suited to achieve one's ascension and security in the field of the *maṇḍala*, the field of agonistic political conflict.[105] The interdependence of *yoga-kṣema* and the *maṇḍala* theory—both central concepts for the *Arthaśāstra*—occasion this moment of attention to the term *yoga-kṣema* here.

One way to understand this passage is to see how terms used here are used elsewhere in the text. We have already done this for yoga above, arriving at "strategy" as the most common meaning of the word in a technical sense. We have also done something similar for the word *kṣema* in chapter 1 as it appears almost exclusively with the word yoga, as outlined above.[106] As noted in chapter 1, Marianna Ferrara argues that the verbal root of *kṣema* (*kṣi*) "develops two meanings": "to stay, dwell, reside" in a state of peace, and also "to have power over, to rule, to possess."[107] While the latter meaning—"to rule"—is only explicitly present in the *Ṛg Veda*, it may be implied within the idea of "dwelling" and "reside," which requires control, security, and protection. In other words, *kṣema* may be interpreted as "residing" in a secure, peaceful, or pacified way, a peace achieved through dominance and governance. This leaves us to understand how *vyāyāma* and *śama* are used in the *Arthaśāstra* and through them, what the text means by yoga and *kṣema* here, as well as the technical compound that the words form together.[108]

There are two places in the *Arthaśāstra* where the word *śama* means a state of "peace."[109] We read that "peace" (*śama*) shares the same "aim/meaning" (*artha*) as "treaty" (*saṃdhi*) and "hostage exchange" (*samādhi*) because all three increase the "faith" (*viśvāsa*) or trust of a king in negotiation with other kings. Peace as *śama* is part of a strategic engagement among kings that also involves the potential for conflict, a negotiated peace. Elsewhere, the word indicates creating peace by pacifying an enemy, rebellion, or other uprising,[110] connotations that are drawn from the word's verbal root *śam*, meaning to pacify, ally, subdue, kill, extinguish, and conquer, as well as become fatigued over such exertions.[111] In this sense, *śama* as "rest" suggests both the exertion and the repose that follows. The aggregate meaning of *śama* in the *Arthaśāstra* is to achieve peace or tranquility, but it carries an implication of the use or threat of violence. It may also mean the tranquility that is the result of pacifying another. In this sense, *śama* would lead to *kṣema* because a population or political entity has been pacified (*śama*) and is now peacefully ruled or controlled, making the territory one of peaceful dwelling (*kṣema*).

The word *vyāyāma*, like *śama*, appears several times in the *Arthaśāstra*, where it refers to activity, exercise, effort, or exertion.[112] For example, it refers to exercise of one's elephants[113] or one's own body.[114] The word also indicates different kinds of effortful activities in general[115] and names an exertion toward an end.[116] In most cases in the *Arthaśāstra*, however, *vyāyāma* is used in the context of military activity, especially in the sense of either moving one's army in a military operation or engaging in military training exercises.[117] In the field of statecraft, which is to say, in the arena of *yoga-kṣema*, the word *vyāyāma* most likely indicates mobilizing one's army.

The definitional passage given above appears in the second book of the sixth chapter, and the title of the chapter itself is, as Olivelle translates it, "On Rest [*śama*] and Exertion [*vyāyāma*]."[118] One of only two chapters in this shortest of the books of the *Arthaśāstra*, it is nonetheless considered an essential statement on statecraft, as noted. It contains the primary theory of the *maṇḍala*, which the text here states is the key concept for the field of politics to which a king must attend. The text explains here that the *maṇḍala* is composed of internal state apparatuses,[119] and that the ring of neighboring kingdoms bordering one's own are either enemy (*śatru*) or ally (*mitra*) at any given moment.[120] These constituent elements of the *maṇḍala* form the internal sphere of the state and its border, the fundamental dialectic of the political theory of this text: the sovereignty of one's state and the distinction between ally and rival are two perennial subjects of political theory in ancient India as well as in the modern West, and *yoga-kṣema* speaks to both concerns.

The words *vyāyāma* and *śama*, when they appear in the *Arthaśāstra*, need to be read in the context of the *maṇḍala* theory, sovereignty, state security, peace and war, and the optimal equilibrium among these things. Likewise, *yoga-kṣema* sits at the core of the text's imagination of the proper use of state power to create the conditions for both stability and prosperity internally and with neighboring states. This power of the state is ensured by the threat or deployment of violent force, however measured and rationalized, which constitutes strategies for "state security," another definition for *yoga-kṣema*.[121]

Building on our analysis above, we may take *vyāyāma* to suggest military "mobilization," the exertion of the king's apparatuses of power and an echo from the Vedic use of yoga to mean harnessing a horse to a chariot for the season of war, that is, mobilizing for battle. We interpret *śama* as peace maintained after such mobilization, after violence or ensured by the threat of state violence, that is, the domestication of violence or peacekeeping. With this in mind, we propose this alternative translation of the passage above that considers how all the key words of this definition relate to their use in other places in the *Arthaśāstra*:

> Peacekeeping [*śama*] and military mobilization [*vyāyāma*] are the basis of state security and welfare [*yoga-kṣema*].
>
> Military mobilization [*vyāyāma*] achieves a state of security [*yoga*] so actions can be undertaken.
>
> Peacekeeping [*śama*] achieves a state of welfare [*kṣema*] so the fruits of actions [*karma-phala*] can be enjoyed.[122]

This passage conveys a prescriptive political logic and symmetry. Mobilization (*vyāyāma*) of one's resources, especially military ones, allows for action, and peacekeeping (*śama*) allows one to enjoy what that action achieves. This process constitutes the cycle of *yoga-kṣema*. The goal of kingship in the

Arthaśāstra is to mobilize and stabilize power successfully and strategically. The idea of yoga is at the core of this political goal. To maintain a state of security and welfare (*yoga-kṣema*) a king must sometimes mobilize for war, take action, as it were, and sometimes keep the peace, a stable political state of security in which he and his constituents can enjoy what was gained in his time of political action. This definition recognizes that *yoga-kṣema* is a compound word composed of two distinct, perhaps even opposite, activities—war and peace. And yet the passage also suggests the synergy and mutual dependence of these two things joined together to describe the scope of state "security and welfare."[123] Without mobilization and political strategy, that is, political action like war, a state does not advance or prosper, but without a period of peacekeeping and security, a state cannot benefit from what it has achieved in that time of advancement and war. Yoga as political action, war, and the assertion of power over another polity is aimless without *kṣema*, a time to enjoy the spoils of war. For the *Arthaśāstra*, this is the point of the state—advance, stabilize, advance again. Yoga is a political concept at the heart of this text's theorization of political power.

The state imagined in the *Arthaśāstra* is enforced, as is the way with states, by the threat of martial power, by *daṇḍanīti*, or what Max Weber describes as "a monopoly of the legitimate use of physical force."[124] Yoga within *yoga-kṣema* as a concept bears the weight of violence, the violence that ensures a state of peaceful governance. This may mark the evolution of *yoga-kṣema* from a concept that described the nomadic seasons of war and settlement in the Vedic period to a term meaning the ultimate political goal of "stability and prosperity" in the *Mahābhārata*, into a political theory for a settled, territorial, and stabilized world envisioned in the *Arthaśāstra*, where the term comes to encompass the core goal of statecraft.

The above passage emphasizes that the goal is to "enjoy the actions," that is, the result of successful and strategic political action. This echoes, but inverts, an essential teaching of *karma-yoga* in the *Bhagavad Gītā*.[125] In the latter text, as we saw, *karma-yoga* is articulated as acting without attachment to the fruits of that action and, as we have shown, this theory of *karma-yoga* is in the service of the politics of conflict that occasions the war in the epic. However, the *Arthaśāstra*'s definition of *yoga-kṣema* enjoins the king not only to act but to enjoy the fruits of those actions, to be attached to action. Walter Ruben argues that at least one concept of yoga in the *Arthaśāstra* is drawn from the epic and specifically the *Bhagavad Gītā*.[126] The

Arthaśāstra is a text with an awareness of the *Mahābhārata* (although there is no mention of the *Bhagavad Gītā* that we can locate), and one finds reference to several of the epic's characters and plot complications, particularly negative ones.[127] If this is an indirect reference to the *Bhagavad Gītā* or the epic, then this passage may appear as a refutation of the *Bhagavad Gītā*'s idea of renouncing one's investment in political action. Instead of acting without attachment to the fruits of one's actions, the *Arthaśāstra*, when it defines yoga and *yoga-kṣema* in terms of political theory and practice, explicitly instructs kings to be attached to their actions and enjoy the fruits of those actions, to be motivated by this very attachment. Why the actions if not for their fruits?

Yoga as Apprehension

We have saved for the end what is perhaps the most enigmatic passage in the *Arthaśāstra* around yoga, and it occurs at the very beginning. As the text opens, it provides an "enumeration of knowledge systems,"[128] of ways of apprehending aspects of state and society crucial to the project of governance. Inaugurating the section on "critical inquiry" is the following line:

> Rational inquiry (*ānvīkṣikī*) is constituted by *sāṃkhya*, *yoga*, and *lokāyata*.[129]

To see *sāṃkhya* and yoga joined in this way suggests the kind of philosophical and perhaps psychophysical traditions that we have said are not evident in this text. If the only yoga of the *Arthaśāstra* is yoga as political thought and practice, as we have argued, then what does this passage mean?

Often scholars assume these three terms name the three well-defined philosophical fields or *darśana* schools to which they would correspond: Lokāyata being the nontheist, empiricist, and materialist philosophy associated with the figure Cārvāka; and Sāṃkhya and Yoga, two distinct but intertwined philosophical schools, typified by the *Yoga Sūtras*.[130] But it is highly unlikely that yoga here refers to the *Yoga Sūtras*, which, as Maas estimates, has its origin around 400 CE, whereas the *Arthaśāstra* is generally situated around 200 CE.[131] Other scholars have argued that yoga here refers to the nascent, evolving, and intertwined intellectual worlds of Yoga and Sāṃkhya that emerge in the epic, not yet as full-blown schools of philosophy.

Others have argued that this is a reference to *karma-yoga* in the *Bhagavad Gītā*,[132] where the intertwining of Sāṃkhya and Yoga as two philosophies, or perhaps one with two expressions, is replete.[133] Because the *Arthaśāstra* does reference the *Mahābhārata*,[134] one can conjecture regarding connections to the epic and to the *Bhagavad Gītā*. As we noted above, if one reads the definition of *yoga-kṣema* as leading to the enjoyment of the fruits of one's actions, then one can see that this as a direct refutation of the *Bhagavad Gītā*'s concept of *karma-yoga*, suggesting just such a connection to the Sāṃkhya Yoga concepts of that text and in the epic.

There are also ways the ideal king is described that correspond to the advice of Krishna to Arjuna and Bhishma to Yudhishthira, especially around psychophysical and meditative yoga. For example, the *Arthaśāstra* tells us that a king who can control the "six enemies" (*ariṣaḍvarga*)[135] and his own senses (*indriya*) can "bring about *yoga-kṣema*" (*yoga-kṣema-sādhana*).[136] This idea of controlling one's senses as well as the "vices" of the "six enemies" is a concept found in the *Bhagavad Gītā* as well as in the *Yoga Sūtras*.[137] A king with this kind of self-control is referred to in the *Arthaśāstra* as a *rājarṣi*, a "sage-king," a king who rules with self-possession, reason, intelligence, proper information and counsel, philosophical training, and knowledge of the science of politics, which is the *Arthaśāstra* itself, all in the service of maintaining *yoga-kṣema*, the growth and stability of the kingdom.[138] At one point, the *Arthaśāstra* tells us that "control of the self" or *ātmavattā* is considered the result of yoga (*yogād ātmavatteti*),[139] that is, an effect of mastery and effort, of discipline in mind and body. These statements about mastery of the self perhaps resonate with psychophysical and meditative yoga, but the examples given above are never described with the term yoga but rather assume the king should control himself just as he would assert political control. These are not special meditative or psychophysical powers; this is just the job description of a good king.

The text tells us that yoga is a form of *ānvīkṣikī*, a way to rationally apprehend or actively perceive (i.e., *īkṣ* or "to observe"). The term suggests a knowledge practice, a way to gather information, rather than a traditional philosophical position.[140] The word *ānvīkṣikī* is introduced at the very beginning of the *Arthaśāstra* and is considered an essential knowledge system (*vidyā*) for kings alongside Vedic religion (*trayī*), economics (*vārttā*), and the "proper conduct of violence" (*daṇḍanīti*), that is, governance of a state.[141] The text also presents *ānvīkṣikī* as a thing kings must learn, along with writing, mathematics, economics, and political practice.[142] This mode of rational empirical inquiry is described, in Olivelle's translation of the *Arthaśāstra*, as "the lamp of all knowledge systems, the right strategy for all activities, and the basis for all Laws."[143] As we have seen, creating the very conditions in which rational inquiry can be carried out is one of the reasons the king must maintain *yoga-kṣema*.[144] In other words, *ānvīkṣikī* is a way of knowing the world, or as Olivelle writes, "rational investigations based on proper logical reasoning."[145] We argue that these investigations in the *Arthaśāstra* are particularly tuned to its subject: the material of the everyday world, information needed in order to govern well, and ways to harness or apprehend information for the aims of a king.

Thus, it is likely that the words *sāṃkhya*, *yoga*, and *lokāyata* here are not naming specific philosophical traditions but rather three key ways of rationally knowing the world and gathering information, things required for statecraft and politics, as the *Arthaśāstra* argues. Karl Potter, citing Paul Hacker, suggests "it is misleading to construe [*ānvīkṣikī*] as referring to philosophy" in this passage of the *Arthaśāstra*.[146] Kangle describes these invocations as references to what is "practically helpful" rather than three traditional fields of philosophy;[147] V. K. Gupta defines *sāṃkhya*, *yoga*, and *lokāyata* as "Understanding . . . action . . . reasoning";[148] and Ramkrishna Bhattacharya calls *lokāyata* "the science of disputation."[149] Jonardon Ganeri refers to *ānvīkṣikī* as "not a body of knowledge but a method of studying the proper aims and methods of knowledge" and states that the *sāṃkhya*, *yoga*, and *lokāyata* in this text "refer to different methods for approaching a critical investigation: a method of listing and enumeration, a method of dividing and reconnecting, and a method of empirical experimentation."[150] Along these lines, we understand the three references above as modes of rational inquiry and action that could be used to guide kings and rule states.

In the *Arthaśāstra*, Sāṃkhya as philosophy does not appear, but *saṃkhyā/sāṃkhya* as calculating or estimating using numerical and mathematical reason is described as a key skill for a king[151] as well as an instrument of governance.[152] Similarly, the text does not explicitly name Lokāyata as a philosophy, but does center the concept of observing the world and drawing conclusions "extending from the world" (*lokāyata*), that is empiricism. A passage we observed above enumerates essential requirements of governance,[153] summarized as the foundation of "worldly affairs" (*lokayātrā*).[154] Apprehending the empirical world and its machinations, being "an expert in worldly affairs," the matter and measure of the *loka* (world) is an essential aspect of governance in the *Arthaśāstra*.[155] In this sense, we could imagine the word "*sāṃkhya*" here means "quantification" and "*lokāyata*" means "empiricism," naming two essential ways for any state to measure, observe, and understand its territory, economy, threats, and opportunities. In our view, then, in the *Arthaśāstra*, the words *sāṃkhya*, *yoga*, and *lokāyata* do not reference three traditional philosophical positions but rather epistemologies befitting the exercise of power, politics, and governance.

It is possible that the yoga of the *Arthaśāstra* here is related to the yoga of the *Mahābhārata* and *Bhagavad Gītā*, and is linked to the yoga of the *Ṛg Veda* as well, but to its use as a term of political thought and practice, an expression of the discipline of governance itself, a rational way to understand and apprehend (*ānvīkṣikī*) statecraft. This is the yoga we have outlined in the last chapter and sustained in this one: yoga as a means to prepare for war and a way of maintaining peace, a way to govern through force but toward a stable prosperity. In this sense, yoga, drawn from the epic and applied in the *Arthaśāstra*, can be considered as a "theory of practice and the practice of theory," to borrow Sheldon Pollock's definition of the genre of *śāstra*, applied to the subject of the world of war, politics, negotiation, and peaceful prosperity.[156] In this sense, *ānvīkṣikī*, the deployment of rational knowledge in statecraft that the *Arthaśāstra* invokes, refers to using qualitative methods based on gathering empirical knowledge drawn from the world (*lokāyata*), quantitative methods based on enumerating and calculating key indicators of one's economy and state power (*saṃkhyā*), and applying these toward the goal of mastering one's political sphere (*yoga*). Together, these three methods, but especially yoga, name a mode of apprehending, of knowledge that is not just understood but grasped, held, contained, controlled—one of the defining features of yoga as a concept of political theory.

Conclusion

In this chapter, we show how yoga in the *Arthaśāstra* names modes of political strategy, including disciplines of information warfare; conjoined with *kṣema*, it describes the ambition of statecraft and indicates ways of apprehension that entail calculation and observation essential to strategies of governance. These concepts are in a genealogical relationship to the idea of yoga in the *Ṛg Veda* and the *Mahābhārata*, we argue. We see yoga consistently referring to the control of force, power, and discipline over and against another within a shared world, which is an intrinsic or emic world view.

While this might strike some as an arcane pursuit, we trace this genealogy of yoga in the field of the political because, when yoga reaches the shores of modernity, it has somehow conveyed these many meanings within its hold. As we discuss in the next chapters, yoga in various forms—the political that is our focus, but also the philosophical and psychophysical—will appear often within nationalist discourse in the colonial and postcolonial periods in India. As we hope to have shown in this chapter and the previous one, when yoga appears within political worlds, it is not an aberration. Instead, this is exactly where yoga has always been, in the middle of politics, at the center of power.

Interlude

PART I OF THE BOOK spans a period from roughly 1400 BCE to around 300 CE. The book's second part begins in the latter decades of the nineteenth century and moves into the middle of the twentieth century. More than a millennium and a half lie between these two time periods. This "interlude," a space between the two halves of the book, is our effort to fill this gap with some very broad strokes by pointing to the excellent work of many scholars. We hope this brief survey shows how the ideas we trace through texts in part I find their way across time to the subjects of part II.

Yoga and politics moved together over the long duration of the late classical, medieval, and early modern periods. Alexis Sanderson refers to a time frame from around the fifth century CE to the thirteenth century as the "Śaiva Age." Numerous kings and polities emerged to fill the void left by the decline of the Gupta Dynasty in the fifth century CE, and worshippers of the deity Shiva adapted their practices of yoga and *tantra* (esoteric ritual text and practice) to the desires of these new kings and rulers.[1] These practices of yoga and *tantra* by Hindus and Buddhists could offer "a body of rituals and theory that legitimated, empowered, and promoted key elements of social, political and economic process that characterizes the early medieval period."[2] Yoga remained a matter of king and court in this era. Benoytosh Bhattacharyya and Patton Burchett also write about this time as a "Tantric Age" from around 600–1200 CE, when yoga and *tantra*, combined with social, public devotionalism (*bhakti*), helped to determine political power and its representation in the "religiopolitical" sphere.[3] Ronald Davidson in his history of *tantra* and Buddhism charts how Buddhist *tantra* practitioners of early medieval India fashioned themselves as divine rulers in relation to the *maṇḍala* theory's political imagination of a king at the center of a feudal agonistic world. Davidson refers to esoteric Tantric Buddhism as "the most politicized form" of Buddhism in India.[4]

Perhaps this was a "Yoga Age" as well when the yoga associated with *tantra* came to dominate most forms of yoga in practice.[5] Yoga flourished in this period, linking Buddhism and Hinduism, as well as idioms of kingship that borrowed from these religious worlds. The emergent and related practice of *haṭha* yoga is attested in Buddhist and Śaiva *tantra* texts from the eleventh century to the early modern period.[6] Key works of the *haṭha* tradition, many of them gathered together and translated in Mallinson and Singleton's *Roots of Yoga*, speak to the ideal conditions for *haṭha* yoga practice.[7] In the main, these texts are concerned with breath control, bodily postures, and meditative techniques, yet several begin with short commentaries on the necessary conditions and contexts for proper practice: the who, where, and how of *haṭha* yoga. These preconditions range from the best time to bathe and ideal foods to consume and avoid, to the correct season in which to commence practice and whether a guru is necessary for initiation. In addition to such mundane subjects, the yogi is also advised to attend to their sociopolitical world. This was perhaps as an effect of the interlinking of yoga and the political world that marked the Śaiva or Tantric Age.

The earliest extant text of *haṭha* yoga appears to be the *Amṛtasiddhi*, a Buddhist text composed in the region of Maharashtra around the eleventh century that Mallinson and Szántó describe as the "first text to teach a system of yoga whose primary method is physical."[8] Among its opening passages, we read:

> In a righteous land of righteous custom where there are good people, alms are easily available and there are no disturbances, [the yogi] should practise the path of yoga.[9]

The text also speaks of its purpose as the "awakening of the civilised" (*susabhya*) for the attainment of "peace" (*śānti*) for the yogi.[10] This very early text of *haṭha* yoga prescribes both a stable, peaceful political condition for its practice as well as an appropriate subject of its yoga, a person who is marked as civilized and lives in a peaceful, righteous land.

This appeal to find a properly ruled place as a sociopolitical condition for the practice of yoga is echoed in the famous *Haṭhapradīpikā* composed a few centuries later, around 1400 CE. This work has become a standard part of the modern yoga teacher training curriculum and a primary focus for yoga studies in general. Its opening notes:

> In a well-ruled, righteous region, with plenty of food and free from upheaval, the Haṭhayogi should live in an isolated hut. It has a small door and is without cracks, holes and bumps. With a small door and no cracks, holes and bumps, neither too high nor too low in size, thickly smeared with cow dung in the proper way, clean, free from all annoyances, pleasing on the outside with a verandah, altar and well, surrounded by a wall: these are the characteristics of the yoga hut as taught by the adept practitioners of Haṭha. Staying in such a hut, free from all worry, in the way taught by his guru [the yogi] should practise nothing but yoga.[11]

This passage of the *Haṭhapradīpikā* is redolent with political implications. That a yogi should live in a well-ruled, righteous land appears the precondition for the lovely yoga hut and verandah the *haṭha* yogi inhabits, a prescription perhaps approximated by contemporary yoga retreats worldwide. Only a properly functioning government can ensure this kind of material stability, this medieval text tells us. A practice of *haṭha* yoga requires a surrounding system of economy, property, agriculture, and security—an operational and beneficial political economy that suggests the ideals of *yoga-kṣema*, we saw in part I. Political stability is a prerequisite for psychophysical yoga in these texts, and so yoga must at some level involve the assessment of politics. If not, how else is the yogi to know the "righteous land" of the "civilized" or the "well-ruled, righteous region"?

This idea that *haṭha* yogis should attend to politics and carry out their practice in a properly governed land appears to endure through the centuries. On the cusp of the early modern period in the eighteenth century, the *Gheraṇḍasamhitā* returns to the same injunctions we have seen in the eleventh-century *Amṛtasiddhi* and the fifteenth-century *Haṭhapradīpikā*. The text prescribes that:

> In a good, devout kingdom where alms are easily available and which is free from upheaval, the yogi should build a hut and encircle it with a wall.[12]

Although a less extensive description and a less bucolic setting than what is contained in the *Haṭhapradīpikā*, the point is the same: the proper practice of *haṭha* yoga can be achieved only within a stable, righteous polity.[13] It is clear that politics has long been on the mind of the yogi.

Over the course of this period, variously called the Saiva Age, Tantra Age, and what we are suggesting could also be called the Yoga Age as well, one can trace a deep line of interest in texts and ideas associated with yoga within Islamic political culture in South Asia from the eleventh century through the period of the Mughals in the eighteenth century. The Persian scholar Al-Biruni visited India in the early eleventh century and translated Patanjali's *Yoga Sūtras* among other texts,[14] what Noémie Verdon describes as the earliest known examples of Indian philosophy translated into Arabic.[15] Carl Ernst's scholarship tells of a now lost Sanskrit text about *haṭha* yoga, the *Amṛtakunda*, that was translated into Arabic sometime between the thirteenth and fifteenth centuries and became the basis for a Persian translation accompanied by illustrations, the *Baḥr al-ḥayāt* by Shaikh Ghawth in sixteenth-century India.[16] When Islam entered the subcontinent as a political power, a literary efflorescence of Sufism and yoga emerged through the genre of the Sufi romance or *premākhyān* literature of northern India. These include texts such as the *Cāndāyan* of Maulana Daud in the fourteenth century, and the sixteenth-century texts *Madhumālati* by Shaikh Manjhan Shattari, the *Mṛgāvatī* by Qutban, and the *Padmāvat* of Malik Muhammad Jayasi.[17] In these narratives, the hero or prince would often travel in the garb of a yogi, encounter yogis, and refine his spirit in light of yoga throughout his quest. In the region of Bengal around this period Shaman Hatley shows how Sufism integrated elements of yoga and tantra into Islamic doctrinal categories. For example, yogic and tantric concepts of the body were mapped onto political worlds of power where "the body itself is likened to a province or a city under the rule of the soul, as king," which rendered "mastery of the external universe possible through yogic technique alone."[18] Ayesha Irani demonstrates how the terminology of yoga is deployed in a seventeenth-century Bengali retelling of the life of Muhammad, a text that is a "missionary and polemical work" and also "pointedly political."[19] Yoga exists beyond techniques of mind and body in these contexts to be folded into and even name political strategies of power.

During the Mughal era, both Mughal and Rajput kings, among others, evinced a fascination and a wariness of practitioners of psychophysical yoga. Art and texts produced at Mughal and Rajput courts document yogis in peaceful, often contorted repose, and bands of yogis embroiled in bloody battles.[20] Yoga for these rulers simultaneously indicated a spiritual philosophy, a set of psychophysical activities, and an organizing principle of politics and power. Paintings from this period capture abstract philosophical concepts drawn from Sāṃkhya philosophy and also document the living practices of yoga, which included ascetic and martial ones, at this time.

The texts discussed in part I, particularly the *Mahābhārata*, continued to circulate in courts and kingdoms throughout this long period. The famous Mughal king Akbar commissioned translations of key Sanskrit works, including those that deal with yoga.[21] As Audrey Truschke suggests, part of Akbar's motivation to devote time, money, and effort on these projects of translation and interpretation was to understand and locate himself within a "tradition of Indian kingship" on the subcontinent.[22] This interest was reflected in the Persian translation of the *Mahābhārata* that Akbar commissioned, titled the *Razmnāma* (ca. 1582 CE), the *Story of War*, which gives outsize importance to the Śāntī Parvan and Anuśāsana Parvan (Books Twelve and Thirteen), respectively, in which Bhishma provides his many "yogas" on governance and politics, as well as equanimity and salvation. An illustration from a version of the *Razmnāma* produced in Moradabad from 1761–1763 shows Bhishma on his bed of arrows delivering his lectures on yoga (figure Inter.1). Whereas these two books make up about 25 percent of the Sanskrit epic, in Persian, they swell to account for 40 percent of the whole.[23] As we note in chapter 1, this is also the part of the epic where the political idea of yoga that we trace appears most frequently.

Akbar's fascination with yoga encompassed both the intellectual and the artistic. He is said to have met with practitioners of psychophysical and philosophic schools of yoga, learned from them, and debated with them. In 1567, he witnessed a pitched battle between yogi groups, recorded both in the *Akbarnāma* (ca. 1590) and in paintings. Scholars like David Lorenzen and William Pinch suggest that, during this period, many of those adept at psychophysical yoga were also "warrior ascetics," yogic figures who influenced India's political and martial worlds, where yoga was both a means of transcendence and of mundane empowerment.[24] These yogis wielded power in the worlds of war, intelligence, and diplomacy. As Bevilacqua and Stuparich

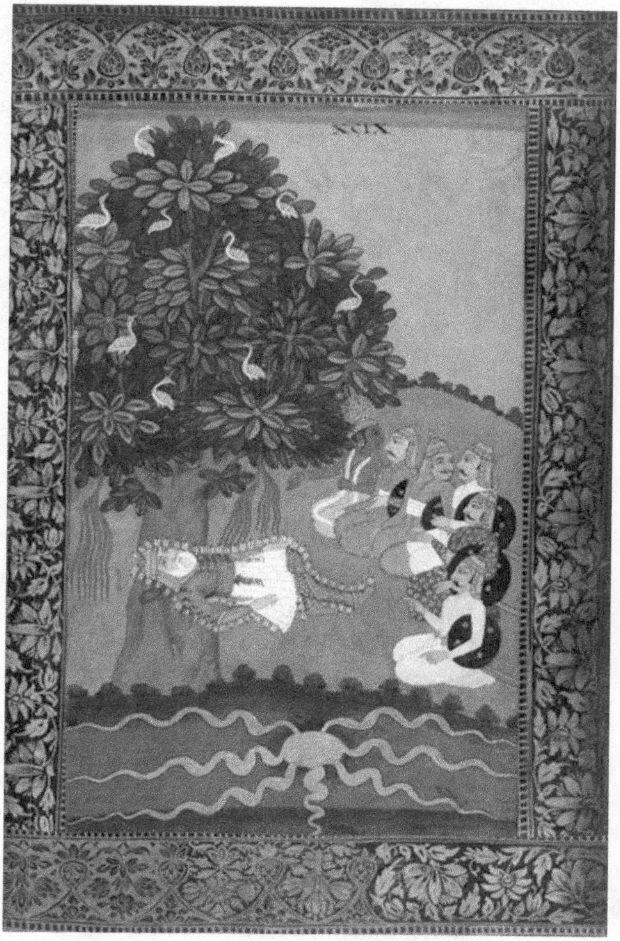

FIGURE INTER.1 Bhishma on a bed of arrows, *Razmnāma*, Moradabad, 1761–1763
Source: The Picture Art Collection / Alamy Stock Photo.

show, this was particularly true of the Nātha yoga communities of northern India from the sixteenth century and into the present.[25]

In social devotional worlds outside courtly contexts, yogis often were viewed as disruptors of hierarchies of power. Famous *bhakti* or devotional figures who challenged social norms were also considered yogis, including figures like Chakradhar (twelfth to the thirteenth centuries CE), Jnandev (thirteenth century CE), Namdev (thirteenth century CE), and Kabir (fifteenth to the sixteenth centuries CE)—a strand particularly powerful in Maharashtra and often associated with the Nāthas.[26] Elsewhere, yogis articulated versions of spirituality and religion linked to martial and political power, such as Samartha Ramdas (1608–1682), a Maharashtrian figure said to have influenced Shivaji (1630–1680) and whose legacy becomes essential to many strands of the region's politics, as Prachi Deshpande shows.[27] The power of yogis in the political field cannot be an accident of history—there are yogis in the political world because yoga itself remained there over centuries, even in the places where it overlapped with philosophy and psychophysical practice.

As the British and European presence on the subcontinent expanded from the sixteenth century onward, the role of yogis in the political sphere was keenly felt by these new actors as well. For seven years beginning in 1770, armed yogis, also called *fakīrs*, both Muslim and Hindu, fought against the forces of the British East India Company in Bengal. This is often called the Saṃnyāsī Rebellion, a reference to an ascetic, or *saṃnyāsī*, who is also called a yogi and *fakīr*. Whether the violent resistance was in response to taxation policies or the effects of a famine, the uprising fixed the figure of the yogi-*fakīr* in the minds of British officials as a threat to their enterprise.[28] And although these events may not have constituted an explicitly anticolonial action, one of the outcomes of this resistance was to lodge the character of the yogi within the rising swell of nationalism, the subject to which we turn in the next chapter of our book. This very brief survey hints at how yoga *as* politics endures through the history we trace here alongside yoga as philosophy and psychophysical practice. Even as we attend to the point where these three spheres meet, we continue to track yoga as political thought and practice as it moves into the modern period in India.

PART II

Modern Period

THREE

Yoga as Revolution in Anticolonial Nationalism

BY THE EIGHTEENTH CENTURY, the political danger of the yogi was apparent. The British understood the yogi to be treacherous because of events such as the Saṃnyāsī Rebellion and because the yogi existed on the periphery of society, an untamed element outside colonial control and surveillance. And perhaps there were echoes of the past, such as the one described in the *Arthaśāstra*, when ascetics—who may have been yogis—were also agents of intelligence gathering, covert action, and disinformation. As a figure who was free of normal society, the yogi was considered a danger to colonial order.

This idea of the yogi registered in English-language media of the nineteenth and early twentieth centuries, where they were often seen as uncontrollable and volatile.[1] The press reported instances of violence at the Kumbha Mela, acts of self-torture that were depicted as grotesque, and legends of yogis snatching and kidnapping people from the streets.[2] In the early decades of the twentieth century, "yoga" would figure as a key word in accounts of sedition, terror, and violence by anticolonial Indian nationalists; it could be a term of abuse as well, as when British prime minister Winston Churchill called M. K. Gandhi a "seditious" and "half-naked *fakir*" that was "a type well-known in the East."[3] Another negative nineteenth-century stereotype of yoga declared it to be an immoral system. Such was the view of the British colonial figure, James Mill, who in his multivolume history of India, disparages as morally objectionable the "yogic detachment"[4] and excessive physical mortification of "Fakeers" and "Yogees."[5]

Holding a space alongside the figure of the seditious yogi and the seditious use of yoga was another narrative, seeded to a great degree by English and European Orientalists, of the "pure" yoga, tied with the religious sentiment of Hinduism and ascetical, peaceful spiritual pursuits that were uncorrupted by and disentangled from the violence of nationalist resistance. This was the yoga of Edwin Arnold, and his poetic rendering of the *Bhagavad Gītā* entitled *The Song Celestial* (1885). This also was the yoga of the *Bhagavad Gītā* as read by the American transcendentalists, Ralph Waldo Emerson, Henry David Thoreau, and Walt Whitman.[6] This kind of yoga was a regular subject of discussion in the English press, where lectures and research praised yoga and yoga societies sprang up from Boston to London and Bombay. This yoga was brought to global attention by the 1896 text, *Raja Yoga*, by Vivekananda, who had entered the global stage during the 1893 Parliament of the World's Religions convened in Chicago.

Scholarship about this explosion of interest in yoga at the end of the nineteenth and in the early twentieth centuries primarily tracks the emergence of the psychophysical and philosophical variants of yoga rather than the political. Elizabeth De Michelis dates modern yoga's origins to the publication of Vivekananda's *Raja Yoga* in 1896 and points to the hybrid milieu of Western and Indian esoteric practices out of which this philosophical stream of yoga emerged.[7] Underscoring another kind of cosmopolitan connection at the birth of modern physical yoga, Mark Singleton writes about the emergence of modern yoga at the intersection of Indian physical culture and European gymnasium practices in the late nineteenth and early twentieth centuries.[8] Yoga in all these instances was a way of psychophysical self-improvement, an ancient mode of spiritual awakening for the modern world, and an opera of philosophical thought stretching over thousands of years. Even Jesus, it was claimed by some in the nineteenth century, may have been a yogi during his "lost years."[9]

These two interpretations of yoga—the seditious and the spiritual—were available for modern Indian political thinkers and activists to draw from in their challenge to British colonialism and their efforts to create a unified vision of Indian nationalism. On the one hand, yoga was dangerous, already filled with politics, and holding a political theory of righteous action, even violence. On the other hand, yoga was a pure, peaceful way to enlightenment and a solution to modern ills that differed from Western imperial and colonial modernity. We suggest that, in many instances, the political thinkers we engage in this chapter were either implicitly or explicitly participating in a discursive battle over the interpretation of yoga—what yoga as a term should mean and how a yogi should be understood. At times their work shows a recognition that yoga as a theory of political action was being sidelined in favor of the philosophical and psychophysical versions of yoga that had found more favor among European and colonial authorities and in the English public sphere.

Our aim in this chapter is to continue the story of yoga as politics, the third sphere of yoga that we have argued is largely occluded both within mainstream yoga studies as well as political theory. We move from a philological and textual approach utilizing Sanskrit texts that marked the first part of this book to a historical and political analysis of materials in Marathi, Hindi, and English from the nineteenth and early twentieth centuries in this second part of the book. In this chapter, we focus on how yoga as political thought and practice appeared in the work of five nationalist leaders: B. G. Tilak (1856–1920), Lala Lajpat Rai (1865–1928), M. K. Gandhi (1869–1948), Aurobindo Ghose (1872–1950), and Dr. B. R. Ambedkar (1891–1956).[10] Many of these thinkers understood yoga, especially its formulation as *karma-yoga*, as a political term interweaving the philosophical, religious, textual, and psychophysical. We argue that they used the term's multiple valences not to disguise or hide their politics under the veil of spirituality but to disrupt colonial, British, and Orientalist conceptions of the political by routing their ideas through the space between the political and the spiritual that yoga occupied. In the process, yoga became a theory of political action and political revolution often passing under the category of "religion" or "spirituality" that was anchored in the political realm of the self as a locus of power, first and foremost, and through the self, into a world that could be envisioned as free despite the yoke of colonial oppression. In contrast to this formulation, we discuss how Ambedkar rejected this use of *karma-yoga* by his contemporaries, seeing it not through the lens of a liberatory theory of political action but as a regressive recovery of caste and religious orthodoxy at odds with his own desire to annihilate caste and its religious justifications in modern India.

The importance of a sound social and political context for yogic success is evident even in texts that are considered core works of psychophysical yoga, as we suggest in the interlude in this book. This chapter delves into a question implicit in the *haṭha* texts we discuss there: What does the yogi do in a land that is not well governed? Drawing from the genealogy of yoga as political thought and practice that we trace in the previous two chapters, we observe here how the concept of yoga enters modern political resistance to British colonial power.

Yoga as Political Art

Arguably the first battle conducted by Indian people against European company colonialism was an uprising, the Saṃnyāsī Rebellion, discussed in the interlude. This armed insurgency was undertaken by "warrior ascetics," as David Lorenzen calls them, organized groups of yogis and *fakīrs* who raided and resisted the rule of the armies and outposts of the British East India Company, perhaps a prelude to the Rebellion/Mutiny of 1857.[11] Roughly one hundred years later, in 1882, the nationalist writer and poet Bankimchandra Chattopadhyay ("Chatterjee") drew on the Saṃnyāsī Rebellion to produce a fictional account of revolutionary heroism and bravery, *Ānandamaṭh*, in which the figure of the yogi is central to the world of political action. The novel also contains the lyrics for what became a nationalist rallying cry, *Vande Mataram* ("I Praise You, Mother").[12] Yoga within the retelling of these events and narratives is at the center of one major mobilization of anticolonial political thought and action in India.

Perhaps for this reason, British colonial officials and British colonial citizens residing in India shared a suspicion of the figure of the yogi or *fakīr* as politically and socially dangerous. If the British sought to dismantle and suppress many of these groups of yogis, they did so—and this is vital to note—because yoga and yogi/*fakīr* groups presented a clear and powerful danger to the British crown and its project of colonialism and economic extraction. We can recall here that the *Arthaśāstra* advised kings to be wary of ascetics as they may be spies or provocateurs, or even double agents, just as a king might himself use ascetics or spies in the guise of ascetics for such purposes. It was not a new idea for the government to be suspicious of yogis. The yogi's position at the periphery of social order provided this ambivalent danger that the British registered and feared.

As we suggest in the previous chapters, the political concept of yoga intersected with psychophysical and philosophical yoga. The *Bhagavad Gītā*, in particular, is an exemplar of how multiple spheres of yoga were drawn together to solve a single political problem—how to fight a civil war. Another way to understand the role of yoga as resistance to colonialism requires turning to the *Bhagavad Gītā* because it conveys the same multiple valences of yoga, even though the political aspects of the text were rarely discussed in the English-language sphere of the time. This oversight on the part of British colonial and imperial authority is at the heart of the curious fact that many Indian nationalists read and wrestled with the meaning of the *Bhagavad Gītā* as a political text while in prison for sedition.

The colonial rules for incarceration appeared to deny access to nationalist political reading materials, but religious materials, and even works of European political theory and philosophy, were considered acceptable; in some cases, prison libraries provided these works to prisoners.[13] The *Bhagavad Gītā* was construed in British liberalism as an allowable text of religion despite its potential as a seditious text of politics, and so the work became a regular companion to nationalists incarcerated for sedition.[14] A heterogenous group of Hindu-oriented nationalist figures found in the *Bhagavad Gītā*'s concept of *karma-yoga* a political theory of action.[15] The text became a touchstone of Swadeshi politics in the late nineteenth and early twentieth centuries, and many of the figures who reformulated and adapted its idea of *karma-yoga* are essential thinkers in various strands of Indian politics today.[16]

Lala Lajpat Rai's Anti-Renunciate Yoga

Lala Lajpat Rai was a key north Indian figure of anticolonial nationalism, a member of both the "extremist" wing of the Indian National Congress (INC) and of the high-caste Hindu reformist Arya Samaj.[17] In 1907, Lajpat Rai was imprisoned in Mandalay Fort, Burma, for his participation in protests in the north Indian town of Rawalpindi, a city in present-day Pakistan. He was released after six months for insufficient evidence against him. Lajpat Rai published a short book about his transportation to Mandalay and his months in prison, where he passed the time reading religious books, including an English translation and Hindi commentary of the *Bhagavad Gītā*, *Message of the Vedas* by Gokul Chand Narang, a Hindi commentary of *Yog Darshan*, Urdu and Persian poetry, English novels, European and English histories, and books about Burma.[18] Of these, he names the Persian poet Hafiz and

Krishna of the *Bhagavad Gītā* as his "two masters," the latter for sharing "words of practical wisdom, pitched in immortal strain."[19]

While in Mandalay, Lajpat Rai also wrote several essays and books of his own, including "The Message of the Bhagwad Gita," an essay originally published in *Modern Review* in 1907. The *Bhagavad Gītā* that he had with him in Mandalay was an English version translated by the anti-imperialist and theosophist, Annie Besant. Mishka Sinha suggests that more so than other contemporary English translations of the *Bhagavad Gītā*, like Edwin Arnold's 1885 poetic *The Song Celestial*, Besant's version of the *Bhagavad Gītā* highlights the similarities between the epic battle therein and the anti-imperial movement for political independence.[20] Whereas Arnold's translation became popular as a text for the "real enquirer, the searcher after truth,"[21] as one review of the book put it, Besant's version remained true to her political commitments toward India's nationalist struggle as an international question of ethics applied to politics. One could say that Arnold's *Bhagavad Gītā* represented the good or spiritual kind of yoga for British colonial authorities, while Besant's *Bhagavad Gītā* represented the dangerous, political, and bad kind. As an anticolonial nationalist, it is clear which one Lajpat Rai preferred.[22]

With Besant's translation as his source material, Lajpat Rai's essay introduces the *Bhagavad Gītā* as "the most beautiful, most sublime, and most popular" portion of the *Mahābhārata*, possibly with the exception of Book Twelve, which he describes as "the last days of the veteran Bhishma after he had received his mortal wounds in the war and was awaiting death on his warrior's bed, *viz.*, the bed of arrows, with its noble disquisition on politics, on war and on the duties of a Kshattriya."[23] As we discuss in chapter 1, this refers to a part of the epic that contains the greatest number of references to yoga as a term and concept. Lajpat Rai begins his essay on the *Bhagavad Gītā* with a brief synopsis and summary of its main ideas before ending with a strong exhortation to his readers as well as an argument about the relevance of Krishna's counsel for the present. He concludes his commentary with an address to his fellow Indians as the "descendants, successors and countrymen of Krishna and Arjuna, swayed as they are, at present, by the forces of ignorance, superstition, chicken-heartedness and false ideas of Dharma and Karma."[24] He and other nationalist leaders saw their task as emboldening a reluctant, complacent, fearful public to join the cause of ending the British Raj, much as Krishna is bound to notify Arjuna of his duty to battle his cousins, the Kauravas.

The penultimate sentence of Lajpat Rai's essay invokes yoga: "It will [be] a shame if the countrymen of Krishna let any false ideas of *Yoga* prevail amongst them or let any false doctrines of renunciation (सन्यास) and relinquishment (त्याग) enfeeble their arms."[25] The false ideas of yoga referenced were the growing tendencies to sequester yoga as a religious, spiritual, or meditative practice, shorn of its potency to name the action of warriors and revolutionaries, as a practice outside society and politics rather than squarely within it. This latter version of yoga—fully enmeshed in the world of politics—is spotlighted by Lajpat Rai and other nationalist figures in their formulations of *karma-yoga*, the yoga of "action." This yoga of action is what Krishna teaches to Arjuna over and against "renunciation" (*saṃnyāsa*) of worldly activity.[26] The dichotomy between renunciation and engagement in political action is exactly the problem addressed by *karma-yoga* in the *Bhagavad Gītā* and in the wider treatment of yoga in the epic as the frame for the war itself. In the two sections of the epic where yoga appears most prominently, the *Bhagavad Gītā* and Book Twelve of the *Mahābhārata*, yoga is taught as a way to compel action rather than retreat from the political field. Lajpat Rai summoned this ancient text of *karma-yoga* to compel his fellow Indians to resist British rule.

Aurobindo's *Karmayogin*

A fellow nationalist and admirer of Rai, Aurobindo Ghose,[27] had a much more extensive engagement with both the *Bhagavad Gītā* and the idea of yoga it expresses. Aurobindo began a practice of *prāṇāyāma* yoga around 1904. However, as one of his biographer's notes, in 1907 "he got involved in politics . . . his *pranayama* became irregular and he fell ill."[28] He was not alone. The political yoga of action came into conflict with the contemplative yoga of stillness for many, including Aurobindo.[29] It is shortly after this period that Aurobindo began to conceive of the meeting of yoga and politics through the *Bhagavad Gītā* and its concept of *karma-yoga*.

After he was arrested in 1908 on suspicions of conspiracy in connection with the Alipore bomb case, Aurobindo was imprisoned in Alipore jail in Calcutta for one year, at least some of which was spent in solitary confinement. The severity of his solitary confinement was lessened somewhat when the jailers allowed him to request from his home clothing and a few books, among which were the *Bhagavad Gītā* and *Upaniṣad* literature.[30] During the trial for which he was imprisoned, Aurobindo and his young codefendants, the accused Bengali revolutionaries, passed the time reading books—a combination of European philosophy, Indian fiction (novels by Bankimchandra Chattopadhyay, for example) that passed colonial censors, and Indian religious texts (*Bhagavad Gītā*, *Purāṇa* literature, Vivekananda's *Raj Yoga* and *Science of Religion*). After his release from prison, Aurobindo wrote about his experiences. Originally published as a series of news articles in the Bengali monthly *Suprabhat* in 1909–1910, the volume was published in book form as *Tales of a Prison Life* (*Kārākāhinī*) in 1920. In the text's preface, Aurobindo notes that he emerged after a year in jail, "as a transformed being with a transformed character, a transformed intellect, a transformed life, a transformed mind." He hailed his jail as a "*yogāśram*," a retreat from quotidian life that "happened to be the British prison."[31] Referring to a British jail as a yoga ashram subverts the kinds of discipline and punishment the British likely hoped to achieve by incarcerating perceived revolutionaries. Aurobindo's word choice emphasizes the production of yoga as political thought formed in this quintessential mode of colonial mastery, the prison.

From 1909 to 1912, after Aurobindo's incarceration, *karma-yoga* and the image of the *karma yogi* or *yogin* became central features of his thought. Shortly after his acquittal in 1909, Aurobindo launched the journal, *Karmayogin: A Weekly Review of National Religion, Literature, Science, Philosophy, &c.*, for which he served as publisher, editor, and primary author (figure 3.1). As the title implies, this journal makes explicit reference to the *Bhagavad Gītā*: the cover depicts the diegetic scene of the field of battle from the *Bhagavad Gītā*, below which is a quotation from chapter 3, verse 30, that reads: "When you have entrusted all actions to me, with thought on the highest self, when you have become free from desire, free from the idea of 'mine,' then fight, with grief gone."[32]

The dyspeptic response that Aurobindo experienced in 1907 trying to combine psychophysical yoga with politics would resolve itself with a focus on the political when Aurobindo combined psychophysical yoga with the yoga of political thought and action of the *Bhagavad Gītā*. In later decades, Aurobindo would write much more about both yoga and the *Bhagavad Gītā*, and would often refer to the entirety of his teaching as "Integral Yoga," especially texts composed with his disciple, Mirra Alfassa, aka "The Mother." Most studies of Aurobindo's ideas about yoga and the *Bhagavad Gītā* draw on

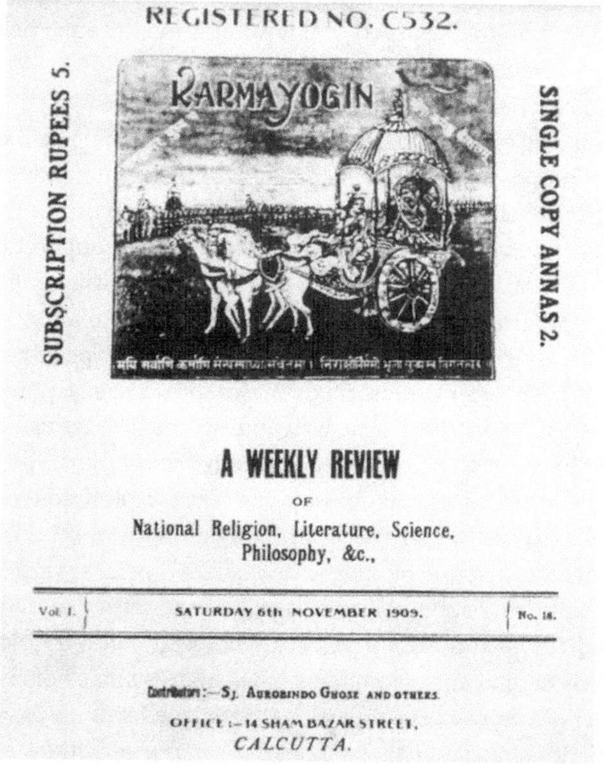

FIGURE 3.1 Cover of *Karmayogin*, 1909

this later, post-political period of his writing,[33] when he sought to express "no views whatever on political questions."[34] Unlike his texts on Integral Yoga and his *Essays on the Gita*, originally published in the journal *Arya* from 1916 to 1918, Aurobindo's essays in *Karmayogin* in 1909–1910 were written just after his release from jail. We propose that for the purpose of exploring yoga as political thought in Aurobindo's work, a key place to look is neither his early, explicitly political writings in the journal *Bande Mataram*, when yoga and the *Bhagavad Gītā* are rarely mentioned, nor his later quietist commentaries on and translation of the *Bhagavad Gītā*.[35] Rather, we look at his writings in *Karmayogin* from May 1909 to March 1910, which contain a distillation of his views on yoga as a political idea more proximate to his time as a political agitator and propagandist. His engagement with yoga and politics crescendos again toward the journal's end around 1910 as Aurobindo eludes British officials who had charged him with sedition for an article published in *Karmayogin* in early 1910.

The first article printed in *Karmayogin* is the text of a speech given by Aurobindo in 1909 on his release from prison, in which he declares his faith as a complex mix of Hindu revivalism, Sanatana Dharma, monotheism, and political activism. He describes "Yoga" as "a mighty truth in this religion" that he sought to practice "to uplift this nation."[36] Throughout the text, he defines *karma-yoga* in relation to the spiritualized quest for Indian political sovereignty.[37] In the opening issue, Aurobindo explains the aims and precepts of the journal. The journal's embrace of such varied topics as "our religion, our society, our philosophy, politics, literature, art, jurisprudence, science, thought, everything that was and is ours"[38] suggests Aurobindo's rejection of the separability of these vast domains of life: "The European is proud of his success in divorcing religion from life. Religion, he says, is all very well in its place, but it has nothing to do with politics or science or commerce, which it spoils by its intrusion."[39] Aurobindo rejects this European disciplining and subdividing of human thought and activity and then instrumentalizes both toward a political end, a common innovation within the political sphere of anticolonial nationalism. His choice of language, separating "ours" from the "European," suggests the intramural, emic quality of yoga as political thought that we describe in our introduction.

The yoga expressed in the *Bhagavad Gītā*, Aurobindo argues, is a technique for combining these varied domains of life into a single internal and therefore nationalistic coherence. For him, like Gandhi, a freedom fighter who couched the struggle against imperialism in spiritual terms, Indian nationalism would not only establish the country's autonomy from British and European political rule but would also enable India to share with the world its unique contributions in the form of *Sanatana Dharma*, the "eternal religion," a moniker increasingly common within modern Hinduism in Aurobindo's time: "India is destined to work out her own independent life and civilization, to stand in the forefront of the world and solve the political, social, economical [*sic*] and moral problems which Europe has failed to solve, yet the pursuit of whose solution and the feverish passage in that pursuit . . . she calls her progress."[40] Aurobindo placed yoga at the center of his vision of India's political future, as we see here: "We believe that it is to make the *yoga* the ideal of human life that India rises today; by the *yoga* she will get the strength to realize her freedom, unity and greatness, by the *yoga* she will keep the strength to preserve it. It is a spiritual revolution we foresee and the material is only its shadow and reflex."[41] He refers to "the yoga" of "perfection in action" as the "whole teaching of the *Gita*"[42] and states: "We believe that the Yoga of the Gita will play a large part in the uplifting of the nation, and this attitude is the first condition of the Yoga of the Gita."[43]

We can see in Aurobindo's words some of the roots of Narendra Modi's speech about yoga to the UN General Assembly in 2014 that we note in our preface. Both frame the unique global contributions that India is poised to make as it takes its place on the world stage, yet yoga will remain "Indian," a feature of the "nation" in this global rise. Aurobindo enjoins the young revolutionaries in his essay "The Ideal of the Karmayogin" to resurface the "patrimony of your forefathers . . . the Vedanta, the Gita, the Yoga."[44] He closes this essay by cautioning that, if his readers follow this path, it will require reconnecting the inner and outer domain into a holistic unity: "you must win back the kingdom of yourselves, the inner Swaraj, before you can win back your outer empire."[45] This concept of political freedom ("Swaraj") emerging from individual acts of sovereignty deeply informs the broad sense of yoga as political thought and practice, both here and in our next chapter; political freedom, when tied to yoga in the colonial period, is a mode of sovereignty that starts with the self but does not end with the self—the self is the fulcrum of a larger political transformation.[46]

Aurobindo returns often to the themes of yoga and the *Bhagavad Gītā* in essays and speeches throughout 1909–1910, which were later published in the pages of *Karmayogin*. Emphasizing his definition of the yoga practitioner as distinct from the figure of the ascetic, Aurobindo says, "When we think of *yoga*, we think of a man who shuts himself up in a cave and subjects himself to certain practices. He frees himself from all bondage. But Srikrishna uses *yoga* in a different sense. He says: Do action in *yoga*."[47] Action in yoga, as we've seen, means acting without attaching oneself to the consequences of that action, but in this way, it has the exact opposite meaning of "not acting" at all. Later underscoring his view that the yoga of the *Bhagavad Gītā* rejects a cloistered life, Aurobindo says, "The teaching of the Gita is a teaching for life, and not a teaching for the life of a closet."[48] Like Lajpat Rai before him, Aurobindo is at pains to emphasize that adhering to the yoga of the *Bhagavad Gītā* requires not isolating oneself from life but rather fully embracing it.

The *Bhagavad Gītā*'s call to follow one's *dharma* becomes for Aurobindo a lesson not just for individuals to pursue their calling but also for the nation as a whole to forge an autonomous route to the modern. In his view of history, nineteenth-century Indian reformers sought to imitate Europe, to pilot the nation's progress using Western metrics and ideals: "European education, European machinery, and European organization and equipment."[49] This "imitative, self-forgetful, artificial" India necessarily failed to achieve emancipation because it ignored Krishna's counsel to Arjuna: "Better the law of one's own being though badly done than an alien *dharma* well-followed; death in one's *dharma* is better, it is a dangerous thing to follow the law of another's nature." "Alien" here is clearly British thought and colonial practice.[50] Where nineteenth-century India failed, Aurobindo believed the twentieth-century version of India would succeed. All around him, he saw signs of an authentic expression of Indian genius—in religion, art, music, and literature alike—as evidence that Indian reformers were no longer imitating the British but instead crafting their own vision of progress. Aurobindo's insistence on authenticity was not wedded to a love of tradition or a conservative nostalgia. He acknowledged that change was required, but held that it should not be imitative: "There is not the slightest doubt that our society will have to undergo a reconstruction which may amount to revolution, but it will not be for Europeanisation as the average reformer blindly hopes, but for a greater and more perfect realisation of the national spirit in society."[51]

On December 25, 1909, Aurobindo published an article, "To My Countrymen," that the British surveillance system deemed seditious, a call for radical political action. Communiqués and inquiries began within the British intelligence apparatus between India and London, and as the pressure mounted to arrest Aurobindo, he went into hiding in the homes of friends in Calcutta. British authorities believed he was on his way to Pondicherry and monitored ports of entry and exit to apprehend the fugitive in transit. Aurobindo published a short piece on March 19, 1910, in the last issue of *Karmayogin* that carried his unique blend of humor, audacity, and political acumen. A report on the whereabouts of "Sri Aurobindo Ghose," most likely written by Aurobindo himself, read: "We are greatly astonished to learn from the local Press that Sri Aurobindo Ghose has disappeared from Calcutta and is now interviewing the Mahatmas in Tibet. We are ourselves unaware of this mysterious disappearance. As a matter of fact, Sri Aurobindo is in our midst and . . . his address is being kept a strict secret."[52] This final message to his readers manages both to poke fun at Western adaptations of yoga and Indian spiritualism (in this case, theosophy) while mocking British colonial law enforcement. Aurobindo's political yoga was always deeply literary and occasionally funny.

Aurobindo stopped publishing *Karmayogin* in early 1910 when he fled Calcutta for Pondicherry, where he remained until his death in 1950. Many things ended at once—the journal itself ended a few months after his departure (many of the broadsheets and pamphlets put out by nationalists for limited readerships had similarly brief lives), and Aurobindo gave up explicitly political nationalist work in favor of a life of spiritual contemplation and exposition, and evading the attention of colonial authorities. His principal writings on the *Bhagavad Gītā* from this later time consist of his "Essays on the *Gita*," which engage philosophical interpretations of the text and include critiques of other interpreters[53] for favoring the *Bhagavad Gītā*'s early chapters and neglecting the "rest of the eighteen chapters with their high philosophy."[54] While the principles of *svarāj* and *svadeśī* nationalism are not absent, his essays are less overtly political and exhortatory in nature, in keeping with his physical and public retreat from the field of nationalist politics. Within Aurobindo's writing after 1910, yoga as political thought and practice is displaced by a view of yoga as individualistic spiritual pursuit of the awareness of the "Divine," what he called "Integral Yoga." His strident impulse to reject European and Western cultural forms seemed softened by his dependence first on the French for political asylum in their colony and later his spiritual partnership with the French mystic Mirra Alfassa—the "Mother"—who founded and ran the spiritual empire that endures in his name, headquartered in Auroville in Tamil Nadu. From a political yogi deeply invested in India's radical nationalist movement, Aurobindo became a reclusive philosopher of personal spiritual transformation.[55] But yoga as political thought was only rising in Indian nationalist practice and rhetoric.

Yoga, the *Bhagavad Gītā*, and the Bomb

Sumit Sarkar, writing about the nationalist movement in Bengal from 1903 to 1908, refers to the "cult of the bomb" that pervaded the political organizations and revolutionary thinking of extremist, violence-oriented nationalists.[56] Sarkar provocatively refers to "the conventional image of the Bengal revolutionary as advancing with a bomb in one hand and the Gita in the other," an image that he believed was "overdrawn."[57] One fascinating illustration of both the fears of the British around "the cult of the bomb" and the political uses of yoga, especially as they exist in the *Bhagavad Gītā*'s modern interpretation, can be found in the public record of two bombings by Indian revolutionaries targeting British officials. Throughout the nineteenth century and until independence in the twentieth, violent resistance to British rule regularly took the form of bombings or attempted bombings.[58] As noted above, Aurobindo was implicated, but acquitted, in just such a bombing plot, the Alipore bomb case of 1908–1909. Some years later, on December 23, 1912, a group of Indian revolutionaries attempted to assassinate the viceroy of India, Lord Hardinge, as he rode an elephant through Chandani Chowk in Delhi in celebration of the transfer of the colonial capital from Calcutta to Delhi. Basanta Kumar Biswas, working under the tutelage and orders of Rash Behari Bose, threw a bomb that struck and injured the viceroy. An investigation began that resulted in the "transportation for life" (life sentence in prison outside India) for one defendant and the execution of four others in October 1914. During this investigation, pamphlets were discovered in the possession of the conspirators that were referred to in court documents and in the press as both "Yoga Pamphlets" or "Yogi Sadhana," and "Liberty Pamphlets."[59] These pamphlets described the yoga of the *Bhagavad Gītā* in philosophical terms, emphasizing *karma-yoga* as a philosophy of acting for others without self-interest. This is a straightforward interpretation of the *Bhagavad Gītā*, as we saw in the last chapter, and its presence here further supports an interpretation of yoga in the *Bhagavad Gītā* as the apotheosis of the philosophy of selfless but nonetheless active political action and even violence.

In the investigation and case that followed, the pamphlets played an important, although highly ambiguous role for the prosecution and the defense. Council for the colonial authority argued that the philosophy of yoga had been "perverted . . . not for spiritual advantage but in order to make [the bombers] passive instruments in the hands of the leaders of the organisation," perhaps a reference to an Orientalist concept (traceable to G. W. F. Hegel and before) that yoga and other modes of Indian spirituality rendered men (in particular) as docile and in spiritual servitude, thus unattuned to the movement of history toward freedom. In relationship to the specific ideas about renunciation in action taken in the pamphlets about yoga, the prosecution argued that "the giving up of the world was to be a means to the end which was the use of the bomb."[60] The British Crown's counsel even suggested that yoga, in its meaning as "self-sacrificing action," became a philosophy to prepare the bombers for their own deaths as revolutionaries and that the very word "yoga" in their writing and communiqués actually stood for the act of bombing itself.[61] Whether or not the term yoga was code for bombing, it is clear that yoga was understood to be a term of political theory and action. One might argue these were modern instances of the classical *yogapuruṣa* discussed in the *Arthaśāstra*.

A second bombing took place at Raja Bazar in Calcutta on March 27, 1913, after which five people were convicted and sentenced to transportation to the Andamans. Among the documents found in the investigation were yoga pamphlets and a note written by one revolutionary, Sharada Charanguha, to his family to inform them that he was going to Benares to "study yoga" for six months. The prosecution argued that this was exactly the time frame for planning and executing the bombing—hence, yoga stood for the period of training and planning for the bombing as well as the entire revolutionary operation in Calcutta.[62] According to the court's evidence, Charanguha further informed his family he would be "incognito" as a "yogi" during this time, a statement reminiscent of the *Arthaśāstra*'s advice on disguises for spies and agents behind enemy lines.[63] In this case, the prosecution, perhaps drawing from the Delhi case, more forthrightly argued that "yoga" was a code word for "violent revolution" itself, even while the defense, as in the Delhi case, insisted these pamphlets were simply spiritual self-help manuals and were unrelated to the politics of their clients. The defense thus also took advantage of the British-European coding of "proper" yoga as quiet, contemplative spirituality in scholarship and popular culture in order to argue their defense.[64] As in the Delhi case a few months earlier, investigation of the revolutionaries' intentions and possessions revealed similar pamphlets on Yoga, "Liberty," and the *Bhagavad Gītā*, one of which was entitled "The Yoga and Its Objects."[65] The prosecuting counsel argued that "the reading of the Geeta [*sic*] had been incorporated into the Yoga pamphlet with a view to political ends" and that "the yoga pamphlet was especially dangerous because it was a call to the [revolutionary] recruits under the garb of higher religious learning."[66] The pamphlet on yoga even referred to Aurobindo as a "True Son of India" from among the ranks of "Self-sacrificing men," who exemplify the yoga of the *Bhagavad Gītā*.[67] The British Crown's counsel consistently argued that such revolutionary and violent readings of yoga and the *Bhagavad Gītā* were "twisted" and were "changed" from their original meaning "to support the cause of anarchism."[68] Thus, both the prosecution and the defense reiterated and strategically used the idea that yoga as political thought and action was not "real" yoga, instead accessing the popular idea that real yoga was passive, meditative, and spiritual. In a report on the Raja Bazar case from the government of Bengal to the Home Office in London in 1915, the two judges who authored the report—Asutosh Mookerjee and Thomas William Richardson—reinforced the idea that yoga as a philosophy or spiritual practice was "innocent" as "even the Bible might be put to a perverted use."[69] Their report distinguished between the "sincere" practice of yoga and the use that revolutionaries made of yoga and the *Bhagavad Gītā*.[70]

One other trial that did not involve an actual bombing but merely the mention of the word "bomb" in publications in Marathi occurred in 1908. In April of that year, some revolutionaries attempted to assassinate, using a bomb, Magistrate Douglas Kingsford in Calcutta. This event prompted the prominent nationalist and public figure, B. G. Tilak, to write a series of articles in his Marathi periodical *Kesarī* reflecting on the meaning of the word "bomb."[71] In these pieces, written in Marathi, Tilak did not argue for the use of bombs—indeed he called bombings "monstrous deeds" that he "repudiated"[72]—but pointed out that the bomb was introduced to India by the British and so it symbolically and practically linked the violence of the colonial state with the violence of the radical anticolonial nationalists willing to kill and die by the bomb.[73] The British government charged Tilak in July 1908 with sedition for these articles, arguing that he was promoting the use of bombs in nationalist activity. In his defense at trial, Tilak suggested that the prosecution did not understand the writing because his essays were in Marathi. No one for the government's case properly knew Marathi so the prosecution and government had to rely on the official court translator, a white British man without a native grasp of the language. Tilak then endeavored to explain in English the nuances of his Marathi prose. He clarified that in his articles he wrote that the word "bomb" had become like a "mantra," that is a "magic spell." The use of the word created a powerful link to the object without requiring the physical object for its use. Instead, he says that "it [the bomb] is a spell-word [*mantra*] for dispelling evil [*toḍagā*]," which is to say, the presence of the British in India. Tilak claims, "The bomb has more the form of knowledge, it is a kind of witchcraft, it is a charm, an amulet."[74] Tilak here plays off of the various meanings, and fears, around yoga by utilizing a term often central to its articulation and practice, the word *mantra*.[75] The bomb is a diabolical device transformed into a powerful term (*mantra*) precisely because of British colonial violence, and the only way to stop it, Tilak argues, is "making a beginning to grant the important rights of *swarajya*" to Indians.[76] The trial, and Tilak's writing and testimony, suggest that in both English but perhaps especially in Marathi and other Indian languages, the word "bomb" had meanings and resonances beyond the ken of British surveillance. As we argue here and in the next chapter, the word "mantra" so closely associated with the practice of yoga, as well as the word yoga itself, had a range of meanings, especially in Indian languages then imported into English, that were not fully comprehended by British authorities and could not easily fit with their understanding of these terms. Despite a robust defense, and even the help of the Bombay lawyer Muhammad Ali Jinnah, the British government sentenced Tilak to six years of rigorous imprisonment in Mandalay.

These bombings and their related cases suggest that yoga maintained its meaning of political thought and action set alongside yoga understood as a quietist, even peaceful philosophy. These events also reveal how the *Bhagavad Gītā* and its concepts, particularly around yoga, existed within colonial surveillance and the police state, as well as within its judicial world, as a possible term of war against the British Crown.[77] The complexities in the interpretation of these ideas of yoga in the *Bhagavad Gītā* show that the colonial authority—either through policy or a lack of imagination—could not fully countenance yoga existing as a term for philosophy, spiritual practice, and self-sacrificing action, on the one hand, and a mode of political violence against the state or anticolonial strategy, on the other. But it is also clear that the Indian nationalist revolutionaries on trial could and did see yoga in this way. As we have shown in the last chapter, all these possibilities coexisted within the term yoga several thousand years before these court trials. And in our discussion of Aurobindo in this chapter, it is just after his acquittal in a similar bombing case in 1908–1909 that he begins to express yoga as a term of political thought and action in the pages of *Karmayogin*. It is our argument that the ancient mingling of meanings for yoga explored in part I of this book underwrote the political thought and action that led to these moments of revolutionary political violence carried out under the sign of yoga.

Tilak's *Karma-Yoga* as a Theory of Political Action

From 1908 to 1914, during Tilak's imprisonment in Mandalay for his writings in *Kesarī*, he studied the *Bhagavad Gītā* extensively. During this time of incarceration, he began writing in Marathi a two-volume book on the *Bhagavad Gītā* that included a lengthy philosophical exposition followed by a stanza-by-stanza translation of the text interspersed with commentary.[78] The titles of the two volumes are worth noting. The first is titled *Rahasya-Vivecan arthāt Gītece Karmayogapar Nirūpaṇ*, or "Analysis of the Secret/Essence or Exposition on the Karma Yoga of the Gītā," and the second is titled *Śrīmadbhagavadgītārahasya*, or "The Essence/Secret of the Sacred Bhagavad Gītā." These titles are similar to one of the articles in 1908 that led to his imprisonment: "The Secret/Essence of the Bomb," or "Bombagolyāce Rahasya." This shared play on the idea of the "secret" or "essence," the *rahasya*, of a subject suggests to us a conceptual continuity, the effort to explain the ramifications of powerful words or texts in political culture that are opaque to others. After its original publication in Marathi in 1915, following Tilak's release from prison, the book was translated and published in several Indian languages. However, an English version was not published until 1935, long after Tilak's death in 1920.[79] The text became known simply as Tilak's *Gītā Rahasya* by its translators and editors, and in popular and political culture.

As Tilak tells it in his preface, his motivation to write the *Gītā Rahasya* was to solve something that had puzzled him since he first encountered a version of the *Bhagavad Gītā* as a teenager: Why should a book that was ostensibly about the urging of a warrior to battle have anything to say about either the paths of knowledge or devotion? In other words, the first sense of the *Bhagavad Gītā* that Tilak had was that it was a text on politics, not religion or philosophy. After he immersed himself directly in the text, freed from the "clutches" of other commentaries and translations,[80] many of which he concluded were erroneous, Tilak found his answer: "the original Gītā did not preach the Philosophy of Renunciation (*nivṛtti*), but of Energism (Karma-Yoga); and that possibly, the single word '*yoga*' used in the *Gītā* had been used to mean Karma-Yoga."[81] Tilak further explains that the *Bhagavad Gītā*'s theory of righteous action did not originate with that text or even with Krishna but is instead part of India's ancient, sacred heritage:

> Such was the doctrine taught by our forefathers, who never intended that the goal of life should be meditation alone. No one can expect Providence to protect one who sits with folded arms and throws his burden on others. God does not help the indolent.[82]

The core of Tilak's aim is to emphasize political action, *karma-yoga*, what his sons, overseeing the translation of the *Gītā Rahasya* into English by B. S. Sukthankar, termed in English his theory of "Energism."[83] Tilak situates the concept of energetic action, of *karma-yoga* in the *Bhagavad Gītā*, in relationship to the Vedic meanings of yoga as discipline in times of war[84] and further argues that the yoga of the *Bhagavad Gītā* is far removed from the philosophical or psychophysical, especially as represented by Patanjali and Shankaracharya.[85] The context of the *Bhagavad Gītā* on the field of battle is both literal and metaphorical for Tilak, but the literal is more heavily emphasized in his analysis.[86] For Tilak, the *rahasya* or "secret" teaching of the *Bhagavad Gītā* is *karma-yoga* itself, potentially violent, revolutionary action in the name of (Hindu) religion, the Indian nation, and political sovereignty.[87]

In establishing the scope and terminology of his commentary on the *Bhagavad Gītā*, Tilak gives considerable attention to defining yoga.[88] His primary motivation is to disentangle the yoga of the *Bhagavad Gītā* from other forms—such as Patanjali's yoga and Sāṃkhya, which he calls the philosophy of "giving up" and associates with renunciation.[89] Tilak argues that in the *Bhagavad Gītā*, almost without exception, the word yoga is an "abbreviation"[90] of *karma-yoga*: a "special device of performing action,"[91] "a particular kind of device, method, or process of performing Action,"[92] and "equability" in action, through all of which he means political action.[93] He anchors this concept of yoga in what he calls "Vedic Karma Yoga," that is, a form of yoga that predates Patanjali or Shankaracharya and instead links yoga to the battlefield at the center of the epic, which is itself informed by the Vedic concept of yoga as war that we analyze in chapter 1.[94] This action is not performed in the abstract or in a field of metaphorical cosmic possibilities but very concretely in the context of war, which is the narrative frame of the *Bhagavad Gītā*. Tilak positions this debate within "the justification of the war on the authority of the Yoga."[95] For Tilak, the most important yoga of the *Bhagavad Gītā* is *karma-yoga*, whether or not that particular term is used. Though he acknowledges that the paths of devotion and knowledge exist in the *Bhagavad Gītā*, he argues that "the *Gītā* enjoins Action even after the perfection of Jnana and Bhakti is attained."[96] Action remains the undisputed point of yoga in the text for him.

Like Lajpat Rai and Aurobindo, Tilak also observed in the *Bhagavad Gītā* an injunction to nationalists, particularly those who identified as Hindu, to act in the world, as opposed to taking the path of renunciation. We might consider that Tilak and other nationalists who favor this interpretation of yoga as political action were engaged in multiple struggles: the material contest with the British for independence, and the effort to draw their fellow Indians into the battle. In this effort, it was essential to establish the *Bhagavad Gītā*'s yoga as primarily a philosophy of action rather than exclusively or primarily for meditation, devotion, or renunciation, that is, a retreat from the battle for independence.

In this text, Tilak makes two related points to explain why the path of renunciation is not a viable one for Indians in the early twentieth century. First, he suggests the message of the *Bhagavad Gītā* may be timeless but must be interpreted anew for each age. Second, he proposes a typology of India's past that divides historical eras into two distinct types. Some eras are what he calls the "Ages of Renunciation," which include the time of the Buddha as well as the centuries during which *bhakti* devotionalism flourished, led by Marathi *sant*-poet figures like Jnandev (ca. thirteenth century) and Tukaram (ca. seventeenth century). During these historical eras, Tilak suggests, it was possible for some to relinquish the field of politics:

> The Rishis who laid down the Law of Duty betook themselves to forests, because the people were already enjoying Swaraj or People's Dominion, which was administered and defended in the first instance by the Kshatriya kings.[97]

Yogis living in such peaceful times had the luxury of retreat, as the *haṭha* yoga texts cited earlier suggested. But the vast majority of India's history is enmeshed in what Tilak calls the "Ages of Action," or of "Karma Yoga." India in the nineteenth and early twentieth centuries is in one of these ages of action, of improper governance that requires redress. Even for those who desire their soul's liberation, Tilak insists that a life of meditative retreat from the material world is not a viable option amid ongoing political and social turmoil. British India does not constitute the kind of well-governed land suitable for that kind of yoga, Tilak argues. He further links liberation in this life and the next, the material and the metaphysical:

> It is my conviction, it is my thesis, that Swaraj in the life to come cannot be the reward of a people who have not enjoyed it in this world.[98]

Perhaps one who seeks liberation during political turmoil must first attend to the mundane world and secure political freedom, and only then can the yogi retreat to find spiritual liberation. Together, Tilak's interpretation of the *Bhagavad Gītā* and the *haṭha* yoga texts we referenced earlier remind their readers that seekers of spiritual freedom must take into account the political conditions in which metaphysical liberation is pursued.

Many of the nationalists who wrote and gave speeches about the *Bhagavad Gītā* focused on the apparent contradiction between an act of killing in the context of war and the desire for spiritual liberation. For Tilak, as for others, the key to resolving this paradox is the *Bhagavad Gītā*'s command to act without attachment or concern for the fruits of those actions. Selfless action could serve as a solvent for the vice of violence. Such action would be deemed righteous, even if it resulted in the deaths of others, as it certainly would in the case of the battle at Kurukshetra, or even in the case of the anti-imperial nationalism that Tilak and his contemporaries were attempting.

> You should not . . . presume that you have to toil that you yourself might reap the fruits of your labours. That cannot always be the case. Let us then try our utmost and leave the generations to come to enjoy that fruit. Remember, it is not you who had planted the mango-trees the fruit whereof you have tasted. Let the advantage now go to our children and their descendants.[99]

What stands out in this passage is Tilak's metaphor of generational inheritance as an explanation for the idea of selfless action. As we saw in the *Arthaśāstra*, the politics of yoga as action is shared between that text and the *Bhagavad Gītā*. However, the *Arthaśāstra*, perhaps in conscious contrast to the *Bhagavad Gītā*, proposes that the fruits of one's actions should be enjoyed, by the king anyway, and a calculation of that benefit should amount to the reason and goal of one's actions in the political realm. Tilak finds a narrow band between these contradictory positions on *karma-yoga*—the *Bhagavad Gītā*'s injunction to renounce the fruit of actions and the *Arthaśāstra*'s insistence that it is the enjoyment of the results of one's actions that should motivate political action itself. He strikes this balance by arguing that the contemporary political actor must renounce the benefits of action for themselves, as the *Bhagavad Gītā* requires, but still should be motivated by the benefits that their actions will produce in the future, for their descendants. The scholar of nationalism, Ernest Renan, writing a few decades before Tilak, proposed that that nation is "a great solidarity constituted by the feeling of sacrifice" in which a "nationalist" acts selflessly for the benefit of future generations.[100] Here, Tilak applies an ancient text to propose a modern solution to the nationalist riddle of selfless action: act not for oneself but for the future nation, his ethics of *karma-yoga*.

Gandhi's *Karma-Yoga* as the Yoking of Violence

Yoga's centrality as an indigenous political theory of action is perhaps best known in relation to the figure of M. K. Gandhi, the most studied of India's nationalists and perhaps any modern Indian figure. Gandhi's adoption of the *Bhagavad Gītā* from the 1920s onward as a political manual of sorts likewise has garnered substantial scholarly attention.[101] Through Gandhi's exhaustively collected writings, we know that he was aware of yoga as psychophysical practice from the 1880s onward, and he appeared to practice some degree of such yoga, particularly some basic form of psychophysical yoga and meditation, during his life. A pivotal moment occurred, however, when he was imprisoned in 1922, accompanied by the *Bhagavad Gītā* along with Tilak's *Gītā Rahasya*—a text, as we have seen, that was in a sense also born in prison. He emerged from imprisonment having fully embraced the term *karma-yoga* for his own style of political action and theory. Like Tilak, Gandhi produced his own commentaries on the *Gītā* from 1926 onward, particularly in his "Discourses on the Gita" from 1926 to 1927. In 1929, he named his Gujarati translation of the *Gītā*, *Anāsakti Yoga* or "The Yoga of Non-Attachment," a reference to the core idea of *karma-yoga* that he sought to draw from the text. In Gandhi's writing from 1926 until his death in 1948, the terms yoga and *karma-yoga* are ubiquitous.[102]

To be sure, the *Bhagavad Gītā* was not Gandhi's only source material; he was eclectic and catholic. To embody "transcendence in the secular world," as Prasanjit Duara puts it, Gandhi drew on everything from yoga and other Indian traditions to the Western critiques of industrial modernity and vegetarian ethics that he encountered through Leo Tolstoy and in London.[103] Gandhi first mentions yoga in his writing in 1908 (the same year of the trials of Aurobindo and Tilak already mentioned in this chapter) as a means to self-control, and here he specifically cites Patanjali.[104] Throughout the early decades of his political career, he seems to understand yoga as it is commonly understood today: a set of meditative techniques, positions, and breathing practices that calm and focus the mind; can heal common ailments; and can help provide resolve in one's undertakings. For example, Gandhi notes in several letters to friends that a particular *āsana* might relieve some illness or another, or that a particular breathing technique might help calm a troubled mind, though he warns his readers from "accepting directions of the next *Hatha Yogi* he may meet with."[105] These do not seem to be political uses specifically but uses of yoga far more in line with the idea—both current and classical—that yoga is a form of medicine. The one place in Gandhi's early writing that we see an opportunity for him to link yoga explicitly with a political end involves not Indian nationalism but British resolve. He refers to Englishmen "who go through the terrible strains of war without collapsing" suggesting that "[they] must be yogis."[106] Given his apparent disdain for the *haṭha* yogi expressed above, Gandhi's laudatory invocation of the Englishman as a yogi points toward the yoga of the warrior, of political action.

The first clear moment where Gandhi explicitly links yoga and his own political ideology occurs when Gandhi calls the tenacity required to master the art of weaving cotton *khādī*, on the *carakhā* or spinning wheel, a form of yoga. Spinning cotton was one of Gandhi's modes of resistance to British colonialism's economic oppression:

> Lastly comes weaving which is purely a matter of practice. One learns the principle in a day. The reader must not be surprised at the ease with which I claim processes can be learnt. All natural and necessary work is easy. Only it requires constant practice to become perfect, and it needs plodding. Ability to plod is *swaraj* [self-rule]. It is yoga.[107]

Yoga is the ability to plod toward self-rule—this phrase foreshadows how Gandhi will draw together his political goal, self-rule for India, with psychophysical yoga to see this practice as inherently political. While this may not strike one as a direct political use of yoga, it is evocative because the spinning of *khādī* and the spinning wheel itself were key political symbols for Gandhi. When he says that spinning *khādī* is a form of yoga, a metonym for self-rule, he is calling one of his most visible modes of public political expression a form of yoga.

In 1922, Gandhi was incarcerated for the crime of sedition against the colonial state, like so many others. And like Nehru, and many other nationalists of his time—Lala Lajput Rai, Sri Aurobindo, B. G. Tilak, K. B. Hedgewar, V. D. Savarkar—Gandhi took the *Bhagavad Gītā* with him to prison. The version he brought with him to the Yerawada jail in Pune was Edwin Arnold's translation, *The Song Celestial*. It was here, behind the bars of a colonial jail, that Gandhi would draw yoga into the core of his politics when he undertook a reading, translation, and commentary on the *Bhagavad Gītā*.[108] When Gandhi drew the *Bhagavad Gītā* fully into his thinking, his idea of *karma-yoga* became the key to his political thought. Through his reading and translation, he linked the *Bhagavad Gītā*'s yoga of action in battle to the idea of *karma-yoga*, action without attachment to the immediate fruits of action. Through this idea, Gandhi accomplished the quite counterintuitive feat of arguing that a text about convincing a man to kill his own family in a civil war was actually a text about nonviolent resistance. For Gandhi, the key to this paradox was unattached self-control that harnesses the self toward political action outside the self. In the *Bhagavad Gītā*, violence was the right outcome, and Arjuna needed to understand selfless action, *karma-yoga*, in order to act. But in the nationalist period, the battle was different, although the need for self-control was the same. Gandhi read the *Bhagavad Gītā*'s message in light of a new conflict and found that self-controlled action, *karma-yoga*, meant refraining from violence in the colonial era and meeting one's enemy with selfless nonviolent force. This political action, also called *satyāgraha* ("grasping truth") and *anāsakti-yoga* ("yoga without attachment"), is what Gandhi named *karma-yoga*. This form of yoga is the very political ideology and action that he advocated and, combined with his idea of "grasping the truth" (*satyāgraha*), seems to echo our argument that yoga is a mode of apprehension, of not only knowing something but also controlling the means of knowledge.

The German political theorist Carl Schmitt argued that the political theology of Judeo-Christian monotheism produces the Western judicial idea of the sovereign, the one who makes the exception. Writing at around the same time, Gandhi argues that the sovereign is the one who has mastered the self rather than others, a concept derived from his reading of yoga.[109] Schmitt's political theology is the politics of domination of others, whereas Gandhi's political theology strives for the freedom of the self in the midst of political subjugation; if Schmitt's sovereign is the political hegemon, Gandhi's sovereign is the detached actor. Gandhi refers to *karma-yoga* as the "sovereign yoga" in his discussions of the second chapter of the *Bhagavad Gītā*, where "yoga means practice" and is a means to "cast off the bondage of action," as a way for people in a colonized context to act as free people.[110] Gandhi, to adapt a phrase from Partha Chatterjee, taught the yoga of the governed,[111] or what Dipesh Chakrabarty and Rochona Majumdar refer to as "politics as it actually was."[112] These are articulations in what J. Barton Scott has called "genealogies of self-rule" in India that intertwine European thought, even liberal thought, with Indian concepts of the ethical self, the "worldly yogi."[113] We agree with Scott when he writes of Gandhi's political philosophy, "a person should govern her body and behavior in much the same way that a nation governs its territory—it being the transferability of technologies of self-rule between these different registers that comes to constitute the domain of the political as such."[114] This aligns with the central concept of yoga in the *Bhagavad Gītā*—that disciplined political action is anchored by a disciplined political self—and it is in accordance with the *Arthaśāstra*—where the *rājarṣi*, the sage-like king, is one who has controlled the self and thereby can control others in the political realm. But where Scott argues for the influence of a nineteenth-century "culture of the self" in the swell of colonial-era political thought, we push for the insertion of a much older, and more endemic, technology of the self marshalled toward the political enemy, colonialism, and toward resolving internal division among Indians.

What differentiates Gandhi's engagement with the ideas of the *Bhagavad Gītā* and of *karma-yoga* from that of Tilak and others is his insistence that the text be read as metaphor. For Gandhi, the battle of Kurukshetra is not a literal war but rather an allegory for the battles waged internally in each individual. In reading the *Bhagavad Gītā* this way, Gandhi set out to reappropriate the text and its interpretations from the "extremist" faction of Indian nationalism—Tilak and Aurobindo included. Chakrabarty and Majumdar suggest that, thanks to his reading of the *Bhagavad Gītā*, Gandhi was able to see politics as it really is—murky and compromised. Far from trying to spiritualize politics, as others have argued, Gandhi finds in the *Bhagavad Gītā*'s lesson of *karma-yoga* a way to inoculate the *satyāgrahī* from the taint of politics by acting selflessly.[115] The key point to note is that, whether nationalists understood the *Bhagavad Gītā* as metaphor like Gandhi or interpreted it literally like Tilak and his fellow extremists, the text and its lesson of *karma-yoga* are understood to be properly in the domain of politics and not concerned with purely religious questions of renunciation, redemption, and spiritual liberation.

Gandhi's interpretation of yoga in the *Bhagavad Gītā* differs from that of his contemporaries in important ways. Perhaps the most distinct difference is Gandhi's rejection of direct violent action, his philosophy of "nonviolence" and "passive resistance." This strident position requires that he read the *Bhagavad Gītā* as a purely allegorical story about the struggles of practical life.[116] This insistence on removing the *Bhagavad Gītā* from its martial history, what Chakrabarty and Majumdar call Gandhi's "antihistory move," might seem strange because the service to which he pressed his allegorical reading was, in essence, another war; this is the very relevance of the text in this time of conflict with colonialism.[117] Of course, Gandhi was not alone in reading the *Bhagavad Gītā* as allegory—this was a common way to read and comment on the *Bhagavad Gītā* in the precolonial period as well. However, Gandhi's insistence on an ahistorical, decontextualized, allegorical reading served his arguments about *karma-yoga* and nonviolence because to accept the historical violence of the *Bhagavad Gītā*'s context was to accept that *karma-yoga* was a way to address the ethics of the inevitability of violent action. Unlike Arjuna, Gandhi did not intend to enter the war for independence by killing others. His antihistorical reading is itself an act of nonviolence because it deletes, literally removes, violence from the narrative of the *Bhagavad Gītā*. In doing so, Gandhi tries to create a cosmic, mythic, allegorical bedrock for a nonviolent political yoga, an *ahimsā* version of *karma-yoga*, his signature political innovation.

Gandhi's position is that yoga is a discipline of nonattachment that allows one to remain ethical amid war. Part of the purity one can achieve through *karma-yoga*, Gandhi argues, is a release from being the agent of violence even in violent conflict. This is Gandhi's concept of *ahimsā* tied to nonattachment, and he draws it directly from the logic of the *Bhagavad Gītā* that argues that the accrual of *karma* is negated when one acts without attachment to the fruits of one's actions. As we have noted, in a significant departure from figures like Tilak and the early writing of Aurobindo, Gandhi rejects violence in the way it is depicted in the *Bhagavad Gītā* and the epic—conventional violent action. Instead, he proposes the idea of passive resistance, where "passive" means "nonviolent" rather than inactive. Despite this disassociation from violence, Gandhi nonetheless marshals a text situated within a war that justifies enacting violence. Gandhi's symbolic interpretation aside, he cannot avoid either the violence in which the text is embedded or the violence in which he is embedded as a political actor amid an often-violent resistance to colonial rule. How can we read yoga in relation to violence in Gandhi's thought in a way that resolves this paradoxical formulation?

While we feel we have accurately portrayed Gandhi's position, our argument differs from that of many commentators on Gandhi, his politics, and his interpretation of yoga in the *Bhagavad Gītā*. Gandhi's approach is conventionally described as non-violent, but we would amend this to suggest that he interprets yoga in the *Bhagavad Gītā* to mean the control of violence, the harnessing of violence for political purposes.[118] In a sense, Gandhi's political yoga is the yoking of violence as a political tool; this is his *karma-yoga*. Just as *yoga-kṣema* came to mean ensuring peace or security through the threat of violence, so we think Gandhi's yoking of violence, his restraint of it, was skillfully used by him to political advantage. This is not the same as saying that Gandhi was violent. Instead, we argue that it was precisely the potential for violence—should Gandhi perish during a fast or a march, or in prison, for example—that gave particular force to his political action. His political theory of this force we argue is found in his interpretation of yoga in the *Bhagavad Gītā*. As we saw in both the *Bhagavad Gītā* and the *Arthaśāstra*, particularly around the term *yoga-kṣema*, yoga also describes a state of peace or stability that is ensured by the threat of violence, that is, a peace secured by violence. Yoga, in Gandhi's formulation through the *Bhagavad Gītā*, both acknowledges the threat of violence and strategically holds it at bay by harnessing the destructive potential of the violence that would follow his death. In this sense of the word *yoga-kṣema*, the state of *kṣema* (peace or pacification) comes *from* yoga (war, violence, forceful control). Indeed, Gandhi's murder at the hands of a Hindu right-wing activist,

Nathuram Godse, in 1948, led to a wave of violence even after India's formal independence from the British.

Many of Gandhi's opponents felt this threat keenly—that he commanded, passively and even perhaps against his will, the massive potential for violence from his followers. As Joseph Alter notes, Gandhi called his fasting a "weapon," another sign that he understood well that the threat of this kind of potential violence was always inherent in his fasts.[119] One such fast forced Dr. B. R. Ambedkar to give up his desire for separate electorates for Dalits in 1932 and agree to the Pune Pact. In Gandhi's hands, yoga as political practice did not advocate violence, but its power was underwritten by the violence that his own death would cause others to enact. The violence contained within Gandhi's nonviolence utilized both psychophysical yoga (arguably expressed through fasting and his ascetical comportment) and the political discipline of controlling an object, in this case, violence itself. Gandhi's yoga is his ability to yoke violence and so to remain in this state of "nonharming," the literal meaning of *ahiṃsā*, a word that also means "security" in classical Sanskrit.[120] This yoga also implies the ability to do the opposite, to loosen the yoke that holds back harm. His opponents, whether the British or other Indians, like Ambedkar, felt the strain of that yoke and responded to it.

Through Gandhi's engagement as well as that of Tilak, Aurobindo, and Lajpat Rai, we can reflect on a larger question: Who did the *Bhagavad Gītā*, a text about fratricide, speak to? In our argument for a classical political theory of yoga in part I, we describe yoga as a discipline of power that is transitive; a subject disciplines and gains power over an object, but it is also intramural, where subject and object share the same political field. The struggle between rivals is agonistic, a contest of power that does not produce a permanent solution but is merely part of a larger unfolding of politics over time represented in the idea of the *maṇḍala*. The people we have discussed so far in this chapter who use the concept of yoga from the *Bhagavad Gītā* do so in a shared political field. Tilak refers to the context of the *Bhagavad Gītā* as a "civil war,"[121] and Annie Besant sees the text encompassing "all souls in East and West . . . for the path is one."[122] Aurobindo and Lajpat Rai speak to their "countrymen" and try to convince them of the oppression they share. This sense of the intramural nature of the *Bhagavad Gītā* is linked to our understanding of yoga as a political idea. In the classical sense, we saw how yoga was applied to the conquest, discipline, and control of others with whom one shared the same system—of ritual, politics, language, battle, family, and so on. Yoga, we argued, yokes things that share a world—it is not a term for the annihilation or subjugation of someone or something wholly other and outside this field of reference. This shared field allows for the possibility for agonism—productive conflict—as opposed to antagonistic annihilation.

Our conjecture around the intramural nature of yoga and the conflict of the *Bhagavad Gītā* is extended to our understanding of what is disciplined, yoked, and harnessed in the political thought of the figures we have studied. In considering early twentieth-century translators and interpreters of the *Bhagavad Gītā*, one striking thing to note is the structural similarity between the battlefield in Kurukshetra and the context of India's freedom struggle. The majority of the roughly 240,000 soldiers in British India in the early twentieth century were recruited within the subcontinent, although the "martial races" theory ensured that some communities were overrepresented compared to others.[123] This fundamentally Indian character of the army, especially at the level of the rank and file, the subaltern, meant the two sides arrayed against one another in the nationalist struggle were brethren in a similar way to the war-wary cousins on either side of the battlefield where the story of the *Bhagavad Gītā* unfolds. The public commentaries and political interpretations of yoga and the *Bhagavad Gītā* discussed so far are premised on an *internal* conflict, a civil cleavage, rather than an external one. In this metaphor, if Arjuna and the Pandavas stand in for the virtuous nationalists, their enemies (the Kauravas) are configured as the Indians who need to be recruited to their side.[124] Colonialism has already fomented civil conflict and separated Indians from one another—a divide-and-rule policy well known to historians and political analysts of colonialism worldwide. One key "yoking" by those who use *karma-yoga* is the joining together of Indians against a common enemy. Yoga here is the effort to define the political field itself, to set the terms and constituents for the field of battle.

The British are outside this field of contest for most of the people we have discussed so far. The political struggle is to control what "India" means, to harness and direct a nationalism of self-identification. The people to be yoked, to be disciplined into action, are their fellow Indians who, in one way or another, are arrayed against their nationalist cause—because they are indifferent, employed by the British, admirers of British liberalism, uninvested in Indian national independence, and even opposed to its success. The *karma-yoga*, the yoga of action, is the compulsion not only for such Indians to take action against the British and form common cause with their fellow nationalists but also to unify. Nationalism was as much about the overthrow of British rule as it was about the consolidation of an Indian identity, a project that endures beyond formal colonialism, a goal of *kṣema* through the yoga that would precede and ensure it. So much has been written about the fractures within this identity—and the people we have discussed here are all part of a very clear "Hindu" social order, and in general one that registers a Brahmanical, "high caste" and normatively male position of power, one often set against Islam in particular, as well as Dalits. The formations of identity around "India" or "Hindu" have never been singular or unified. Social, political, and religious divisions, and especially, the practices of caste patriarchy, have long fractured a singular identity in India. The extramural question of the violence and repression of European colonialism was not more important than the intramural question of what forms of culture and society could be possible within a nation-state free of colonial rule.

Ambedkar on the *Bhagavad Gītā*, *Karma-Yoga*, and the Buddha's Despair

The ideas and leadership of Lajpat Rai, Aurobindo, Tilak, and Gandhi were important and influential, but they did not represent all Indians. Political identities formed around religion, gender, class, region, and caste complicated the nationalist views outlined above, particularly those that went against the grain of a perspective that was largely elite caste, male, and Hindu. Alongside a mode of nationalism that sought as its primary aim freedom from British rule was a long history of political thinkers and activists who strove for freedom from the systems of Hindu-oriented caste patriarchy that they identified as having their own colonizing effects on the majority of the people of India over thousands of years, well before the arrival of British and other European powers to the subcontinent. Thinkers like Savitribai Phule (1831–1897), Jotirao Phule (1827–1890), Iyothee Thass (1845–1914), and Erode Venkatappa Ramasamy "Periyar" (1879–1973) felt that the end of British rule risked bringing the return of another colonial-like form, that of Brahmanical, elite caste, patriarchal rule. To forestall that outcome required leveraging the presence of the British to establish laws and protections for India's women, religious minorities, Shudras or Bahujans, and Dalits. Those who held such positions were often described as "radical" or "anti-national" or "pro-British" because they argued that the underlying normative structures of caste and gender hierarchy had to be eradicated for any idea of freedom or equality to have meaning in a postcolonial future. Many male, elite-caste nationalists, including those discussed in this chapter, also expressed their opposition to these same hierarchies. These assurances, however, could not allay the fears of non-caste-elite thinkers whose own contemporary experiences of caste and gender, and understanding of history, provided a potent counterpoint.

Dr. B. R. Ambedkar, one of the most important political leaders of modern India, critiqued the uses of the *Bhagavad Gītā* and *karma-yoga* by these other leaders but nevertheless instrumentalized a core concept at the heart of this line of thought: that the power of religious discourse should be harnessed strategically to craft a modern political theology of freedom. Among the vital political thinkers critiquing the normative, orthodox structures of caste and gender, Ambedkar stands out. Born into a Maharashtrian Dalit community considered "Untouchable" in orthodox Hindu society, Ambedkar lacked the religious, social, economic, and political capital enjoyed by the figures discussed in this chapter so far, all of whom were Brahman men, except for Gandhi, who comes from an elite-caste Modh Bania community, coded as *vaiśya* or "merchant" in the classic *varṇa*-caste typology. Despite the disadvantages accrued to him by birth, Ambedkar pursued an education that included graduate degrees, and a law degree, from Columbia University and the London School of Economics. His education was supported in part by the Raja of Baroda, the Maratha ruler of a Princely State outside direct British control, much like the state of Aundh discussed in the next chapter. Notably, Princely Baroda was one of the first states in India to implement a reservation policy for Dalits and other disadvantaged communities. Ambedkar became the Chair of the Drafting Committee for the Indian Constitution. Though Gandhi is often remembered as the "Father" ("Bapu") of the Indian nation, we might speak of Ambedkar as the Father ("Babasaheb") of the Indian state so far as a modern state is composed of laws and founded by a constitution, the sovereign rule of law. Gandhi had little or no involvement in the drafting of the Indian constitution, although he, along with many of his compatriots, played a pivotal role in the consolidation of Indian nationalism. Ambedkar did not place his faith in the moral imagination of the nation, but in the legal structure of the state and human rights. As the chief architect of the constitution, Ambedkar is considered a key builder of the Indian state.

Ambedkar may have shared with the people we have studied the view that political power could be drawn from religious contexts and concepts, and that a political theology of freedom in the modern world might use the material of the premodern period to craft a new vision. However, Ambedkar felt that the materials, traditions, views, rituals, and texts that make up "Hinduism" could not serve this purpose for Bahujans and Dalits and for most women. Ambedkar famously converted from Hinduism to Buddhism in 1956, with perhaps half a million others. Much of Ambedkar's work directly engages Hindu texts, often in Sanskrit, particularly those that provide religious or philosophical justification for caste oppression.[125] In this vein, Ambedkar understood that the reason the *Bhagavad Gītā* was used so extensively by elite nationalists was because it represented *their* patrimony, as Aurobindo wrote in 1909.[126] Ambedkar's point was that this was not the patrimony of most Indians. As elite caste Hindu men, for the most part, Aurobindo and the other leaders that dominated the nationalist movement inherited the traditions that produced and sustained the *Bhagavad Gītā*.

Aishwarya Kumar notes that, at one time, perhaps around 1926 and 1927, Ambedkar considered the *Bhagavad Gītā* "a basis for our demand for equal rights," referring to equal rights for "Untouchables" in India attainable through the instrument of *saytāgraha*.[127] This was around the same time that Gandhi was formulating his political commentary on the *Bhagavad Gītā*. Within a few months, Ambedkar's position on the *Bhagavad Gītā* as an emancipatory text appears to have changed dramatically, and he began in 1927 to write "Essays on the Bhagwat Gita: Philosophic Defence of Counter-Revolution: Krishna and His Gita," a work he never finished or published in his lifetime.[128]

In "Essays on the Bhagwat Gita," Ambedkar does not mention Gandhi's work at all; rather, he focuses his attention on Tilak's *Gītā Rahasya*, likely the Marathi original because the English version would not be published until later.[129] Ambedkar argues that the concept of *karma-yoga* drawn from the *Bhagavad Gītā* by the kinds of elite caste, Hindu male nationalists that Tilak represents does not refer to selfless action in the service of the national good. Instead, Ambedkar argues that the text upholds "the dogma of karma kanda as propounded by Jaimini," which is a reference to Pūrva Mimāṃsa.[130] Attributed to a figure named Jaimini, Pūrva Mimāṃsa is one of the classical

Hindu schools of philosophy rooted in the ritualism of the Vedas and an orthodox vision of social order. Here *karma kāṇḍa* refers to the portions of the Vedic texts that detail rituals to be performed by Brahman men for compensation (*dakṣiṇā*). In other words, Ambedkar argues that the *karma-yoga* of the *Bhagavad Gītā* refers to making society conform to ancient, regressive, and ritualistic hierarchies around caste and gender, construing social norms as a way to provide "compensation" to elite caste Hindu men. It is a "philosophic defense" of classical caste and gender typologies and hierarchies.[131] Ambedkar not only sees in *karma-yoga* a reference to a deep-seated and regressive position about caste patriarchy, he also sees it as a modern defense of casteism. Krishna tells Arjuna it is his duty as a male member of the warrior caste (*kṣatriya*) to fight but that he should relinquish attachment to his own actions. Ambedkar suggests that this serves as a justification for the "dogma" of caste—act according to caste rules without attachment to one's own freedom or civil rights.[132]

One reason Ambedkar converted to Buddhism was that he viewed it as a historical, social, religious, moral, and political revolution against caste oppression. He describes the *Bhagavad Gītā* as a "counter-revolutionary" text because, he argues, it was created by orthodox Hindu thinkers to counter the revolution of Buddhism, to "save" caste patriarchal Hindus from "the attack of Buddhism."[133] Ambedkar held that Buddhism presented the true concept of nonviolence and a rejection of caste distinctions and hierarchy. The *Bhagavad Gītā*, on the other hand, supported violence and valorized the caste status of elite caste men. Ambedkar dismisses Tilak's writings on the *Bhagavad Gītā*, suggesting that he represents an "orthodox" point of view,[134] and argues that Tilak's use of the text set off a chain of such engagements among other nationalists that amounts to "a trick of patriotic Indians."[135] In his view, these efforts hid, in the guise of a philosophical call to political action and freedom, an actual defense of Hindu caste patriarchy as a social norm.[136] Ambedkar therefore could find no political emancipatory potential in either *karma-yoga* or the *Bhagavad Gītā*, both of which he considered to be regressive attempts to shore up caste-patriarchal normativity. For him, they represented a modern return of the counterrevolution against the emancipation of India's non-Brahman communities from the thrall of caste patriarchy through the ritual and caste ideas of *karma*.

While Ambedkar ultimately rejected the *Bhagavad Gītā* as a source for a politically empowering thought or practice, concepts from the text nonetheless may have influenced his thinking in significant ways. As part of his conversion, Ambedkar wrote one of the most important texts of modern Buddhism, a treatise on the Buddha's life and teaching called *The Buddha and His Dhamma*, published in 1957, the year after his death. One can view *The Buddha and His Dhamma* as an iteration in the long history in India of control over concepts and power in which Ambedkar situates the *Bhagavad Gītā* and its modern interpreters as well. Ambedkar's work is a counter to this counterrevolution, a return to the original revolutionary impulse of Buddhism now relevant in the modern period, as he saw it, revised and rearticulated for a new political age with many of the same old political battles around caste and gender yet unresolved.

Within this renewal of the Buddhist challenge to Hindu caste patriarchy, we can find one of the very few invocations of yoga anywhere in Ambedkar's work. Ambedkar narrates the despondency the Buddha faces after his enlightenment when he contemplates spreading his teaching, his *dhamma*, to a world that may not be prepared to accept it.[137] Writing in English, Ambedkar titles this section of the text with a compound Sanskrit word. He calls it "The Buddha and His Vishad Yoga."[138] For anyone attuned to the *Bhagavad Gītā* and its commentarial tradition—both classical and modern—the Sanskrit compound word *viṣāda-yoga*, "the yoga of despair," is suggestive. It appears in the title of the first book of the *Bhagavad Gītā* in both the commentarial tradition and in many English translations.[139] Each chapter of the *Bhagavad Gītā* presents a different technique or subject by which Arjuna is yoked by Krishna in the effort to get Arjuna to fight. For example, chapter 2 of the *Bhagavad Gītā*, in which Krishna uses the philosophy of Sāṃkhya to compel Arjuna to fight, is called *sāṃkhya-yoga*, "the yoking of Sāṃkhya," and so on. The word yoga in these cases is often referred to as "teaching" or "reflection" on a given subject. The active, transitive nature of yoga that we have outlined suggests, however, that each title tells us by what object (philosophy, thought, feeling, concept) Arjuna is controlled. The first object, "despair" (*viṣāda*), occurs before Krishna can counsel Arjuna—all the other "yogas" occur as part of Krishna's teaching. Here, Arjuna is yoked, controlled, by his own despair, and thus he acts out of that despair. The remaining chapters of the *Bhagavad Gītā* show Krishna offering other strategies, other means of control, to replace the inaction occasioned by despair.

We can find no comment by Ambedkar on why he chose this title. Though it appears to us to resonate with the *Bhagavad Gītā*, he may have intended no resonance at all. Given his deep knowledge of and critique of the *Bhagavad Gītā* and multiple other Sanskrit texts of Hinduism, it seems unlikely, however, that such a symmetry would have been an accident. Ambedkar was too brilliant and careful a scholar to select such a redolent phrase without intention. If this echo of the *Bhagavad Gītā* was purposeful, and if we can consider *The Buddha and His Dhamma* as a "counter counterrevolutionary" text set against the *Bhagavad Gītā* in some way, then we might interpret this "yoga of despair" through these interconnections and critiques that marked Ambedkar's thought.

In the text, Ambedkar imagines the Buddha feeling despair about teaching his *dhamma* to the world. Speaking to himself, the Buddha says, "It is hard for mankind to liberate itself from the entanglements of God and Soul. It is hard for mankind to give up its belief in rites and ceremonies. It is hard for mankind to give up its belief in Karma."[140] We might imagine that Ambedkar combines the idea of *karma* as the mechanism of transmigration in Hindu and Buddhist thought with his political critique of this term in relationship to *karma-yoga* in the *Bhagavad Gītā* and in its modern uses. In both cases, *karma* underwrites caste-gender hierarchy, he has argued, either as the "law" that determines status in one's next life or as the "ritual" of social order encoded in Vedic literature. Here, in relation to Ambedkar's thinking, *karma* may indicate the caste-gender complex of oppression. The Buddha of Ambedkar's text worries that people are too attached to these ideas of superiority, hierarchy, and normative Hindu social order assigned at birth to understand the "radical equality" of the Buddha's thought.[141] The idea that humanity is yoked to a political order of inequality and so unable to comprehend the *dhamma* is at the root of the Buddha's *viṣāda-yoga* as expressed by Ambedkar here. In other words, Ambedkar, through his re-creation of the Buddha's life, expresses perhaps his own despair that a caste-ridden society is not yet ready for the equality intended in a constitutional democracy. As much as the writers discussed in this chapter could appeal to their imagined emic cultural world comprised of fellow Indians, Ambedkar saw himself as outside this world because of the structures of caste patriarchy that often configured him, as a Dalit man, as outside the conventional fold of Hinduism.

Like Arjuna and Yudhishthira in the *Mahābhārata*, the Buddha considers a life of ascetical renunciation rather than active engagement with the world: "Why not remain a sanyasi away from the world, and use my gospel to perfect my own self?"[142] As in the epic and the *Bhagavad Gītā*, someone else helps the Buddha see the right decision. This is the Buddhist figure Brahmā Sahampati, a kind of divine mortal who appears to convince the Buddha to preach the *dhamma*. While Ambedkar receives this story from established Buddhist narratives, he tells it in his own way. The title "*viṣāda-yoga*" does not seem to exist in any other retelling of this moment from the life of the Buddha in any source.[143] Ambedkar seems to depart significantly, and we suggest purposefully, from centuries of previous Buddhist biography that appears not to use this title. Ambedkar may have adopted this term in order to gesture toward his critique of the *Bhagavad Gītā* as a counterrevolutionary text renewed for a pernicious modern politics.

The Buddha resolves, Ambedkar writes, to do "his duty to return to the world and serve it, and not sit silent as the personification of inactive passivity."[144] Ambedkar thought the *Bhagavad Gītā* was designed not only to counter the revolution of Buddhism but also to co-opt its terms and ideas, bending them toward a regressive end. This statement by the Buddha that he will remain "active" acts as a countermove, taking the same kind of language around engaging in activity—like the "energism" of *karma-yoga* in Tilak's text—but placing it in the service of a revival of Buddhism as a religion for a people seeking equality in a modern, rational, liberal state. We speculate that Ambedkar chose the terms he did, invoking forms of *karma* and yoga, to leave a legacy of challenge to the kinds of narratives around yoga as political thought and action discussed in this chapter.

Conclusion

The people that populate this chapter all sought sovereignty in a colonized world. They marshalled ideas from the past, situated within a politico-religious history, and deployed these ideas to inspire political action. Yet a parallel world existed alongside the formal colonized spaces of British India. Covering almost half of India's landmass and constituting almost a third of its population were a collection of around 550 semi-sovereign Princely States. The engagement with the *Bhagavad Gītā* by the nationalists we discuss in this chapter represents an expression of political yoga among revolutionaries who were explicitly opposed to British rule. However, the delicate political liminality of the Princely States made overt antinationalist expression a fraught endeavor. Just as the *Bhagavad Gītā* and its idea of *karma-yoga* provided a covert means of political expression, another variant of yoga as politics would emerge in a Princely State in India to claim sovereignty under the yoke of colonialism.

While yoga as political thought and practice remains our chief interest throughout this book, we also pay attention to where the three spheres of yoga intersect and overlap. This chapter emphasizes the intersection of yoga as political thought and action with yoga as philosophy in the context of nationalist politics, specifically the idea of *karma-yoga* in the *Bhagavad Gītā*. The next chapter explores the intersection of yoga as politics with yoga as psychophysical practice, where we trace the emergence of the Surya Namaskar within the Princely State of Aundh.

FOUR

Yoga as Sovereignty in Princely India

A MONUMENTAL SCULPTURE greets those who arrive at the Indira Gandhi International Airport in New Delhi. Bronze figures arrayed in a spiral depict each position of the Surya Namaskar, a series of movements that is one of the signature sequences of modern yoga. This sculpture, completed in 2011 during the government led by Manmohan Singh of the Indian National Congress party, transmits to the visitor—especially the foreign one—a visual presentation of political soft power. It stands as a reminder to all who pass by that yoga traditions, and especially the Surya Namaskar, are of Indian origin, a point of pride for the Indian nation. The location of this sculpture, at the international gateway to India's national capital, is apt because the Surya Namaskar has long existed within the worlds of politics and power.

In parallel with the emergence of *karma-yoga* as a key political theory for nationalist figures, which we discuss in chapter 3, was the codification and spread of yoga as psychophysical practice, the early roots of what are today's *āsanas* and yoga studios. One key site for the development of psychophysical yoga as a health intervention was colonial Bombay, where two institutions, Kaivalyadam in Lonavala and the Yoga Institute in Bombay, were founded in the early twentieth century and carried out extensive research on the scientific principles and effects of various aspects of postural yoga, yogic breathing, and meditation.

What is more germane to our study of yoga's political entanglements in the colonial period, however, are modern postural yoga's origins in various

Princely States. The Princely, Native, or "subimperial" state was something like a vassal state that was allowed to exist in various degrees of domestic sovereign rule as long as its ruler declared allegiance to the British Crown.[1] These were the subjects of "indirect rule" in India. Not all Princely States or their sovereign rulers were the same; their greater autonomy, coupled with a concentration of royal financial and political power in these locales, both enabled exploitation and made possible novel, more salutary experiments.[2] In this chapter, we examine a set of interlinked transformations in sovereign rule in the Princely State of Aundh, at the center of which we position the practice of the Surya Namaskar. We argue that the Surya Namaskar was understood by its chief proponent, Bhawanrao Shriniwasrao Pant Pratinidhi (1868–1951, hereafter "the Raja"), to be a physical practice within a discourse emerging from an elite martial tradition of yoga as both psychophysical technique and political strategy, a way to claim sovereignty through the governance of the self amid the liminal freedoms afforded by indirect rule. The importance of the Surya Namaskar as a practice of sovereignty began with the actual psychophysical exercise but radiated outward and ultimately reverberated through Aundh's political, educational, economic, social, and penal domains.

Aundh and Its Raja

It is known by some but not often noted that the place that played an important role in introducing the world to the Surya Namaskar was also one where there were early models of universal suffrage, a liberal democratic constitution, an independent judiciary, and the open-concept prison. Located 150 kilometers southeast of Pune in western India, the Princely State of Aundh was made up of a scant seventy-two villages, a small territory of roughly five hundred square miles that was dispersed in roughly twenty-four discontinuous patches across the modern districts of Satara and Sangli in Maharashtra and Vijayapura in northern Karnataka. This "crazy quilt"[3] was the result of a series of annexation agreements between the British East India Company, the rulers of the much larger Satara State, and the principality of Aundh over the course of the nineteenth century. Given the small size of Aundh, the Raja's purse was likewise modest, especially compared to the larger and wealthier polities both in the Deccan (Satara, Kolhapur,

Baroda) and elsewhere (Travancore, Mysore, Hyderabad). It was even further constrained because, of Aundh's seventy-two villages, full revenue from twelve villages and partial revenue from another four were given as *inām*, or grants, to separate individuals. In one important respect, however, Aundh had a freedom that few other principalities could claim because it paid tribute to no other political power, neither the British nor other Deccan states.[4] In this sense, its sovereignty was more robust than that of other Princely or Native States in British India.

In the early twentieth century, Aundh entered spheres of political contention that tested the limits of its political sovereignty on a few occasions.[5] In the first decade of the century, Aundh's ruler at the time, Gopalkrishnarao Parashuram "Nanasaheb," who was the Raja's nephew, was charged by the British with plotting to murder his own prime minister. The British often found ways to depose or otherwise bypass rulers who were problematic or whose actions ran counter to their interests, although it is unclear if that was the case here. The public protested what was perceived to be a "secret and unfair trial,"[6] but swift litigation resulted in Nanasaheb's removal and replacement with his uncle, the Raja, whose reign began in 1909 and ended when he voluntarily abdicated his rule with the institution of a democratic constitution in 1939. The political strategies of the Raja, even the Surya Namaskar, need to be seen in relation to the precarity of his installment as the ruler of Aundh as well as the capricious nature of colonial control of the Princely States.

Just a year after the Raja assumed charge, Aundh was again in political jeopardy. Four young men, two of whom were from Aundh and were teachers in Aundh schools, were implicated in what became known in the press variously as the Aundh Conspiracy Case and the Satara Conspiracy Case. The four were accused of joining an effort in 1906 to collect arms and establish a local branch of a nationalist secret society, Abhinav Bharat, which was started by the Hindu nationalist leader V. D. Savarkar and his brother with the aim of overthrowing the British. The prosecution alleged that the young men were connected to the wider networks of revolutionary nationalists in eastern and western India and claimed to have found in their possession the writings of Savarkar, instructions for bomb making, and pamphlets about how the Russians organized revolution. In addition, they noted the presence of the *Dāsbodh*, a seventeenth-century text attributed to the Maharashtrian figure Samartha Ramdas (ca. 1608–1681) that includes discussions of a form of Surya Namaskar, yoga, regional nationalism, and political power.[7] Of the four accused, three were found guilty and sentenced to between three and eight years of imprisonment.[8]

Despite these scandals, the Raja was perceived by the British to be a loyal subject, one who contributed money to and otherwise supported the British war effort (as did M. K. Gandhi and other nationalists) and encouraged his subjects to do the same. He regularly attended gatherings to honor visiting imperial dignitaries in Bombay, Pune, and the resort town of Mahabaleshwar. The Raja thus excelled in the social role of a loyal Indian prince.

He was also the architect of a series of reforms that we suggest are emblematic of yoga as political practice. These included incorporating Surya Namaskar training throughout Aundh, reforms to the educational system, administrative and judicial devolution, initiatives to achieve economic self-sufficiency, and penal reform. The pinnacle of Aundh's political reforms was the Raja's abdication of his royal privileges in favor of a constitutional democracy in 1938–1939, eight years ahead of India's declaration of independence from British rule and more than a decade before India's own democratic constitution would come into effect in 1951. He also played a leading role in social, educational, political, and cultural reform movements outside Aundh. For example, he was the first major patron of the Bhandarkar Oriental Research Institute's project to compose a critical edition of the *Mahābhāratha*, for which he also painted illustrations and commissioned art from other artists.[9] Although he was a Brahman by birth, he was critical of religious and caste practices that discriminated against women and non-elite castes alike and that, in his view, were responsible for social decline; he did not strictly obey the norm common for men of his community of wearing the sacred thread, either.[10] In many senses, he can be considered an example of a "Brahmin double," someone who, by virtue of his caste and gender position, could afford to mount criticisms of the very structures that upheld his authority.[11] These various political, social, and ethical stances informed how he deployed his practice of the Surya Namaskar to speak to and effect his political positions.

The Surya Namaskar and Yoga

The origins of the Surya Namaskar are fuzzy. Neither the sequence, nor its famous central component, the "downward dog" pose, have been found in any known premodern *haṭha* or other text on yoga, including the most famous one, the *Haṭhapradīpikā*.[12] In Western India, however, the sequence of movements and postures is closely associated with the early modern political elite of Maharashtra. One commonly understood focal point for the Surya Namaskar in western India is the religious and political figure, Samartha Ramdas, who espoused a mixture of psychophysical and philosophical yoga, Hinduism, Maharashtrian pride, martial strength, and physical exercise.[13] The key work attributed to Ramdas, the *Dāsbodh* (ca. 1654), mentions performing "salutations to the sun" (*sūryās namaskār*) in several places.[14] These salutations appear to be a form of yoga for Ramdas, although his only instruction on how to do this *namaskār* is to perform *sāṣṭāṅga*, a prone prostration performed "with eight limbs" on the ground.[15] This is also one origin point for the interchangeability of the Surya Namaskar with the *sāṣṭāṅga namaskār* (*namaskār* with eight limbs [touching the ground]) in the Raja's writing and practice, as well as in other texts, and in common parlance in Marathi.

The elite ruling communities of the Maratha Confederacy, particularly those of Brahman and Maratha castes, appear to have practiced the Surya Namaskar/*sāṣṭāṅga namaskār* as a form of martial exercise. Sadashivrao Bhau, a member of the powerful Brahman Peshwa lineage that ruled from Pune, wrote to the Peshwa Balaji Bajirao, his uncle, in December 1759 to complain that he could not perform his usual exercise of *daṇḍa namaskār* because of a wound in his back from being recently injured.[16] The *daṇḍa namaskār* (making the body "like a staff") is often used as a description of the *sāṣṭāṅga namaskār* and largely interchangeable with it, and also the Surya Namaskar, in Marathi. There appears to be a thread running from the *sūryās namaskār*/*sāṣṭāṅga namaskār* of Ramdas in the seventeenth century through the practices of the Maratha/Brahman ruling elite of the eighteenth century and to the Surya Namaskar of the nineteenth and twentieth centuries that the Raja of Aundh describes.

The *Encyclopedia of Indian Physical Culture*, published in 1950 and where these various forms of *namaskār* and much else are discussed, was funded by three royal Maratha families—the Rajas of Baroda, Sangli, and Phaltan. The preface to the *Encyclopedia*, which was written by the Raja of Aundh, declares that "of all the exercise, Indian and foreign . . . the Surya Namaskar is the first and foremost," a declaration apparently blessed and approved by the many Maratha and Brahman princes and princesses featured in the book's dedication.[17] As we will see, the Raja himself attributes his practice of Surya Namaskar both to his own father and to the influence of the Raja of Miraj, another Princely State. Indeed, some important roots of the contemporary practice of psychophysical yoga started within Princely States like Aundh and Mysore, and thus outside the formal structures of the colonial state. And central to this process was the Raja of Aundh, who is sometimes remembered as the creator of the modern Surya Namaskar but is more aptly described as its major twentieth-century publicist.

Formerly a practice perhaps exclusive to the ruling elite of the region, the Raja took this embodied demonstration of elite power and not only institutionalized its custom within his state but shared it with the world. The Raja sought to transfer a concept of elite political sovereignty, corporeally expressed in the Surya Namaskar and elite political power, to the citizens of his state, the citizens of India, and far beyond. More than any other modern figure, the Raja modeled the pathway for yoga in this form to be invested with a somatic mode of political sovereignty that would enter the modern bureaucratic state, seamlessly interweaving modern concepts of secularism, liberalism, and democracy. Together the example he set in Aundh would provide a blueprint for independent India's absorption of yoga into its statist project, a subject we take up in this book's conclusion. For the Raja, the Surya Namaskar was equally a psychophysical practice and a political strategy.

Scholars seem to agree that the Raja of Aundh was the first person to present, refine, and propagate the Surya Namaskar in the modern period.[18] There is disagreement, however, about whether his Surya Namaskar practice was considered to be a form of yoga and part of yoga *āsanas* either by the Raja himself or by others who surrounded him—practitioners, scholars, his family, the general public. The prevailing consensus among scholars of yoga is that neither the Raja nor other key figures of his day considered the Surya Namaskar to be a form of yoga or *āsanas* at that time.[19] However, through a reading of his Marathi and Hindi writings and the reaction to his work by others in his time and later, we offer a different point of view.

As a child, the Raja's father instructed him and his siblings in a regime of training that included various Indian physical practices, like wrestling and the Surya Namaskar. He recalls in his autobiography that, from the age of twelve, his father began teaching him the Surya Namaskar, but the young prince instead preferred spending his time bodybuilding under the tutelage of a Muslim wrestler and bodybuilder named Imamuddin Pailavan hired by the Raja's father to put his sons through their regimens of physical fitness. The Raja recalls lying to his father that he had done 150 Surya Namaskars, when he had really done only eight.[20] In 1897, he acquired the necessary weights to follow the bodybuilding techniques of Eugen Sandow (a pseudonym of the eastern European bodybuilder Friedrich Wilhelm Müller), and began an exercise regime that would last for the next ten years.[21] Things turned sharply in 1908, just before he would be appointed to the throne.[22] The young prince had an encounter with the prince of neighboring Miraj, who chastised him: "Why do you do these foreign exercises and not our Surya Namaskar? It is the Raja of all exercise.... Why do you do the Sandow-Müller exercises? Do our Namaskar! It is scientific and enjoyable."[23] From this point onward, the Raja tells us in his autobiography, he abandoned all other forms of exercise, including the Sandow methods, and performed only Surya Namaskars.

Over the next several decades, the Raja used a variety of media to tell the world about the Surya Namaskar. Around 1920, he published his first articles in a Marathi weekly, *Puruṣārth*, that describe how to perform the movements, under the title "Sāṣṭaṇga Namaskār" rather than Surya Namaskar—another indication of the interchangeability of these two terms in Marathi and in the Raja's own genealogy of practice.[24] The popularity of these writings led him to publish a Marathi book on the subject in 1922 entitled *Sūryanamaskār*.[25] The Raja's Marathi book, he claims, spread from "Kashmir to Lanka-Ceylon" but remained largely inaccessible to people who did not read Marathi. This prompted him to complete a version in English so the Surya Namaskar practice could spread "outside India" and be made accessible to the widest audience in the British Empire, including Britain and Europe.[26] This first English version, titled *Surya Namaskars*, was published in 1928 by the Aundh State press, with circulation throughout British India, where it was widely read.[27] The English *Surya Namaskars*, which was reissued in five editions from 1928 to 1940, also circulated throughout global English-language public spheres, from the United States, Canada, and the United Kingdom to British India and Australia.[28] Throughout this time, the Raja either wrote or commissioned versions of the book in Hindi, Kannada, Telugu, Tamil, Gujarati, and Bangla and planned versions in Urdu and Malayalam.[29]

In all of his texts on the *sūrya namaskār* in several languages, special sections emphasize the practice by and for women. From 1922 onward, the Raja specifically addressed a kind of gender equality when writing about and teaching the Surya Namaskar, a point that both presages the global future of modern postural yoga, which is dominated by women in terms of participation, and also distinguishes the Raja's text from that of others who wrote in later years about the Surya Namaskar, such as Krishnamacharya's *Yoga Makaranda*.[30] One may also note, in this vein of egalitarian access, that unlike other emergent yoga systems or even many traditional *haṭha* yoga systems, the Raja never asserted the need for a guru or formal instructor, nor did he call himself a guru or suggest his practice required adherence to past texts or teachers.[31]

Yoga on Film

Around 1928, the Raja created a silent film of just under eleven minutes on the practice of the Surya Namaskar.[32] He either showed the film himself or arranged screenings of the film throughout British and Princely India as well as during his travels abroad. The film, entitled *Surya Namaskar* in both English and Hindi (figure 4.1: top left), is attributed to the Raja and has bilingual placards in English and Hindi that are interspersed with moving images of people performing the Surya Namaskar sequence. Given the great importance the Raja placed on performing and converting others to the practice of Surya Namaskars and the high cost of making a film almost a century ago, we consider each element of the film to be a deliberate choice on the part of the Raja and those close to him.

After a few introductory placards, the first images of the film show the Raja emerging from his palace in full regalia, with a turban on his head and a sword hanging at his side (figure 4.1: top right). In the next scenes, the Raja is shorn of all regalia, wears shorts with a bare chest, and performs several rounds of the Surya Namaskar sequence of movements (figure 4.1: middle row, left and right; bottom row, left and right). Although the Raja was a Brahman, as were so many of the princes of the fragmented Peshwa dynasty throughout western India, he does not wear a sacred thread, nor does his son, who appears in subsequent frames (figure 4.2: top row, left; top row, center). Neither wears any other marker of religion or caste, in keeping with the Raja's broader social reform commitments. This contrasts with other photographs of the Raja from this time, in which he does wear a

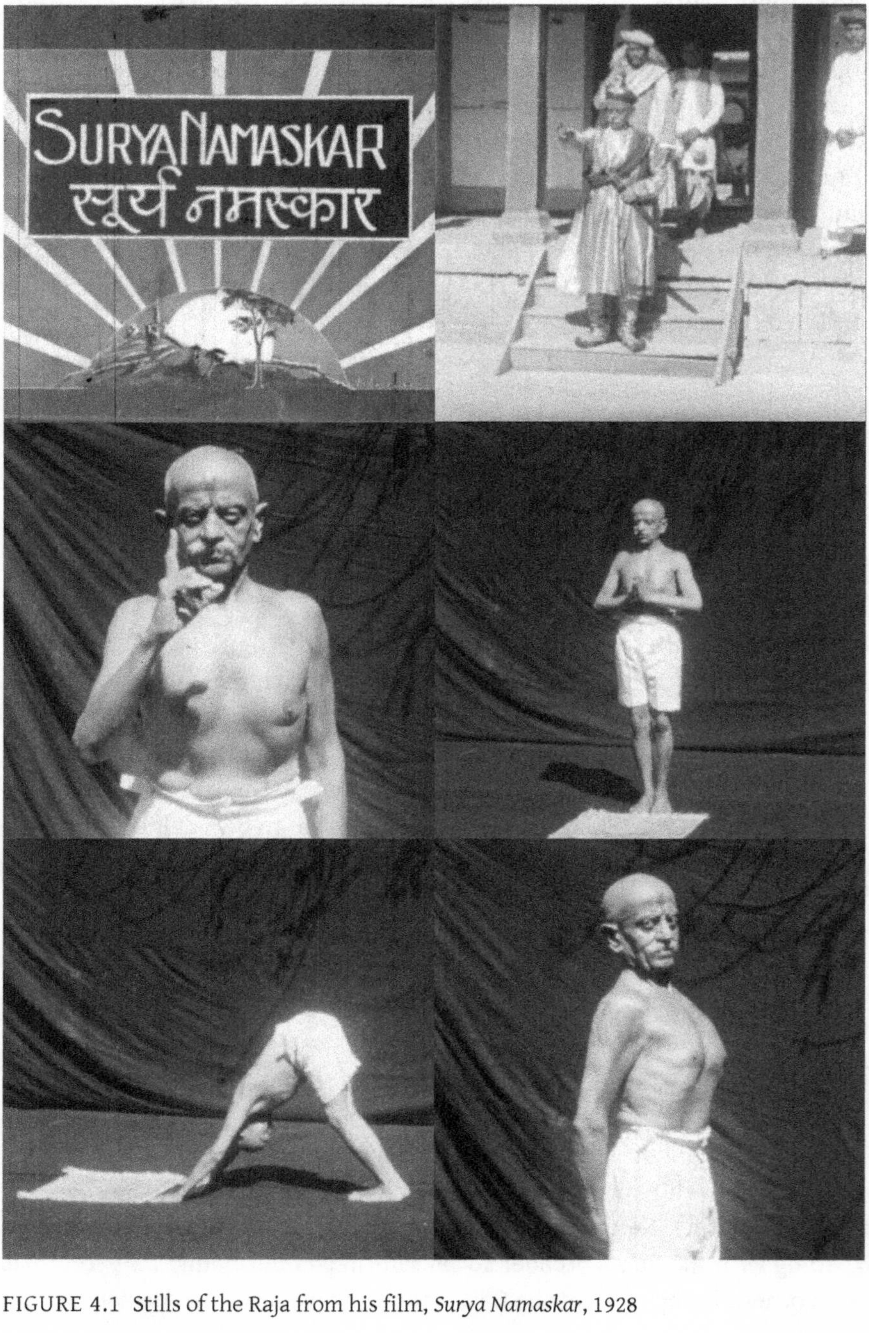

FIGURE 4.1 Stills of the Raja from his film, *Surya Namaskar*, 1928

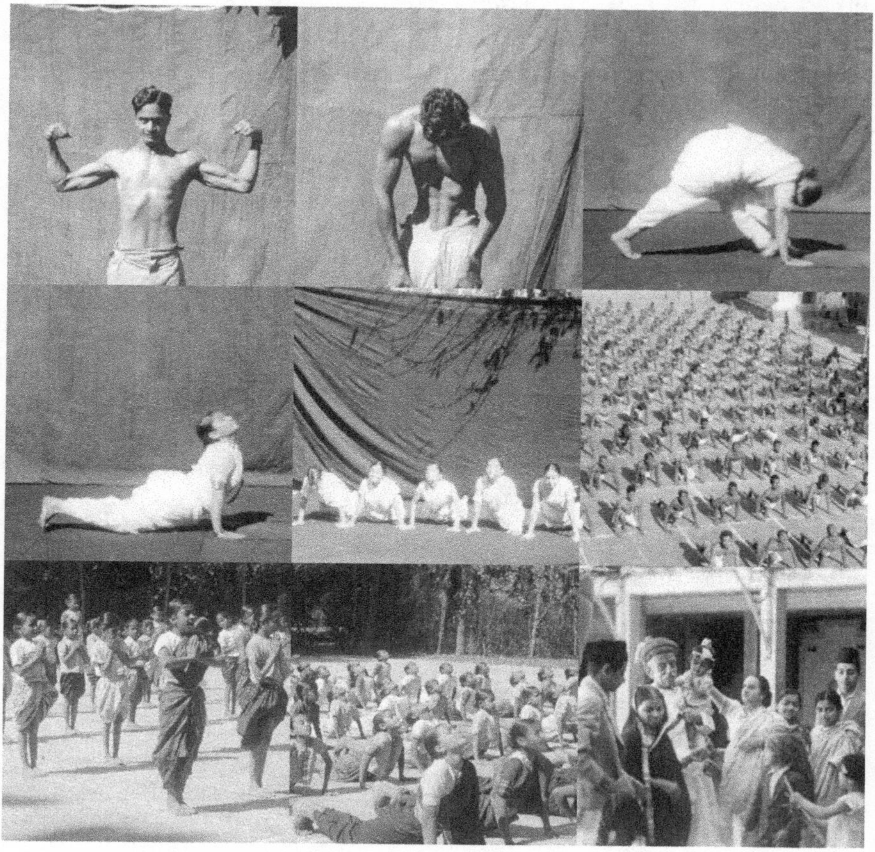

FIGURE 4.2 Stills from the *Surya Namaskar* film

sacred thread, and is also a notable difference from the yoga teacher Krishnamacharya in Mysore, who first appears in a film performing yoga in 1938, with a prominent sacred thread across his chest and a vertical Hindu Vaishnava mark (*ṭiḷak*) on his forehead.

The form of the Surya Namaskar depicted in the 1928 film is a swift, flowing movement with a pause only at the first and last positions (which are the same), with the downward dog position occurring in the middle. While the term *vinyāsa* is not used by the Raja, as far as we can tell, the idea of a flowing set of movements or steps is clearly evident in the way the Raja and others demonstrate the Surya Namaskar in this film.[33] Alongside the Surya Namaskar, the Raja's son, Apa Pant, also demonstrates the classic *haṭha* yoga technique of *naulī*, which involves manipulating the stomach and intestines through a dynamic movement of the abdominal muscles (figure 4.2: top row, center).[34] In addition, the Raja and everyone else who performs the Surya Namaskar in the film can be seen speaking before beginning each new sequence. They are likely chanting the *mantras* that the Raja felt were integral to the practice and about which he writes in all his books, another key aspect of many forms of psychophysical yoga.

The word yoga does not appear in English or Hindi in the film; instead, the Surya Namaskar is described as an "exercise" in English and *vyāyām* in Hindi. As we will see, however, the Raja makes no distinction between yoga and exercise/*vyāyām* in his writing in English, Marathi, or Hindi, and yoga is described as both exercise and *vyāyām* in these languages in India as well. Likewise, the placards for the Surya Namaskar sculpture in the Indira Gandhi International Airport in New Delhi that we mention at the start of the chapter describe the Surya Namaskar in Hindi as both yoga and *vyāyām*. There is here perhaps an echo of the association between yoga and *vyāyāma* that we explore in the *Arthaśāstra* in chapter 2. Later in this chapter, we dwell extensively on the Raja's choice of words to describe his practice, especially when addressing an English audience.

A gender balance appears important in the film. Following the demonstration of Surya Namaskar and *naulī* by the Raja's son, the Raja's wife, the Ranisaheb, performs the Surya Namaskar in a nine-yard sari (the men are in shorts) (figure 4.2: top row, right; middle row, left). This way of draping a sari was common throughout western India at the time (and still is in many parts of the region) and, unlike the five-yard draping method, makes it possible for a woman to perform the Surya Namaskar properly, with legs spread apart rather than always kept together. After the Ranisaheb's demonstration, the film shows the five princesses of Aundh performing the Surya Namaskar in synchronized sequence (figure 4.2: center), following which the youngest members of the Raja's household are shown making a brave and disorderly attempt to perform the sequence under the watchful tutelage of the Raja and later the Rani, who enters the scene to assist.

The next two scenes capture groups of schoolchildren performing Surya Namaskar. The film notes that requiring students to practice the Surya Namaskar is "one of many reforms introduced by the Chiefsahib in his

State," suggesting again that the Surya Namaskar was a component of other social and political reforms undertaken by the Raja.[35] It appears that boys (figure 4.2: middle row, right) and girls (figure 4.2: bottom row, left; bottom row, center) practiced separately because they were likely divided by gender in schools generally; one last placard emphasizes that "school girls are taught" the Surya Namaskar as well.

The film ends with a rather chaotic family montage (figure 4.2: bottom row, right) as the Raja tries to arrange his children and grandchildren for a family photo. This final scene emphasizes the very personal nature of the Surya Namaskar practice for the Raja and his family and its rootedness in the genealogy of his own political lineage, and the opening of this lineage to the general public.

In 1936, the Raja toured Europe, bringing with him his English text and his Surya Namaskar film. The Raja's stop in London in July was covered by several London papers, whose articles describe how the Raja's Surya Namaskars could "make mothers look younger than daughters" and bring litheness to aging bodies.[36] The Raja and his son Apa Pant, then a law student at Oxford, were interviewed by a prominent journalist, Louise Morgan, who published a series of four articles that describe in detail how to perform the Surya Namaskar as instructed by the Raja, with photos of the positions that feature the Raja's son and the claim that the Surya Namaskar will cure "bad temper" (figure 4.3).[37] In a method echoing the publication of his first book in Marathi on this subject, these articles were subsequently combined with numerous sections from the Raja's English *Surya Namaskars* to form a new book,[38] *The Ten-Point Way to Health*, published in 1938, the same year that the fourth edition of the English *Surya Namaskars* was published in India and throughout "English speaking countries."[39]

By the 1930s, the Raja's fame in Maharashtra for his promotion of the Surya Namaskar was sufficiently great that he found himself the subject of a satirical play. In 1933, P. K. Atre or "Acharya Atre"—who would become one of twentieth-century Maharashtra's most famous authors—wrote a play based on the Raja and his fascination with the Surya Namaskar, entitled *Sāṣṭāṅga Namaskār*.[40] In the foreword to the play, Atre says, "I decided to write a satirical play, at the center of which is the ludicrous propaganda the Chief of Aundh was spreading [about the Surya Namaskar], and around this I placed cultural idiosyncrasies found in Maharashtra."[41] The play tells the story of a Brahman man who is a minor noble and his children, to whom he

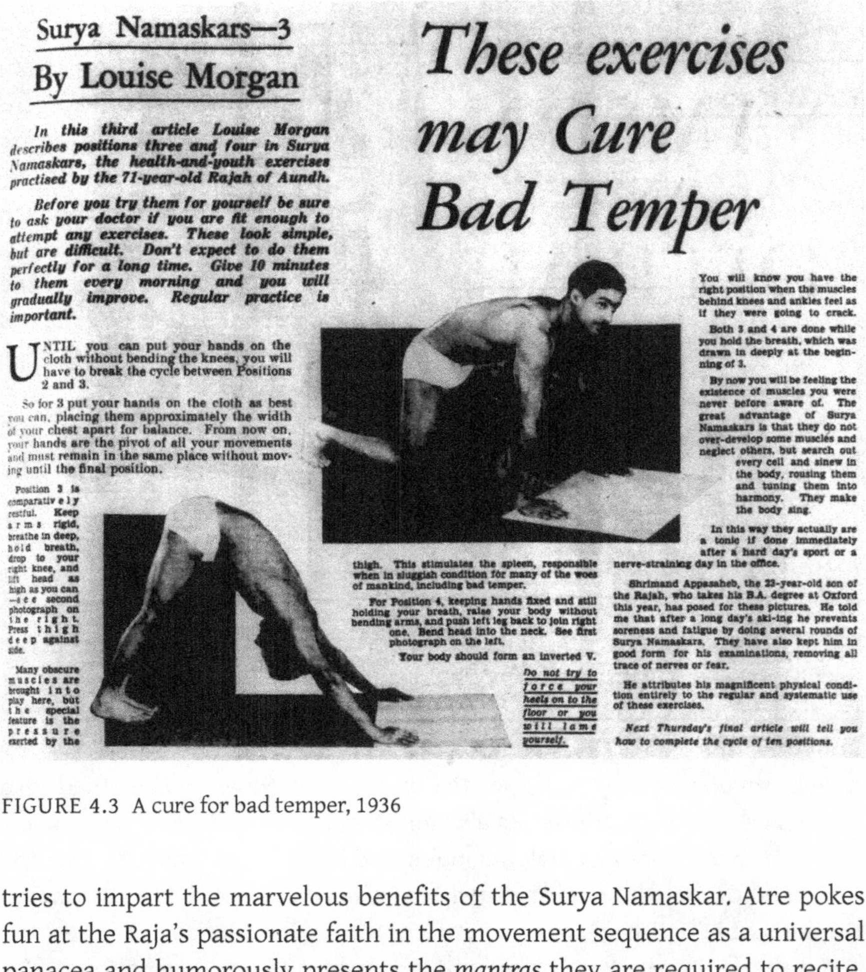

Surya Namaskars—3

By Louise Morgan

These exercises may Cure Bad Temper

In this third article Louise Morgan describes positions three and four in Surya Namaskars, the health-and-youth exercises practised by the 71-year-old Rajah of Aundh.

Before you try them for yourself be sure to ask your doctor if you are fit enough to attempt any exercises. These look simple, but are difficult. Don't expect to do them perfectly for a long time. Give 10 minutes to them every morning and you will gradually improve. Regular practice is important.

UNTIL you can put your hands on the cloth without bending the knees, you will have to break the cycle between Positions 2 and 3.

So for 3 put your hands on the cloth as best you can, placing them approximately the width of your chest apart for balance. From now on, your hands are the pivot of all your movements and must remain in the same place without moving until the final position.

Position 3 is comparatively restful. Keep arms rigid, breathe in deep, hold breath, drop to your right knee, and lift head as high as you can—see second photograph on the right. Press thigh deep against side.

Many obscure muscles are brought into play here, but the special feature is the pressure exerted by the thigh. This stimulates the spleen, responsible when in sluggish condition for many of the woes of mankind, including bad temper.

For Position 4, keeping hands fixed and still holding your breath, raise your body without bending arms, and push left leg back to join right one. Bend head into the neck. See first photograph on the left.

Your body should form an inverted V.

Do not try to force your heels on to the floor or you will lame yourself.

You will know you have the right position when the muscles behind knees and ankles feel as if they were going to crack.

Both 3 and 4 are done while you hold the breath, which was drawn in deeply at the beginning of 3.

By now you will be feeling the existence of muscles you were never before aware of. The great advantage of Surya Namaskars is that they do not over-develop some muscles and neglect others, but search out every cell and sinew in the body, rousing them and tuning them into harmony. They make the body sing.

In this way they actually are a tonic if done immediately after a hard day's sport or a nerve-straining day in the office.

Shrimand Appasaheb, the 23-year-old son of the Rajah, who takes his B.A. degree at Oxford this year, has posed for these pictures. He told me that after a long day's ski-ing he prevents soreness and fatigue by doing several rounds of Surya Namaskars. They have also kept him in good form for his examinations, removing all trace of nerves or fear.

He attributes his magnificent physical condition entirely to the regular and systematic use of these exercises.

Next Thursday's final article will tell you how to complete the cycle of ten positions.

FIGURE 4.3 A cure for bad temper, 1936

tries to impart the marvelous benefits of the Surya Namaskar. Atre pokes fun at the Raja's passionate faith in the movement sequence as a universal panacea and humorously presents the *mantras* they are required to recite. The fictional Raja of the play—Rao Bahadur Sheshadri—speaks of the great Maharashtrian Brahman *sants* and yogis—Samartha Ramdas and Jnandev (ca. thirteenth century CE)—as model proponents of the Surya Namaskar, which gave them superior health and strength, and also links the practice in the play to texts that also expound yoga of various kinds.[42] Atre, himself a Brahman, here extends a longer tradition in Maharashtra of Brahman male performers, artists, and public figures critiquing Brahmanical cultural forms, often in juxtaposition to the quotidian, non-elite world, which arguably is a trait Atre shared with the subject of his satire.[43] The fictional Raja's children reject the Surya Namaskar and its *mantras* as the outdated stuff that fathers do.[44] At the play's denouement, the young princess's suitor ingratiates himself to her father by enthusiastically joining him to perform Surya Namaskars while chanting the required *mantras*. The play comically expresses the enduring affect of Maharashtra's minor nobility of the time, especially in and around Pune, linking it to stereotypes around Brahmanism, caste, masculinity, and the waning elitism of the bygone Peshwa era, all expressed through the Surya Namaskar. The popularity of the play suggests the currency that the Raja's work and persona had in Maharashtrian popular culture of the 1930s, where the Surya Namaskar was indelibly linked to the Raja's own, sometimes quirky, fame.

The Problem with "Yoga" in English

Conspicuously absent in the several iterations of the Raja's English books—*Surya Namaskars* and *The Ten-Point Way to Health*—is the word yoga. This absence is part of the reason most scholars do not think the Raja himself understood his practice to be a form of yoga. However, the Raja's engagements with the Surya Namaskar were often described by others in English as yoga. The *Daily Mirror* published a piece on the Raja of Aundh and his Surya Namaskar method, which came out just before Morgan's series of didactic articles. The first line of the article read: "The *Daily Mirror* publishes to-day for the first time in England part of the ritual of Surya Namaskars" and goes on to describe these exercises as "traditional Indian or Yoga exercises." The title of the piece reiterates the claim that the Surya Namaskar is a form of yoga: "The Yoga Way to Fitness for Men, Slimness for Women" (see figure 4.4).[45]

The Ten-Point Way to Health does not explicitly describe the practice as yoga, but does describe the first position of the Surya Namaskar as "the stance taught by the ancient Yogis of India" that "is being taught to thousands of school children in Great Britain to-day in accordance with the Board of Education's most recent syllabus."[46] In 1970, Apa Pant wrote a book in English with the same title his father had used, *Surya Namaskars*, which has a complicated byline: "By Bhawanrao Pant Pratinidhi, Raja of Aundh . . . As explained to his son, Apa Pant, High Commissioner of India in U.K."[47] Although authored by Apa Pant, the text yet claims to be the intention, if

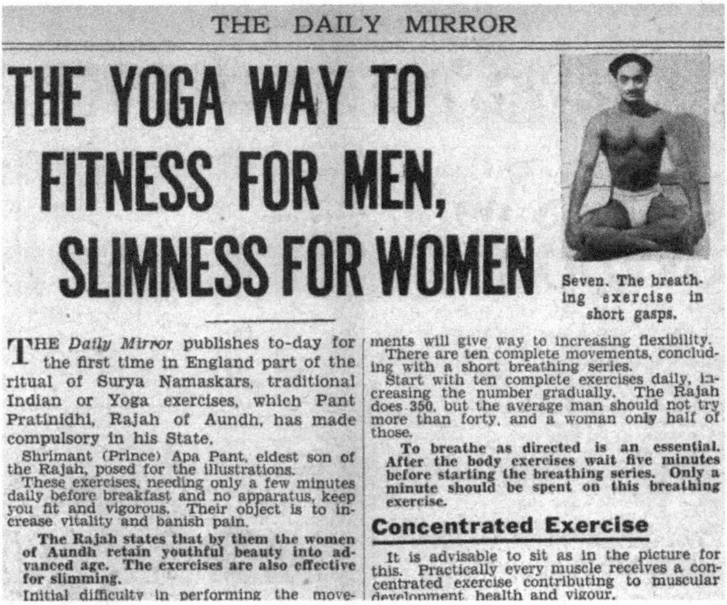

THE DAILY MIRROR

THE YOGA WAY TO FITNESS FOR MEN, SLIMNESS FOR WOMEN

Seven. The breathing exercise in short gasps.

THE *Daily Mirror* publishes to-day for the first time in England part of the ritual of Surya Namaskars, traditional Indian or Yoga exercises, which Pant Pratinidhi, Rajah of Aundh, has made compulsory in his State.

Shrimant (Prince) Apa Pant, eldest son of the Rajah, posed for the illustrations.

These exercises, needing only a few minutes daily before breakfast and no apparatus, keep you fit and vigorous. Their object is to increase vitality and banish pain.

The Rajah states that by them the women of Aundh retain youthful beauty into advanced age. The exercises are also effective for slimming.

Initial difficulty in performing the movements will give way to increasing flexibility.

There are ten complete movements, concluding with a short breathing series.

Start with ten complete exercises daily, increasing the number gradually. The Rajah does 350, but the average man should not try more than forty, and a woman only half of those.

To breathe as directed is an essential. After the body exercises wait five minutes before starting the breathing series. Only a minute should be spent on this breathing exercise.

Concentrated Exercise

It is advisable to sit as in the picture for this. Practically every muscle receives a concentrated exercise contributing to muscular development, health and vigour.

FIGURE 4.4 "The Yoga Way to Fitness for Men, Slimness for Women," 1936

not the actual words, of his father. The work states: "This exercise [Surya Namaskar], a form of yoga, has been practiced in India from antiquity." The book concludes with a long treatment on "the life of a yogi" and the method of "yoga" as descriptions of the Surya Namaskar.[48] Whether these are the actual words and thoughts of the Raja or, more likely, his son's memories, Apa Pant certainly understood himself in a genealogy of practice with his father (as the Raja felt about his own father, and so on). In other words, even if the Raja did not directly describe the Surya Namaskar as yoga in English, others around him clearly understood the exercise of Surya Namaskar to be a form of yoga.[49] However, in his Marathi and Hindi writings, the Raja is far more explicit in describing his beloved Surya Namaskar to be a part of yoga.

As noted, key scholars of the roots of modern yoga have argued that the Surya Namaskar taught by the Raja was "not considered to be *asanas* at the time"[50] or "was not yet considered part of *yogāsana*,"[51] and specifically, "for Pratinidhi [the Raja of Aundh] . . . and those who practiced and taught their techniques, *sūryanamaskār* was not yet considered a part of yoga."[52] Perhaps scholars and practitioners of *haṭha* yoga specifically rejected the Surya Namaskar as a legitimate form of yoga in *their* system of *haṭha* yoga, but this does not account for or represent all forms of yoga. For example, a century earlier, Brahmananda, writing a commentary on the *Haṭhapradīpikā* in 1837, warned *haṭha* yogis to avoid "multiple repetitions of practices such as the sun salutation."[53] Mark Singleton has clearly shown that Krishnamacharya and others who situated their practice within the genealogy of *haṭha* yoga did not consider the Surya Namaskar to be part of their practice of yoga as late as 1935.[54] Our claim is not that the Surya Namaskar was considered part of *haṭha* yoga by either the modern custodians of that tradition (like Brahmananda, Krishnamacharya, Yogendra, or others) or by the Raja or others who practiced the Surya Namaskar. Instead, we argue that the scholarly assessment about whether the Surya Namaskar is considered a form of yoga has allowed their specific genealogies and understandings of *haṭha* yoga to stand in for all forms of psychophysical yoga. But the traditions of yoga as psychophysical practice exceed the specific boundaries of any particular form of *haṭha* yoga, as the Raja of Aundh's Surya Namaskar demonstrates. Furthermore, a host of terms intersected in non-English worlds. For example, the distinctions between yoga and *vyāyāma* (exercise, mobilization) often blurred, especially for psychophysical traditions rooted in the Princely States.[55] The Raja articulates a genealogy for the Surya Namaskar as yoga that might be separate from any stream of *haṭha* yoga. As a *rājā*, as a sovereign king, he did not rely on the canonical power of a given yoga tradition to lend authority for his own practice. Instead, his Surya Namaskar is rooted in an entirely separate, royal genealogy of psychophysical practice that consistently describes the Surya Namaskar as yoga, especially in his Marathi writings.

Throughout the Marathi and Hindi texts of *Surya Namaskar* starting in 1922, the only word used to describe the ten positions of the Surya Namaskar is *āsana*. This word, *āsana*, is rendered as "position" throughout the English texts *Surya Namaskars* and *The Ten-Point Way to Health*. When the Raja's son, Apa Pant, refers to the Surya Namaskar, as taught to him by his father, as yoga, he does so probably because this was a word used by his father himself. It is apparent that the Raja understood the positions of the Surya Namaskar to be *āsana* and a form of yoga (although perhaps not *haṭha* yoga).

The Raja explicitly uses the term yoga to describe the Surya Namaskar and aspects of its practice in several places in Marathi and Hindi. In two sections—one on the control of sight (*dṛṣṭi*) and another on the control of speech (*vāṇī*)—the Raja uses the term yoga to describe the method of control of each: *dṛṣṭi-yoga* and *vāṇī-yoga*.[56] These same sections appear in the English version as well, but here they are rendered "The Application of Sight and Speech."[57] While the translation of yoga as "application" may not appear at first to signal psychophysical or philosophical yoga, this section of the Raja's English book is prefaced with a quotation from chapter 6 of the *Bhagavad Gītā*, a chapter that famously addresses how to perform psychophysical yoga and yogic meditation.[58] In other words, for the Raja, the yoga of sight and voice here is the same as the yoga of chapter 6 of the *Bhagavad Gītā*, which is commonly accepted as a reference to psychophysical yoga.[59] In the Hindi text, he concludes this instruction by writing, "When this *āsana* is fully settled, then one can commence the practice of yoga" (*yoga-abhyās*).[60] By the practice (*abhyās*) of yoga, he means the Surya Namaskar.

In the Marathi version, rather than *yogābhyās*, the Raja writes, "By this yoga [*yogāne*] the mind will be fully assisted in reaching concentration [*cittaikāgrya*]" in *sāṣṭāṅga namaskār*.[61] The Raja recounts in his autobiography the comments of a medical doctor who oversaw a nursing home in Bombay in 1934. Speaking of the adverse side effects of the various medications taken by his residents, the doctor commented: "If we are to be spared from these terrifying poisons [Western medicines], then it is only by the disease-preventing power of the yoga of the Surya Namaskar [*sūryanamaskārācyā yogāne*]."[62] In his discussion of sound, he refers to the technique of *mantra* as a yoga that will purify blood, stimulate the sinuses, and open the chest.[63] The Raja also integrates *prāṇāyāma* throughout his Marathi and Hindi writing about the Surya Namaskar, which he renders as "breathing" in his English prose.[64] While discussing the practice of the Surya Namaskar by schoolchildren in Aundh, the Raja writes that they became healthy "by the yoga of the Surya Namaskar" (*sūryanamaskārāṃcā yogāne*).[65] In a section in which the Raja is discussing the Surya Namaskar, exercise in general, and a proper diet, he again invokes the *Bhagavad Gītā*:[66] "For one who is joined to yoga, yoga destroys all pain—in food and sport, in the undertaking of action, and in sleeping and awakening."[67] The Raja is clearly referring to the Surya Namaskar by the term yoga in this quotation. One might argue that the Raja's use of the word yoga here merely means "way" or "application," but this would ignore the many contexts that give this word meaning here that embed the term in both psychophysical and philosophical understandings of yoga. The

Raja not only considers the Surya Namaskar to be a form of psychophysical yoga, as those described in the *Bhagavad Gītā*, but also as a form of *karma-yoga*. We have already discussed this term's laden political meanings in chapter 3. Here, it appears that, for the Raja, the Surya Namaskar is both a mode of *karma-yoga* and a form of psychophysical yoga described by Krishna in the quotation from the *Bhagavad Gītā*. The resonance with the political uses of this term, especially in Marathi, would not have been lost on the Raja, who attended carefully to the activities and writings of all key nationalists.

If one reads the Raja's writing in Marathi and Hindi, a few things become clear. One is that the Raja certainly understood the Surya Namaskar to be a form of *āsana* and a form of yoga, although he never claims a genealogy of *haṭha* yoga for his practice. However, what he can convey by describing the Surya Namaskar in Marathi and Hindi as "yoga" exceeds the boundaries of this term's restricted meaning in English. In Marathi and Hindi and other non-English Indian languages, yoga retains its very wide semantic meaning, moving from the general sense of application, use, method, strategy, union, and technique to psychophysical practices and philosophical positions.[68] Several of these meanings converge in the passages above, where yoga refers to a particular technique, but specifically a technique consonant with what is described in chapter 6 of the *Bhagavad Gītā* and with other techniques that employ terminology like *āsana* and *prāṇāyāma*. What other "yoga" could these references indicate, other than the psychophysical and philosophical form that is the primary subject of most uses of "yoga" in English over the past two centuries?

In the nineteenth and early twentieth centuries, the scholarly world of yoga studies (although not named as such then) was a field of knowledge well known to the Raja. The Raja's personal library included all the literature that encompassed the ancient, classical, and medieval fields of psychophysical and philosophical yoga.[69] His copies of Patanjali's *Yoga Sūtras* and the *Haṭhapradīpikā*—texts cited in his English, Marathi, and Hindi writing on the Surya Namaskar—sit alongside a robust collection of periodicals from organizations like Kaivalyadham in Lonavala and the Yoga Institute in Bombay.[70] The Raja's understanding of yoga as well as the contemporaneous popularity of yoga was evident as well in his published work beyond his books on the Surya Namaskar. In his illustrated book on his travels and photography at the caves at Ellora, the Raja describes the Buddha as commonly seated in the "Yogic pose called padmasana, sitting cross-legged with the eyes fixed on the point of the nose."[71] And in his illustrated work on the Ajanta caves written in 1932, the Raja, commenting on images of Buddhist monks practicing yoga, describes "the system of yoga" as "experiencing a revival of which is taking place in our own times."[72] When the Raja articulates his Surya Namaskar as yoga, he is fully aware of *haṭha* yoga and other forms of psychophysical and philosophical yoga, including the emergent forms of modern yoga, and their representation in multiple languages. His use of the term yoga is highly informed. Alongside these many texts on yoga as psychophysical practice, the Raja's library also contained the complete works of Swami Vivekananda as well as early editions of Tilak's and Gandhi's translations and commentaries on the *Bhagavad Gītā*, where they name *karma-yoga* as a philosophy of political action. The Raja seemed to be well-aware of all three of the spheres of yoga that we discuss in the introduction to our book—yoga as psychophysical practice, yoga as philosophy, and yoga as politics—and all are well-represented in his library collection.

Yoga was all around the Raja in the English public sphere to which he constantly paid attention; it could hardly be ignored. By the 1920s and especially by the 1930s, yoga was a familiar term in all major European and American metropoles. Yoga societies had existed in London since the late nineteenth century, and one can point to the lasting effect of Vivekananda and the interests in yoga held by figures like Henry David Thoreau (1817–1862) in the United States, who referred to himself in 1849 as a "yogi," a term already highly resonant with meaning in the American public sphere in his time.[73] In India, foreign and Indian experts lectured on yoga regularly, and yoga demonstrations—of both the health variety and the supernatural kind—were common in places like Bombay at this time. Even the idea that yoga would improve your health, make your skin glow, fight off the middle-age bulge, and otherwise improve the self was commonplace in the 1920s, when the Raja of Aundh began publishing in English about Surya Namaskar. In other words, the absence of the word "yoga" to describe the Surya Namaskar system was hardly inadvertent—he omitted the word in English while being fully aware of the term's cachet for a global English-speaking audience and the worldwide spread of yoga in the latter nineteenth and early twentieth centuries. We suspect that he left out "yoga" in his English works on purpose, and we think the reason is political.

As we discuss in chapter 3, alongside its many associations described above, terms like yoga and *karma-yoga* had been associated with violent antinationalism, attempts at assassinating British officials, the sway of revolutionaries like B. G. Tilak and Aurobindo Ghose, and the growing threat to the British posed by Gandhi's popularity. As we note below, the Raja's nationalism did not work against British colonialism in ways as direct as these, nor did he acquiesce entirely either. He threaded a fine needle, and this delicate strategy might have been jeopardized by the use of the term yoga in English given its politically dangerous associations. The Raja also would have been constantly aware of his own fraught position given how he came to the throne.

Beyond these concerns, the term yoga had several additional associations in the global English public sphere that the Raja may also have hoped to avoid. The Raja may not have wanted to be associated with contemporary tales of yogis swallowing poison or sharp objects, being buried alive, or enduring beds of nails, all common stories carried in the Indian English press. Witness the 1902 film by Thomas Edison, *Hindoo Fakir*, often described as the first film to capture yoga and a portrayal of a "yogi."[74] The film does not feature psychophysical yoga, nor does it show anything resembling the usual depiction of a "yogi" of this kind. Instead, the film is a fairly common magic show, suggesting that yoga and associated terms, like "Hindoo fakir," circulated in a highly Orientalized field of fantasy in the Raja's time. There was also a swelling "business" of yoga already underway in England and the United States, where yoga teachers—Indian and non-Indian—sought students and student fees and published their own books that sometimes included fantastic tales of encountering yogis and sometimes included didactic texts on performing yoga. The Raja may not have called the Surya Namaskar "yoga" in English because he wanted to avoid entering what was a burgeoning capitalist, guru-oriented enterprise, an association that would not match his vision or approach to the spread of the Surya Namaskar.[75]

The sexualization of yoga was also fully in place in the 1920s. The conflation between the "positions" of the Surya Namaskar and other forms of yoga, and the "positions" of the *Kāmasūtra* led John Campbell Oman, writing in 1903 about India's "yogis," to clarify for his reader that: "there are *âsans* and *âsans* known to the Indian people, and they are not all connected with *sadhuism* nor with religious practices; many of them quite the reverse . . . [a] book descriptive of these latter exists, but it is, I believe, on the Index *liborurum prohibitorum* of the Indian police."[76] Oman is likely referencing the *Kāmasūtra*, which was first published with vivid illustrations in England and

India in 1883, when it was promptly banned (until as late as 1968 in the United Kingdom and 1962 in the United States).

Despite avoiding the term yoga in his English writings on the Surya Namaskar, the Raja could not escape the snare of sexualized Orientalist fantasies: a British tabloid article in January 1937 lampooned the Raja and his Surya Namaskar, describing it as the Raja's strategy to select and groom women for his harem.[77] The Raja, through the efforts of his son, won a libel case against the publisher in July 1937. But for us, the associations that led to the article suggest another reason the Raja may have wished to avoid the semantic field of "yoga" in English in the 1920s and 1930s and its politics of sexuality, Orientalist fantasy, and the body.[78]

The brief study we have undertaken here of the Raja's writing about the Surya Namaskar and yoga in multiple languages reveals not only that he understood the Surya Namaskar to be a form of yoga—a *yoga-abhyās* and *yoga-āsana*—but that a politics of culture, power, and representation might have motivated his choices about when and how to talk about this signature set of movements. Given the importance of the Surya Namaskar to all aspects of the Raja's understanding of himself as a political and physical being, we now undertake an analysis of the Surya Namaskar *as yoga* in his political thought, that is, as a strategy for political sovereignty located at the nexus where mind and body meet society and political power.

The "Aundh Experiment" in Sovereignty

Of the many reforms that the Raja undertook in Aundh, the one that has received the greatest attention, for good reason, is the undoing of royal privileges that began in a piecemeal way in 1917 and continued until the Aundh Constitution was adopted in 1938 and came into force the following year.[79] The first step on this journey was the creation of the Aundh Pratinidhik Sabha, or the Aundh Representative Assembly, which had been convened in an ad-hoc way as early as 1917 but was formed officially in 1923 and played an advisory role in its early years. Although initially composed of nominated members, on the Raja's birthday in 1922, he announced that the assembly would be at least partially elected in order to better represent villagers' interests. The assembly had thirty-five members, of which eighteen were elected, ten were state officials, and seven were nominated non-officials.

That same year, he announced that the state budget would be placed before the assembly for discussion and approval.[80] An important reform taken in those early years was the separation of judicial from executive functions, with parallel decentralization of both functions to village- and district-level bodies. To equip citizens with legal understanding, Aundh Act VI of 1932 allowed villagers to be appointed as assessors to help justices with some criminal and civil cases, which "prepared the ground for the introduction of the jury system."[81] The judicial system was tailored to meet the smaller size and dispersed nature of the state, with the villages organized into three talukas, or divisions. In Gandhi's view, the cumulative effect of these changes was to make justice in Aundh "cheap, swift, and effective."[82]

By 1928, the assembly was given the right to elect its own president and the authority to pass a budget. The next year, the Raja announced "his intention to grant responsible government to his subjects within five years,"[83] although this was an optimistic pledge, and representative government would take some years longer. The new constitution was formally adopted by the legislative assembly on January 21, 1939.

A great number of individuals played important roles in what several authors have named the "Aundh Experiment," the long process of devolving power to the people of Aundh and forming a democratic state in the middle of colonial India.[84] One was the Raja's firstborn son, Trimbak, who returned from England as a trained barrister and carried out extensive administrative reforms and departmental reorganization but died while still a young man. The Raja's second eldest son, Apa Pant, played a decisive role in the state's administration, the devolution of power, the creation of a constitutional democracy, and a variety of other reforms in Aundh, and wrote about many of these experiences.[85] In the first (and still only) substantial study of the democratic constitution of Aundh, Indira Rothermund attributes much of the spirit of it, the "immediate cause" of it, to another individual, Maurice Frydman (1901–1976), a Jewish refugee from Warsaw who was an electrical engineer by training.[86] While still a young man in Europe, Frydman had a chance meeting with J. Krishnamurti and encountered the writings of Ramana Maharshi.[87] He became fascinated by Indian systems of philosophy and spirituality, and accepted with alacrity when he was invited in 1935 to work as managing director of the newly established Mysore Electrical Factory. There, Frydman met Apa Pant, who was touring Mysore's growing industrial undertakings in 1937 for inspiration to take back to Aundh.

Frydman's admiration for Indian nationalism and his budding friendship with Apa Pant led him to leave Mysore to invest his energies in Aundh at a critical moment when the details of the constitution were being worked out.

Two years before his move to Aundh, Frydman was initiated into a spiritual tradition by an Indian guru, Swami Ramdas, at Anandashram in Kanhangad in what is now Kerala, where he was given the Sanskrit name Swami Bharatananda ("One Who Finds the 'Joy of India'") to reflect his new status as a spiritual seeker.[88] Frydman spent the remainder of his life in India, and over that time met and interacted with a number of other political and spiritual figures, including Ramana Maharshi, M. K. Gandhi, and Nisargadatta Maharaj (1897–1981). In his final years in Bombay, Frydman spent time recording and translating conversations that took place between Nisargadatta and the many devotees who visited him. Based on the texts of those conversations, Frydman and Nisargadatta compiled a book in 1973, *I Am That*, in which they develop what they called "Nisarga Yoga" or "the Natural Yoga." They describe yoga itself as "a chain of experiments . . . to realise independence."[89] Later, the text records Nisargadatta saying, "The cause of suffering is dependence and independence is the remedy. Yoga is the science and the art of self-liberation through self-understanding."[90] Frydman's identity as a yogi and a purveyor of a form of yoga should be considered when one understands his close relationship to the Raja, his political role in the formation of Aundh's constitution, and much else in its political formation, particularly the penal reforms that we discuss at the end of this chapter.

As a devotee of Gandhi, Frydman linked the Raja to Gandhi and with Frydman's encouragement, the Raja visited Gandhi's ashram in Sevagram from November 29 to December 1, 1938.[91] Gandhi says of his own role in Aundh's constitution, that he "[hammered] into shape the Aundh Constitution."[92] The meeting with Gandhi led to some key points that would be included in the document, which was drafted in partnership with Apa Pant and ratified by the Raja.[93] With respect to the issue of suffrage, for example, Gandhi insisted that the constitution include a literacy test for voters, a regressive position given that the first plan for the constitution did not include a literacy requirement and that Aundh did not have universal literacy among adults.[94] Frydman and Gandhi undoubtedly helped to work out constitutional details, but the political revolution in Aundh had already been underway for two decades, which is perhaps what drew their attention and energy to the place.[95]

Aundh has received very little scholarly attention in the English-language academy. Aside from newer work by Deepti Mulgund (2016, 2017) on the Raja of Aundh as an artist, art collector, patron, and museum builder, we have the scholarship of Rothermund and work by Joseph Alter (2000), both of whom come to the subject of Aundh by way of a deeper interest in Gandhi and his politics and legacies, as well as through an attention to physical culture in Alter's case. Our account emphasizes that these political, social, and economic changes were underway several decades before any direct involvement on the part of Gandhi, and so naming them Gandhian or attributing too much weight to his influence distorts the actual role of the Raja, his collaborators, and the people of Aundh. As a scholar of Gandhian politics, Rothermund, for example, focuses considerable attention on cottage industries in the state that relied on the *carakhā*, or spinning wheel, an emblem of productive household labor closely linked to Gandhi.[96] As early as the 1920s, however, the state's departments of industries and chemistry were developing technologies that would diversify farm income, both small-scale ones like household yarn-spinning and weaving that Gandhi would have approved of, as well as industrial-scale experiments in metal forging and chemical dyes that Gandhi might have found antithetical to his political economic model of small-scale enterprises and village self-sufficiency. Rather than view Aundh as derivative of Gandhian self-rule or village democracy, we argue that one should view the state and its leader as theoretical innovators of an indigenous sovereignty, one that yoked together physical, educational, economic, humanitarian, carceral, and political reforms in a novel package that presages the aspirations of the future Republic of India.

Education was at the heart of the state project in Aundh. More than anything else, it was the broad commitment to education in Aundh over thirty years that accounts for the success of its later democratic experiment and may also be one of its lasting influences on postcolonial India. Once the 1939 constitution gave over administrative and judicial powers to village bodies (*pañcāyat*), it was the grassroots educational infrastructure that was in place throughout the state—the "village teachers with their dedicated, competent, versatile and cultured approach"—that enabled the democratic vision of Aundh to flourish.[97] This is also the site of the Raja's most visible and durable implementation of the Surya Namaskar within government policy. We turn to the experiment in educational reform next.

Schoolhouse Yoga

The administrative reports from the Raja's early years as ruler contain careful accounting of the spread of education and literacy and demonstrate the subject's importance in Aundh's annual budget (see table 4.1). In 1909–1910, the year that the Raja took the throne, education spending was roughly 3 percent of the state's total budget while royal expenses (which included the *khāsagī*, or private royal purse; allowances made for other members of the royal household; and the *pāgā*, funds to pay the royal foot soldiers) were 18 percent of the state budget.[98]

Education spending as a share of the total budget grew with each subsequent decade. By 1942–1943, as befitting a democracy, the state budget had tilted in favor of public goods like education, which took up nearly 10 percent of the total budget, and away from the royal family. Education was made compulsory and free for all children up to the fourth standard, school supplies were provided for students from poor families, and there were scholarships available for poorer students who wanted to pursue higher education.[99] Beyond direct funding for schools, the budget also included other expenditures to support education, including funds to hire women to summon delinquent children to school as well as funds for adult education, an effort that grew in significance after the 1938 constitution imposed a literacy requirement for voting.[100]

Rather than mimicking what was found in the surrounding British province, Aundh's educational curricula were distinct, embracing a wide variety of educational and extracurricular pathways. In the middle schools, drawing and English were compulsory, and debating unions were set up for both teachers and students. Carpentry, singing, and weaving were other optional

TABLE 4.1
Budget allocations for education and royal expenses in Aundh State

	1909–1910	1916–1917	1923–1924	1935–1936	1942–1943
Total royal expenses	18.3%*	17.7%	13.7%	12.9%	7.2%
Education	2.9%	6.1%	8.6%	8.5%	9.8%

Source: *Annual Administration Report of the Aundh State*, various years.
*Percentages calculated by the authors of this book.

subjects. Children of artisans were allowed to learn their craft with their families but were still required to attend school for reading and writing.[101] The Raja's philosophy of education embraced technical education and hands-on experience rather than purely book learning and rote memorization. The lone high school in Aundh had a large collection of scientific instruments, imported from Europe, that the *Times of India* noted "would put to shame the laboratory outfit of many of the large colleges in British territory."[102] These various educational commitments fed directly into the vision for economic progress through technological innovation that was likewise reflected in the state budget.[103]

Perhaps the most distinctive feature of Aundh's school curricula was its emphasis on the Surya Namaskar. By 1927, all students performed daily Surya Namaskars, and the Raja made annual visits to appraise the Surya Namaskar practice of students throughout the state. In addition to the physical practice of Surya Namaskar, *Bhagavad Gītā* instruction was mandatory in high school, and during a *Bhagavad Gītā* celebration, the Raja reminded the students: "The business is with the actions only, never with its fruits, so let not the fruit of action be thy motive nor be thou to inaction attached," echoing the lessons being drawn by prominent nationalists like Tilak and Gandhi.[104] By 1935, the Raja had issued a standing order that 1 crore [ten million] Surya Namaskars be performed during the four Hindu sacred months of the lunar calendar, which roughly correspond to the monsoon season, beginning sometime in June or July and ending in September or October.[105]

For the Raja, the collective practice of the Surya Namaskar was both a way of enabling physical and mental strength and also a mode of social reform. In the Raja's Marathi autobiography of 1946, he writes (translation ours):

> Today there is no Untouchability in any of Aundh's institutions. Wherever I can go, men and women who are considered Untouchable can also go. In the Shri Yamai pavilion, the children of Brahmans, Marathas, Muslims, Mahars, Chambars, Mangs, all the various castes [*jāti*] do the ritual of Surya Namaskar together every day. This is also in all the other village institutions of Aundh as well. Hindu children, but also Muslim children, recite Om while performing the Namaskar. No one complains. Rani Saheb is partially responsible for this. Therefore, it can clearly be stated that today Untouchability does not exist in the institutions of Aundh.[106]

We have no way to verify if Muslim children really performed the Surya Namaskar and recited Om without complaint, or that the presence of all castes at the Shri Yamai Pavilion proved the eradication of untouchability in Aundh, although Gandhi also praises him as unique among princes for his efforts around untouchability.[107] But what we can see is that the Raja used the collective practice of Surya Namaskar among children, in educational contexts and also more generally during gatherings and celebrations in Aundh, to enact, consolidate, and then highlight Aundh's progressive social and political approach to caste, religion, and social justice. The social frame was avowedly Hindu rather than secular: the chanting of Om; the collective performance on Hindu holy days; the location within a space consecrated to the *kuladevī* or family goddess of the Raja's family, Shri Yamai. Yet in the Raja's conceptualization, the Surya Namaskar was as much a practice of mind and body as a practice of social politics, a strategy for creating bonds across caste and religious difference. The Raja here appears to articulate clearly a position that we might call a liberal Hindu secularism, one that was liberal and secular in its intentions but Hindu in its cultural frame. This liberal Hindu secularist point of view would also come to characterize the public attitude of Jawaharlal Nehru and some other Congress leaders after independence. Whatever the actuality or success of these efforts, clearly the Raja made political use of the Surya Namaskar.

The Raja's Surya Namaskar advocacy was also an important means for him to press for the health and empowerment of women. He consistently wrote that "boys and girls," and "men and women" should practice the Surya Namaskar, and all his books in all languages note that the Surya Namaskar can address the special concerns of women. In 1925, the Raja delivered the presidential address to students at the Maharshi Karve Women's College, founded by Dhondo Keshav "Maharshi" Karve, in Hingani near Pune. The Raja appealed to the assembled students to rid themselves of what he described as "slave mentality," something to which their parents were still subject. He argued that education for female students needed to place a great deal of importance on what were traditionally considered men's subjects: history and economics, social and political conditions.[108] The following year, while attending the anniversary and prize distribution ceremonies at Shreemati Nathibai Damodar Thackersey (SNDT) Women's University in Pune, he condemned the quality of education in British India as something that is "preparing a class of beggars," which, if repeated in women's colleges, would merely produce the same mentality.[109] He lamented the disempowerment of women in his society and ascribed at least partial responsibility to the "physical and mental degeneration" caused by "early marriages." In response, he enacted a law in Aundh to end childhood marriage. He argued that hundreds of years of unfair treatment had meant that many women believed themselves to be weak, something for which he blamed "the community and the framers of the Hindu religious code." Now the time had come that "the fact of social injustice should be impressed on the minds of girls so that they should be prepared to resist all kinds of injustice." He then appealed to "all Hindu women to prepare themselves both physically and mentally for the important task of preserving their rights." While distributing prizes at the end of the day, he repeated the same advice, basing his comments this time on the *Bhagavad Gītā*, and urged daily exercises so that girls and women would become physically strong.

His views on the place of women in society underwrote his sense that the Surya Namaskar was a physical practice that could shore up personal strength and self-defined sovereignty. Such emphases on women and on their health and empowerment are apparent in the articles published in England in 1936 by Louise Morgan, which underscore this gendered component but, given that the audience for this book would have been British, leave out the concomitant political angle. His awareness of gender and power remained a consistent aspect of his teaching, a commitment to gender equality that was instituted in the practice of the Surya Namaskar and the field of education, and likewise enshrined in the principle of universal suffrage for the literate, regardless of caste or gender.

At some points, the Raja's politics in relation to the Surya Namaskar were yet more plainly expressed. The English *Surya Namaskars* opens with the Raja emphasizing the importance of the practice as "indispensable to every modern individual so that in the present struggle for existence he be able to protect himself, his community and his nation."[110] Pointing toward the royal practice of the Surya Namaskar, the Raja writes, "With the Peshwas disappeared the hardy race of the Bapu Gokhales, the Bhawanrao Pratinidhis and the Mahadji Shindes . . . [a] conquered nation gradually loses its self-confidence and ultimately becomes almost a blind follower of the conquering nation in its superficial forms of conduct and vices and not in its characteristic virtues such as patriotism, self-sacrifice, unity, self-respect, etc."[111] Consider this passage along with his references to his encounter with Raja of Miraj and Samartha Ramdas, and one can see here that the Raja charts out his own "lineage" of yoga, through the Surya Namaskar, one that has its origin not in classical texts of *haṭha* yoga or traditional gurus but in elite Maratha politics. The Raja points to the faded glory of the Maratha Empire, in which his family was once a key player, as the last sovereign rulers in the region of Maharashtra prior to their defeat by the British in the early 1800s amid their own internal strife.

For the Raja, however, the Surya Namaskar is not part of a revival of this religious-caste-gender power (he seems to feel that that time has passed); rather, it is a preparation for a struggle that the people of Aundh, perhaps all Indian people, were already amid. The Surya Namaskar became a means of ensuring that the movement for self-rule would take root in the political and administrative institutions that he could tweak and control as Raja as well as through the individual bodies and minds of his subjects on their way to becoming citizens of some still-dreamed-of sovereign state. In a kind of inversion of Michel Foucault's concept of biopower, the Raja here hoped to instill within his people a biopower technology of liberation rather than a means of control. The Raja was passing on his genealogy of political yoga—of the Surya Namaskar as a means to embody sovereignty—to the people of Aundh and beyond, to the people of India writ large.

We have already established the emphasis placed on Surya Namaskars throughout Aundh's educational system, from elementary school through high school. The Raja promoted the exercise outside Aundh as well, visiting Satara annually to award prizes to winners of Surya Namaskar competitions at Kanya Shala and the New English School.[112] In 1930, the Raja served as president of the Physical Culture Institute of Pune, which held free training classes for physical education instruction. During that year, he toured throughout Maharashtra and Mysore, where he delivered lectures and screened his 1928 film *Surya Namaskar*.[113] By 1933, Aundh had an official "Namaskar Demonstrator," G. D. Lale, who was deputed to Mussoorie and other towns in North India to give demonstrations of the Surya Namaskar.[114] The Raja wrote to the mayor of Bombay in 1934 to urge him to adopt Surya Namaskar practice in the Bombay municipal schools, and offered to send someone who could demonstrate proper technique. The Bombay schools welcomed the Surya Namaskar trainer from Aundh and agreed to try the practice in a few schools.[115] Some of this outreach was finding traction in Pune as well, where colleges in the city made physical training mandatory for all students and gave them an option of eight practices, one of which was Surya Namaskar.[116] The Raja's outreach also extended to colonial administrators and even to those in the metropole. Whenever given a platform, it seemed he took the opportunity to lecture on the Surya Namaskar, demonstrate its proper form, and screen the film that showed its correct execution and many positive effects. He showed the film in his royal bungalow in Mahabaleshwar in March 1933, at a tea party he hosted for the governor of Bombay, Frederick Hugh Sykes, and other officials, and again in September 1935 at the Hotel Cecil in Shimla, at a lunch he hosted for the viceroy and countess of Willingdon.[117]

The Surya Namaskar was gaining popularity in Mysore as well, the place where most studies of the Surya Namaskar's inclusion into modern yoga are situated. A 1929 *Times of India* article notes the following:

> The Mysore Government have realised the urgent need of improving the physical condition of the youth of Mysore. They have deputed for this purpose Mr. S. N. Simha, a gentleman well-versed in the Surya namaskar system of physical culture brought into vogue by the Sri Bala Saheb Pant Prathinidhi of Aundh.[118]

Surya Namaskar is now central to the practice of many contemporary forms of psychophysical yoga, yet there is still no clear sense of how it came to be so. Mark Singleton emphasizes that Surya Namaskar was not yet considered part of yoga as understood by Krishnamacharya and others emerging out of Mysore in the early 1930s. Instead, the Surya Namaskar and yoga are portrayed as operating in close parallel: while the Surya Namaskar was taught as part of the physical instruction class, Krishnamacharya started his *yogaśāla* (yoga school) to orient the royal youth to yoga as a separate system of exercises.[119] Elliott Goldberg argues that Krishnamacharya could have absorbed knowledge of the Surya Namaskar from one of the local gymnasia, where it was already popular by the time Krishnamacharya wrote his book *Yoga Makaranda* in 1934.[120] Jason Birch and Mark Singleton argue that Krishnamacharya's particular form of the Surya Namaskar may be related to the Kannada *Vyāyāmadīpike* (1896) itself drawing from the Sanskrit text they refer to as the *Haṭhābhyāsapaddhati*, an extant version of which is from the nineteenth-century from Maharashtra.[121] Another possibility is that Krishnamacharya knew of the Raja's work in Marathi and English, had seen his film, read his books, and so on. Anyone attuned to yoga in the public spheres of India in multiple languages would have had knowledge of the Raja and his Surya Namaskar system. The proximity of a local gymnasium where the Surya Namaskar was being practiced is likely not the source (or the only source) of Krishnamacharya's familiarity but more probably a sign of the deep saturation of the Raja's Surya Namaskar within the physical cultural worlds shared with Krishnamacharya. If Krishnamacharya did not consider the Surya Namaskar part of yoga as late as 1935, this was probably because he did not view this practice as rooted in *haṭha* yoga, did not recognize it as *his* genealogy. In any case, as we describe above, Aundh's administrative reports and the press coverage of the Raja's travels and lectures suggest instead that at least one of the lines connecting the Surya Namaskar to Mysore was a product of the Raja's efforts to spread the practice as widely as possible. At least fifteen years before the publication of Krishnamacharya's *Yoga Makaranda*, starting with his first Marathi writings on the Surya Namaskar, the Raja had begun to forge a connection in print between the Surya Namaskar, yoga, and *āsana* practice.[122] And if we consider the Raja's autobiographical recollections of learning the Surya Namaskar from his father, these connections were already widespread among the Deccan states in the early nineteenth century and possibly earlier. Unlike Krishnamacharya, as we have seen, the Raja did not explicitly connect his practices with *haṭha* yoga, and so we would not place him in a genealogy of the "new *haṭha yoga* syntheses" in the modern period. As his son's demonstration of the *haṭha* yoga technique *naulī* in the *Surya Namaskar* film suggests, however, there already was at least some integration of *haṭha* yoga into the Raja's practice of the Surya Namaskar.[123] We argue that he positioned himself within a different genealogy of yoga practice, one traced from Samartha Ramdas to the royal Maratha sphere. This genealogy places the Surya Namaskar at the center of an interlinked set of political, martial, and ritual practices.[124]

Whatever the route and history of the Surya Namaskar into the future canon of modern yoga, we can see that this creative cultural adaption between two (or more) Princely States shows how these semi-sovereign locations within the general context of British colonialism bypassed their colonial observers; integrated the new frontiers of their emerging notion of political, economic, scientific, and corporeal "modernity"; and used modern postural yoga—yoga as psychophysical practice—in line with the broader use of yoga as political thought and action in the heterogeneous sphere of Indian nationalist public debate.

Economic Nationalism

One of the most influential and consistent critiques of the British Empire to emerge in the late nineteenth and early twentieth centuries centered on colonialism as a set of extractive economic practices. Writers like M. G. Ranade, Dadabhai Naoroji, and R. C. Dutt attributed India's consistent poverty and episodic famine to the way that imperial tax and tariff policies drained India of its wealth, systematically decimated existing industries, and failed to use public monies to stimulate new industrial technologies. Many of these Indian critiques of empire self-consciously drew from and resonated with intellectual and scientific streams from Germany, the United States, and Japan as a way to "break free from the London-centric imperial straightjacket" as Kris Manjapra puts it.[125] German nationalist economists like Friedrich List and others proposed a model of economic governance in which the state would play a foundational role rather than leaving initiatives to the market, as advocated by British liberal economic theorists of the day.[126] "Late industrializers," as Alexander Gerschenkron later named them, were all those who came to the project of industrial transformation after other economies were already dominant and therefore had to catch up quickly or else be relegated to trade relations from which others would always gain more.[127] Successful late industrializers like Germany leaned on the state as banker and coordinator to encourage domestic industries in sectors where none existed, helping to position German capitalists to compete with firms from globally dominant centers like imperial Britain. In India, as in Germany, economic nationalist ideas provided a potent counterpoint to British liberal economic assertions that were increasingly seen as, in the words of Mahadev Govind Ranade, "English and Insular."[128] Unlike in Germany, however, in British India, where governance remained firmly linked to imperial interests, there was limited opportunity to enact such policies. The situation was different among India's Princely States, in particular, those governed by ambitious and progressive rulers and advisers, which could seize their greater autonomy to experiment with a range of policies inspired by these critiques of empire.

Like the prince of Mysore, the Raja of Aundh developed a holistic vision of Indian modernity that existed alongside colonial Western modernity and also in contradistinction to it. In Aundh, as in Mysore, there were early efforts to use state funds and resources to catalyze economic transformation—with public spending on electric works, land and capital given to indigenous industrialists, and efforts in public education and health that far exceeded those in the neighboring villages and towns of British India. To entrepreneurs, the Raja was generous with land and capital, both from his personal wealth as investment capital and also as loans through the State Bank of Aundh, which was set up for this purpose. By 1938–1939, companies started with the Raja's support by the Kirloskars and the Ogales and headquartered in Aundh had become thriving operations. The Ogale Glass Works won contracts to supply lanterns and globes to the government of India and glass bottles to the Tata Industries for their cosmetic goods, and carried out extensive research on newer glass technologies.[129] Eventually, the Ogale brothers set up factories abroad, in the Princely States of Mysore and Travancore and in colonial Ceylon as well.[130] Kirloskar Brothers, the pump and machine manufacturers incorporated in 1920, would become one of independent India's most significant industrial houses. The Raja gave the Kirloskars land on which to establish their factories, which became known as Kirloskarwadi, and in addition to supplying capital, also served on its first board of directors.[131] Within a few decades of its founding, the company had expanded from its initial production of farming tools to manufacture power looms, lathes, and a variety of power pumps, as well as manage its own company town within Aundh State.[132]

Aundh also encouraged industrial growth by seeding new technologies and combining industrial training and entrepreneurship in high schools throughout the state. Aundh had its own director of industries to manage initiatives that would diversify farm income—by far the mainstay of livelihoods in Aundh as in most of British and Princely India. In the 1920s, Director P. A. Inamdar, along with the state research chemist, Mulay, were sent on tours throughout India and the European continent to learn about various cottage industries and consider their potential application in Aundh. At various points in the 1920s and 1930s, Mulay's laboratory studied ways to manufacture sugar from jaggery; increase the sugar content of Indian red carrot and vegetable dyes; and manufacture waterproof textiles, paper, and matches.[133] In 1922 alone, the state bank gave loans to Ogale Glass Works, Aundh Weaving Mill, Aundh Chemical Works, and a new cutlery factory.[134] The state bank also held prize competitions to encourage entrepreneurship and organized industrial exhibitions to award prizes to high school students.

The Raja conveyed his political economic philosophy through a Marathi phrase, *kaccā māl vikū nakā, pakkā māl gheū nakā* [don't sell raw things, don't buy ripe things]. In his autobiography, the Marathi writer G. D. Madgulkar, who grew up and went to school in Aundh, recounts the Raja giving this advice to a group of students.[135] Madgulkar also recollects the Raja's dismay when learning that a student wanted to be a bureaucrat or administrator and his delight when hearing of another's ambition to set up a glass bangle factory. In the Raja's estimation, the people of Aundh should use their raw materials to make things, their cotton to spin cloth and their sugarcane to manufacture sugar, and only export finished products. The Raja was not opposed to trade with other territories per se, only certain kinds of trade that, in his view, would keep Aundh and its people poor. His economic philosophy extended as well to his personal choices. He wore cloth spun only in Aundh's villages and ate only grains and vegetables grown in Aundh's fields.[136] He sought to embody the political and economic sovereignty he strove to realize for Aundh.

In Asia, decades before the successful developmental states of Taiwan and South Korea used related strategies to effect economic revolutions, these tactics were embraced by Meiji Japan and Princely States in India like Mysore and Aundh, anywhere with enough autonomy to craft independent policies. That such a program would even be attempted, let alone find some success in this modestly sized state of Aundh, is perhaps surprising. We suggest that one reason for this success is because these efforts in the economic domain were part of a larger package of technologies to make the self and, by extension, the nation, sovereign.

"City of the Free"

As we noted in chapter 3, the prison was an ambivalent site for Indian nationalism. It was both a marker of the power of the colonial state and, as a site where many nationalist revolutionaries spent many months and even years, an emblem of resistance, sacrifice, and stoic patriotism. In prison, many of the nationalist leaders turned to the *Bhagavad Gītā* as a political text and formulated their ideas of yoga, particularly *karma-yoga*, as a way to resist colonial rule. The prison had come to represent the power of the British as well as the power to resist the British. How would this dual meaning of the prison in political ideology of the time be read in the context of Aundh? And how does this relate to yoga as a political concept?

One of the more extraordinary features of Aundh was that it was the site of one of the first open prisons in India. Named Swatantrapur, which Apa Pant translates as "City of the Free," it was founded in 1939, the same year as the constitution came into force.[137] The Raja donated a piece of land for the prison that was located about three kilometers from the town of Atpadi, one of the larger towns in Aundh State. One strong advocate of this penal reform was Aundh's yogi advisor, Frydman, who conceived of Swatantrapur as a place where model prisoners could spend their last years in semi-freedom. Even before this, the Raja had carried out other efforts at penal reform; he launched a program to teach skills to prisoners so that they could support themselves after their release, and in October 1944, he marked his birthday by abolishing the death penalty in Aundh.[138] The first inmates of Swatantrapur were prisoners drawn from other jails in Aundh.[139] The prisoners—all of them men—could come and go freely from the grounds of the prison and were permitted to bring their wives and children. They worked on the prison farms (for modest pay) but were also given small plots of land for their own use. The fact that the concept of the open prison was conceived of and flourished in this Princely State, we argue, is both a metonym for the constrained sovereignty of Princely States like Aundh and a veiled critique of colonial power and the conditions of control it placed on the people of India. We view the open prison much like the Surya Namaskar: as a political strategy of sovereignty, a way to harness a measure of freedom in an unfree world.

A Princely State that is under the control of British colonial rule is not unlike an open prison. People in the state are free to come and go, but with permission, under surveillance, and in the name of whatever might be considered "productive" by the "Paramount Power," the term used in the Aundh constitution to refer to British authority. And it is a right earned by "good behavior," the opposite of which earns their removal from power (as happened to the Raja's nephew in 1909) or the full assimilation of the Princely State into the empire. This fact was likely not lost on the Raja, Frydman, or others who endeavored to create Swatantrapur. The annual reports from Aundh to the British authority evince the constant constraint and surveillance of the state by the British in parallel with a mode of political imprisonment. Each annual report was secretly vetted by a political agent for the

British Crown, and that agent's adjudication of the veracity of the annual report is appended to each one, meaning each report written by a Princely State was also a test of its loyalty and transparency, especially in political matters. Just as the Surya Namaskar provided a means of empowerment amid the disempowerment of colonial rule, so too we read Swatantrapur as a technique to control the self, a way to build a sense of self-possession and determination that the Raja hints at in his Surya Namaskar book by invoking "the present struggle for existence." In a society under constant colonial watch, the open prison was a direct metaphor for this mode of indirect rule by the British Crown and the political conditions under which the Raja practiced and promulgated the Surya Namaskar.

During research we visited Swatantrapur, which is now one of several open prisons in India. The sixty-one acres of land, once "barren, waterless, drought-stricken wasteland," have been transformed thanks to the labor of generations of prisoners who have passed through.[140] The site remains out of the way still. We stopped in Atpadi town to inquire of several fruit vendors about the location of Swatantrapur until someone could point us in the right direction, although it is only a few kilometers from the town's center. As for memories of Swatantrapur in Aundh, we encountered few. Neither the curators at the Aundh Museum nor the librarians at the royal library nor the caretakers of the royal residence located in the town of Aundh had any clear idea if Swatantrapur still existed, and in some cases had no knowledge of it at all. At Swatantrapur itself, there is no plaque or statue commemorating its origins in a Princely State or that it was established by the Raja and Frydman. The prison's warden, aware of this history, several times suggested that we should contact the royal family to propose that some commemoration be established. At the entrance to the prison, into which we could drive directly, is a sign that describes the place as an "open colony" (figure 4.5). The original dwellings are still standing, but the twelve prisoners who were serving their sentences at Swatantrapur at the time of our visit lived in a large modern building that can house twenty-eight prisoners and their families. Each accommodation opens onto a central courtyard and consists of a large studio that combines living space and a kitchen with a private bathroom in the corner. The warden explained that the prisoners work eight hours daily on the prison lands, on which they grow and harvest corn, pumpkin, and other vegetables that are sent to feed inmates at other prisons in Maharashtra. Each prisoner is given two *guṇṭās* of land

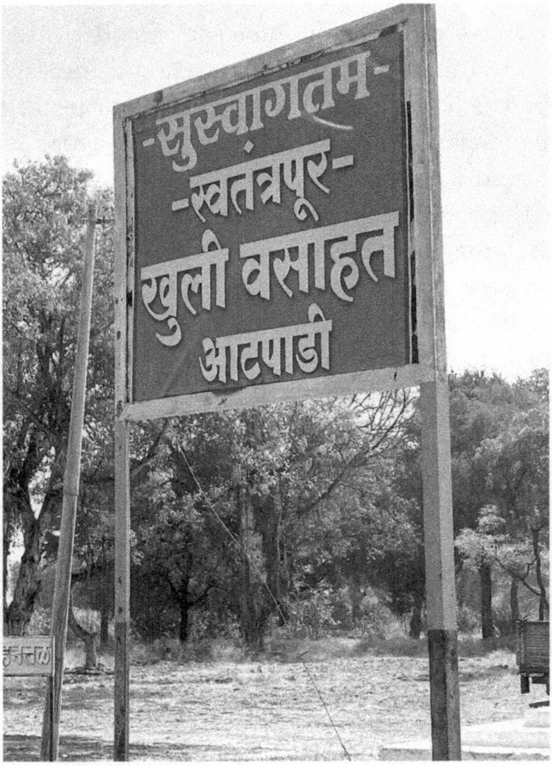

FIGURE 4.5 Signpost for Swatantrapur that reads "Welcome—Swatantrapur—An Open Colony, Atapadi"

(one-twentieth of an acre) to raise crops for their own consumption or to sell in the market, as they choose, and during our visit we saw tomato and chili plants thriving in these plots. Swatantrapur remains unfettered by fences or walls of any kind. The warden and his staff wear only plain clothes, and when we asked why, were told that this was to ensure that no *vāīt pariṇām* ("bad effect") falls on the prisoners' families, especially the small children.

We were surprised that only a few people with whom we spoke in Aundh seemed to know of Swatantrapur's existence. It is occasionally written about in Indian newspapers, where it is described as the result of Gandhi's influence and rarely connected to Aundh, the Raja, or Frydman.[141] Its story, though, is already well-known, if indirectly, in Indian popular culture

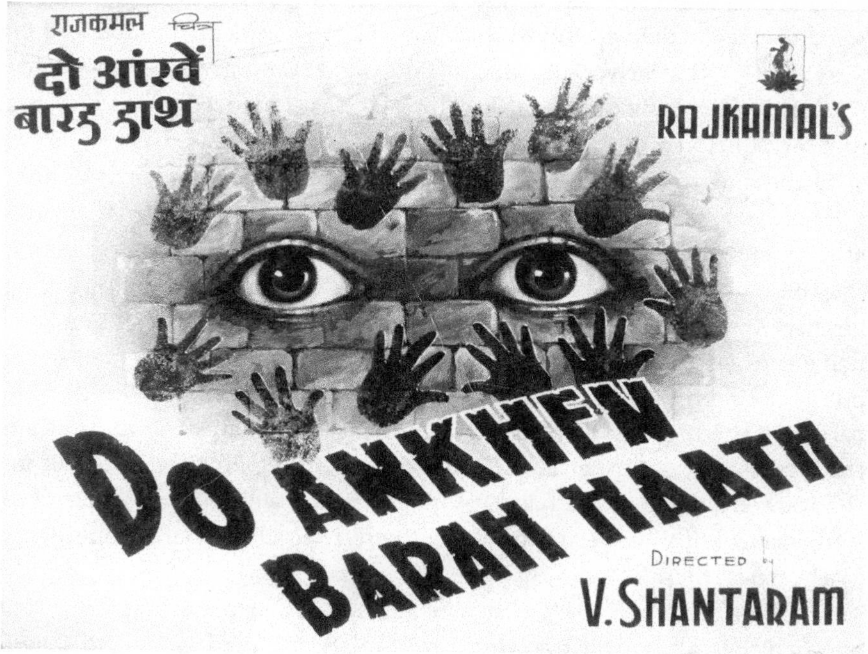

FIGURE 4.6 Publicity poster for the film *Do Ankhen Barah Haath*, 1957

through the famous 1957 Hindi film, *Do Ankhen Barah Haath* [*Do Ānkhe Bārā Hāth*] (*Two Eyes Twelve Hands*), the first foreign film to win a Golden Globe in 1959. It was directed by V. Shantaram, who also acted as the film's male lead.[142] The title refers to the two eyes of the warden and the twelve hands of the six inmates around whom the story revolves (figure 4.6). Imagine Foucauldian panopticism turned into a musical and you get a sense of the film. It opens by declaring itself based on actual historical events described in Hindi and English this way: "Almost twenty years ago, in a small state of India, an idealist started on a great experiment. . . . The story of this motion picture is based on his real experiences." The film tells of a visionary warden who convinces his superior within a colonial-style prison to allow him to take six hardened murderers to a barren patch of land and create the first open prison in India. Although Aundh is not explicitly mentioned in the opening sequence, the reference to a "state" in India around 1937 must be to the State of Aundh. The film's scriptwriter was G. D. Madgulkar, a celebrated Marathi poet, playwright, and screenwriter who grew up in Aundh State, studied at Aundh High School, and was deeply influenced by the Raja.[143] In the early 1950s, Madgulkar visited Swatantrapur and resolved to write a short book on the place, which he was convinced to produce as a film script instead.[144]

In the film, the warden is heavily influenced by Gandhian ideals of nonviolence, self-sacrifice, productive service to others, and the idea that nonattachment to the self can allow one to transcend the limits imposed on the self by others. The prisoners refer to him as "Bapu," a word meaning "father" that Gandhi's many followers and friends used for him. The warden ensures the cooperation of the jailed not by threats to their well-being but by noting the threat to his own self—the warden has staked his life and career on the good behavior of his inmates. If the inmates transgress, then they harm him, not themselves. The film makes the point many times that the warden's life is in the hands of his prisoners, who may do violence to him or may fulfill his desire to reform them. Their choices are limited only by their own morality.

This is a kind of karmic debt, an internalization of responsibility for another that alters the traditional etic relationship of jailer and jailed, transforming it into an emic one, which we have argued is emblematic of yoga as a political idea. The jailer has "yoked" his prisoners by transferring to them a responsibility for him and his well-being, much as Gandhi uses his own body through fasting to harness the violence of revolution. One can view this as the transition from a statist colonial mentality—the state is not of the people but rather confines and controls the people—to the mentality of the sovereign representative state—the people are responsible for the well-being of the state, even above themselves. While the yoke is still a strategy to control, it is transformed from control of the other in colonialism to control of the self in the semi-sovereign state, the precursor to the fully independent state after 1947. However one interprets the film, the story of an open jail in the heart of a Princely State walled in by the structures of colonialism can be nothing if not a commentary on independence and freedom.

We read the project of Swatantrapur as a metaphor for how to find and achieve sovereignty in the context of empire. One option is to make the prison walls themselves the conditions for freedom, as with Aurobindo who described his British jail as his *yogāśrāma*. In Aundh's Swatantrapur, the walls of the jail were removed to collapse the difference between prison life and the outer world, allowing inmates a level of independence that even those who were technically free perhaps may not have felt in other parts of British India at the time. For Foucault, the prison is emblematic of the way that power in modern states operates by forcing the self and the very nature of social being into a particular form, causing people to internalize surveillance. *Do Ankhen Barah Haath* follows this theme with very little subtlety—there will be no external control, only internalized surveillance. When the warden dies at the end of the film trying to save his prisoners from a raging bull, the inmates grasp their heads and scream that they can see his eyes still, searing into them. But it is not the intrusion of surveillance that causes them anguish; it is the death of a beloved warden who had taught them self-control, leaving them with the internalization of his moralizing gaze.

Conclusion

The school, the hospital, the prison—these are the institutions that, for Foucault, are emblematic of the discipline of modern states. What do we make of the open prison in the context of Aundh and what it envisions for the working of modern power, the likes of which we have linked to the Raja's practice and expansion of the Surya Namaskar? Perhaps this is a continuation of Foucault's argument to its logical extreme; the imperatives for discipline are so thoroughly internalized by the subjects of power that not only is the panopticon obsolete, but the very walls and fences of prison become redundant because all barriers are now internalized. Or perhaps what Aundh represents is an alternative genealogy of sovereignty, an ideal "Indian governmentality" that does not flow through a central, totalizing figure but rather moves through subjects as individuals, properly self-disciplined through years of education and techniques of self-control such as the Surya Namaskar.[145] In pointing out how yoga enabled the Raja to redefine the locus of sovereignty, we agree with Shruti Kapila's contention that many of India's early twentieth-century political thinkers were engaged in rethinking foundational political categories like sovereignty. As she notes, Tilak, like Gandhi, insisted on an "anti-statist political subject" and a "subject-oriented horizon of the political."[146] We suggest that the repertoire for this political articulation draws on an older genealogy of sovereignty rooted in the individual as expressed through the idiom of yoga. Yoga requires a subject, as we argue in our definition of yoga in the introduction, and that subject is either a sovereign actor already or an actor who aspires to sovereignty.

The Raja's experiment with the sovereign possibilities of the state in the confines of colonial-era semi-autonomy was not limited to political structures like constitutions and representative legislatures or to economic structures like the state bank: it also deeply involved the human body. As the Raja proclaimed in celebration of Aundh's constitution, "We have to urge the people of Aundh to remember always that government being control, self-government implies self-control and self-sacrifice."[147] One form this mode of "self-control" took was the institution of the Surya Namaskar, as we discuss here. We build on the insights of Joseph Alter about the connection between the Raja's interest in bodily discipline and his political reformism, but we suggest that the link connecting these two is *yoga as politics*, where we see a comingling of yoga's multiple valences—particularly political thought and psychophysical practice.

Chapter 3's focus is on nationalist insurgency, revolutionary opposition to colonial power, and an expression of individual activism coordinated for a shared political end, but in this chapter, we see political sovereignty instituted in an "experimental" state in which yoga, through the Surya Namaskar, plays a major role both as psychophysical practice and political strategy. In other words, if someone like Gandhi, Tilak, or Aurobindo used yoga to express a politics of individual resistance to British rule, the case of Aundh suggests this strategy of individual sovereignty has been elevated to the level of the state, the constitution, the people, and a nascent modern bureaucracy. The history of Aundh, its Raja, and the Surya Namaskar also serves to suggest the routes of yoga—as education and public health—in the postcolonial Indian state and its well-grooved bureaucratic pathways, the subject of our conclusion.

Conclusion

Yoga Infrastructure in India's Bureaucracy

THE RAJA OF AUNDH passed away in 1951 in a sovereign, democratic India. His beloved Surya Namaskar would become part of the global phenomenon of modern yoga, even if the Raja was largely muted in this history. Although the concept of yoga as political thought and practice was sublimated, still it remained always tucked just under the surface of the ubiquitous proliferation of yoga mats and yoga studios, a force underwriting yoga's new pathway in modern states and modes of capitalism and neoliberalism. When studies of these new formations examine the intersection of yoga and politics, they position the practice of modern psychophysical yoga within political contexts rather than consider how yoga itself might name political thought and practice, the broad project of this book. Most studies of psychophysical yoga since Indian independence in 1947 study its presence outside India, and especially in Europe and North America.[1] These studies across multiple disciplines and fields of knowledge engage the political world in different ways, taking up questions of colonialism, cultural appropriation, penal regimes, race, class, body normativity, sex and sexuality, religious practice, and capitalist consumerism. After the 2014 parliamentary elections brought to power the Bharatiya Janata Party (BJP), an avowedly Hindu right-wing political party, and Narendra Modi as prime minister, yoga assumed a new prominence in Indian politics and political life, and scholars, too, have shifted their attention back to India.[2]

These two bodies of scholarship—one focused outside of India from the 1950s to 2014, and the other within India from 2014 onward—leave a gap, a lack of attention to the period between 1947 and 2014 within India, and to what we call yoga infrastructure. By this, we mean how the Indian state implemented yoga, usually psychophysical yoga, within its bureaucratic regimes after 1950. We've sought to fill this gap in earlier work, and here we build on that work to offer a brief history of what happened to yoga in India from 1947 onward.[3] Our aim is to show how the Indian bureaucratic state harnessed the power of yoga as psychophysical practice, performed yoga upon yoga as it were. Our hope is thus to link together the many streams of yoga analyzed in this book, namely, its conceptualizations as philosophy, psychophysical practice, and political strategy. Underwriting the bureaucratic control of psychophysical yoga as a state enterprise in India over the last seventy years is the implicit political concept of yoga. The bureaucratic state itself is a "yoking" force applied to psychophysical yoga and deployed for the "people," the constituting subject of the secular democratic republic of India. This conclusion to our book draws together what we have discussed so far about yoga as political thought and practice into the contemporary period to contextualize the strategy of the current Indian state. As we will see, the story of yoga infrastructure in postcolonial India begins well before the 2014 politics of Modi and the BJP.

Yoga's Bureaucratic Infrastructure for Education

In debates about educational curricula in the late colonial period, a consensus emerged that psychophysical yoga, alongside wrestling and other physical practices (especially those involving competition and martial arts) should be considered part of the physical cultural heritage of India and should be incorporated into public school curricula in British India.[4] This consensus was influenced by and even perhaps patterned after the Raja of Aundh's implementation of the Surya Namaskar in the schools of Aundh and elsewhere in British India. Indeed, a bureaucrat from the Ministry of Education with whom we spoke referred to the Raja's *Surya Namaskars* as an early model and form of the *Common Yoga Protocol*, the standard government-authorized textbook on how to perform physical yoga, published by the Indian government since 2015.

The legacy of these early debates about yoga's place in public schools persisted into the postcolonial period. Physical education, and particularly teaching yoga in school, was seen as a mode of public health and, over time, the postcolonial state would introduce yoga into both its education and health bureaucracies. To address the dearth of qualified teachers required to teach yoga comprehensively in Indian schools in the 1950s, the central government began awarding grants to support yoga training at the National College of Physical Education in Gwalior and subsidizing the cost of yoga certification for schoolteachers. Instructors and curricula were sourced from India's premier institutions of instruction and research in psychophysical yoga and meditation, such as the Yoga Institute of Santa Cruz founded by Shri Yogendra in 1918 and Kaivalyadhama in Lonavala founded by Swami Kuvalayananda in 1924.[5]

The Indian state supported the creation of new institutes to train yoga teachers as well. For example, in 1959 the government gave financial support and land to the yoga guru Dhirendra Brahmachari, an influential figure during the prime ministership of Indira Gandhi in the 1970s, to establish the All-India Yoga Teachers' Training Institute in Kashmir.[6] Another effort was the result of the Yoga Health Department run by the Bharat Sevak Samaj (BSS). The BSS had been established in 1951 by the Indian Planning Commission as part of the country's First Five-Year Plan to serve as a vehicle for ordinary citizens to participate in the country's planned development.[7] It is significant for us that one of its early departments was devoted to yoga. In 1956, Prime Minister Nehru himself awarded certificates of completion to a batch of forty-five yoga teachers trained by the BSS's Yoga Health Department. At the event, which was held at the prime minister's residence, Nehru remarked that unlike other forms of exercise, yoga could produce "a kind of alertness of mind and elasticity of body" and that he hoped that a "large number of yogic exercise training centers were opened all over the country."[8] The government's efforts to promote yoga training continued for the next three decades. Education ministers pledged periodically to incorporate yoga instruction in school materials, but progress toward this goal was confined to sporadic experiments in select schools rather than wholesale curricular implementation.[9]

After several decades of helping to facilitate yoga teacher training, the Indian government began to institute yoga in public school curricula in 1986 during Rajiv Gandhi's government. We track this process through two educational policy statements that are issued periodically by the Indian government: the National Policy on Education (NPE) and the National Curriculum Framework (NCF). Both documents take up the subject of yoga in the 1980s, during Rajiv Gandhi's time in office. The NPE, which is issued by the Ministry of Education, first discusses yoga in the 1986 policy statement, which contains a separate section entitled simply "Yoga."[10] The text reads:

> As a system, which promotes an integrated development of body and mind, Yoga will receive special attention. Efforts will be made to introduce Yoga in all schools. To this end, it will be introduced in teacher training courses.

Based on the directives from this document, the central government, again under the leadership of the Indian National Congress (INC), began expanding on its efforts to train yoga teachers and build infrastructure suitable for sustaining yoga instruction, a necessary prelude to instituting yoga in Indian state schools, especially through the newly formed National Institute of Yoga.[11] Rajiv Gandhi and his party lost power in 1989 to a coalition government headed by V. P. Singh of the Janata Dal, and shortly after this, Rajiv Gandhi was assassinated. In 1991, a new INC-led coalition government was at the helm, headed by P. V. Narasimha Rao, and India issued its first set of stamps to commemorate yoga (figure C.1); it seemed psychophysical yoga

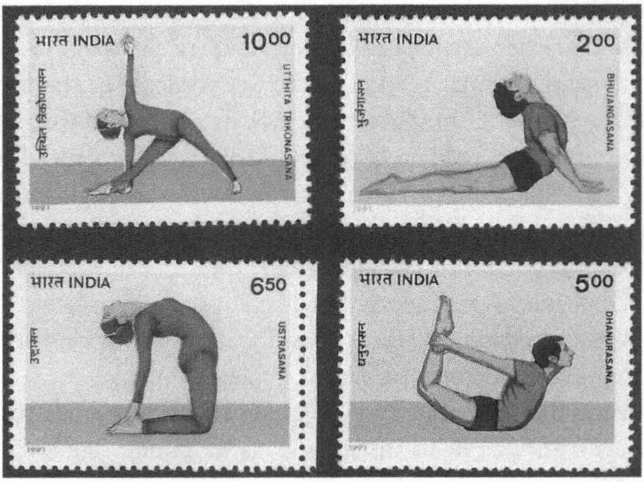

Figure C.1 Yoga stamps, 1991

was in the political sphere in many ways.[12] A year later, the government put out a new NPE that reworked the earlier version and again mentioned yoga.

The NCF is another important policy articulation for public education and, like the NPE, its release is episodic. The first mention of yoga in an NCF document that we have been able to trace occurs in 1988, and here the language is very brief and appears to quote directly (without attribution) the NPE of 1986: "As a system which promotes an integral development of body and mind, yoga should receive special attention."[13] Other than this reiteration, yoga only appears as one of many kinds of exercises and martial arts along with "gymnastics, calisthenics, athletics, aquatics, judo, . . . drill and marching, scouting, camping, and various team games."[14]

The next iteration of the NCF, in 2000, is notable as the first articulation of education policy under a BJP-led government, in this case led by Atal Bihari Vajpayee as prime minister. Much of the document echoes the NCF of 1988 under Rajiv Gandhi, where yoga is coupled with physical exercise and martial arts, though the 2000 version departs from its predecessor in several significant ways.[15] First, yoga is no longer confined to the context of physical education but is included in a section on "Indigenous Knowledge and India's Contribution to Mankind."[16] The document states:

> Paradoxical as it may sound, while our children know about Newton, they do not know about Aryabhatta, they do know about computers but do not know about the advent of the concept of zero or the decimal system. Mention may also have to be made, for instance, of Yoga and Yogic practices as well as the Indian Systems of Medicine (ISM) like the Ayurvedic and Unani systems which are now being recognised and practised all over the world. The country's curriculum shall have to correct such imbalances.[17]

This invocation is notable for several reasons. Although articulated by a Hindu right-wing government, it mentions a traditional medicine system associated with Islam, that is Unani, and the text emphasizes the global spread of yoga, yogic practices, and Ayurvedic medicine.

The document also correlates Sanskrit and yoga, expressing a more strident call for Sanskrit to be taught in public schools:

> A major shift in designing Samskrit [*sic*] courses and transacting curriculum in the subject is that the language is to be treated as a living phenomenon which is

> still relevant to the general life needs of the people of India, and which has caught international attention because of the global interest in subjects like yoga.[18]

As with the passage above, the language of the "global" and "international" sits side by side with "Indigenous," presaging how the Indian government beginning in 2014 under Narendra Modi would lay claim to the worldwide practice of yoga. The document recognizes how Sanskrit words and related terms travel along with yoga around the globe. This is the first time that Sanskrit is coupled explicitly with yoga in an official Indian government education policy document, to our knowledge. People of many religions have used Sanskrit over its long history, yet its primary association in popular imagination is with Hinduism.[19] The alignment of yoga and Sanskrit then implies a Hindu perspective even while this and every other government document about Sanskrit and yoga, to our knowledge, point out the multireligious, pan-Indian nature of both. In other words, for those who associate Sanskrit primarily with Hinduism—arguably a majority of those with a cursory knowledge of either subject—yoga here might follow those same associations and become encoded as "Hindu."

This pattern was repeated after the 2014 election in India: a preexisting bureaucratic infrastructure for yoga was elevated by a Hindu right-wing government and associated with Sanskrit and other indicators of "Hindu" identity, even while official government documents and public statements studiously avoided claiming yoga as an exclusively Hindu practice. As we note in other work, this is a purposeful and even legal strategy because to claim something like yoga or Sanskrit to be exclusively "Hindu" and to implement its instruction in public schools would violate Article 28 of India's constitution, which forbids "religious instruction" in any state-funded school.[20] This is one of the reasons that Hindu nationalist figures like Modi, Baba Ramdev, and Yogi Adityanath do not claim in public contexts that yoga is Hindu or even religious; rather, they speak of yoga as "secular," a "carrier of India's spiritual tradition," and a practice that "has no religion."[21] As with the implementation of Sanskrit in relationship to yoga, a connection to Hinduism may be implied, but is not overtly stated in order to avoid a constitutional contest for state policy around yoga. A third interesting point to note about the 2000 NCF is that it places yoga side by side with environmental concerns. In a section on possible "Elective Courses," the "emergent" courses that are proposed are: "computer science, bio-technology, genomics, yoga and environmental education."[22] This precedes by almost a decade and a half Modi's similar invocation in his first speech to the United Nations General Assembly in 2014, in which he called for an international yoga day. In that speech, Modi describe yoga as something that "can help us deal with climate change."[23]

Perhaps the most foundational government policy statement on yoga and education is the 2005 NCF, issued under an INC-led United Progressive Alliance coalition government headed by Prime Minister Manmohan Singh. The text of the 2005 NCF adds very little that is new, however it has been cited in cases presented before India's Supreme Court in 2016 around teaching yoga in schools,[24] and it is referenced by many other proponents of instituting yoga in Indian public schools.[25] In an interview with an official from the National Council of Educational Research and Training (NCERT)—the body tasked with producing textbooks for Indian government schools—we were told that the watershed moment for teaching yoga in schools only came after this NCF in 2005.[26] Like the first official educational policy document to champion yoga in schools (NPE of 1986), the NCF of 2005 was composed under an INC-led government, and this may be the reason that the text is often cited after 2014 as expressing "nonpartisan" politics around the importance of yoga in Indian government schools.

Beginning in 2014, BJP-led governments revised both the NCF and the NPE, which was renamed the National Education Policy (NEP). A new NEP issued in 2016 gives ample time and authority to the 1986 and 1992 NPEs, both drafted under INC governments. In making policy recommendations for yoga under the directions of "Sports and Physical Education," the text states:

> Yoga is an art from ancient India, which the whole world is increasingly adopting for healthy development of the body and the mind. The United Nations has recently declared an annual International Yoga Day, recognizing its potential vital role in nurturing the body and the spirit. Every school, both public and private, should be encouraged to bring Yoga in as part of the schooling process, and facilitate every child to learn the basics of Yoga. Particularly in urban schools, where there is shortage of playground facilities, Yoga can play a significant part in the development of a young student.[27]

The document declares that yoga should be taught in both public and private schools but does so in the form of an "encouragement" rather than a mandate. It echoes both the sense of yoga's place within a globalized sphere and its Indian origins. On these points, the 2016 document aligns with the NCF of the previous BJP government a decade and a half earlier. Since 2016, several Supreme Court petitions and cases have sought to press for the full realization of these policies around teaching yoga in government schools, a subject about which we have written, though its full implementation appears still to be mere aspiration.[28]

In a new NEP issued in 2020, yoga is referred to as a product of India's premodern "education system" and is listed as a subject within the "Knowledge of India" category of education.[29] Instruction in yoga is cited as a mode of "internationalization" by way of a subject that has global recognition and therefore provides a way to promote Indian culture in general.[30] It is also referred to as a means of "health care."[31] Echoing earlier associations between Sanskrit and yoga, the 2020 NEP mentions that among the subjects to be taught through Sanskrit is yoga.[32]

In 2023, a new NCF was issued that reflects many of the same themes charted already, but in an expanded and detailed manner.[33] Yoga is predominantly associated with sports, as well as physical and mental well-being.[34] However this NCF also cites key thinkers like Aurobindo on "the science of Yoga" and concentration, and B. K. S. Iyengar on yoga as a physical-educational route to ethical living.[35] Yoga remains a subject of history and cultural diversity and notably is described for the first time as part of "Indian martial arts,"[36] where it is mentioned alongside the Chinese martial and meditative art, Tai Chi, along with Indian martial arts forms such as "wrestling, *mallkhāṃb*, archery."[37] There is also a curious association of yoga with "chariot racing." The text concludes by noting that for all these activities, including chariot racing, "regular practice of yoga" is essential. To our knowledge, no previous NEPs, NPEs, or NCFs mentioned chariot racing, and this association is, among other things, an unexpected recurrence of a theme as old as the *Ṛg Veda*. Yoga here retains a martial and hence political valence.[38]

Yoga Infrastructure for Public Health

Alongside this emphasis on yoga and education, the Indian state, from the 1950s onward, treated yoga, as one government official told us, as "a free method of public health" and therefore also a way to "fight poverty." Yoga was conceived as a mode of public health and even medical intervention, ideas that echo the Raja of Aundh's understanding of the Surya Namaskar as medicine, an antidote to the side effects of Western allopathic medicine, applied to the body politic of a state.[39]

Beginning in the 1970s, INC-led governments made space for yoga within the bureaucratic state's public health infrastructure. The government established the Central Council for Research in Indian Systems of Medicine and Homeopathy in 1969–1970 under Indira Gandhi. This was meant to institutionalize not just psychophysical yoga but also a host of other indigenous health and physical training systems. In 1976, the Vishwayatan Yoga Ashram and Trust for the Promotion of Yoga was rechristened the Indian government's Central Research Institute for Yoga. In 1988, under the leadership of Indira Gandhi's son, Rajiv Gandhi, the government again renamed the institute the Morarji Desai National Institute of Yoga (MDNIY) in honor of another political leader, Morarji Desai.[40] The renaming of the institute after Desai is apparently related to his interest in nonallopathic forms of medicine and, in particular, his practice of *śivāmbu*, or "auto-urine therapy," a practice loosely associated with *haṭha* yoga where it appears as *amarolī mudrā*.[41] MDNIY is now the primary government agency overseeing yoga teacher training for Indian public schools as well as for private yoga instructors.

The Vishwayatan Yoga Ashram had been founded by the yoga guru Dhirendra Brahmachari (Dhirendra Choudhary) in 1959. From the start, the institute received annual funding from the Ministry of Education, and Brahmachari himself was allotted a government bungalow.[42] From the late 1950s, when the charismatic guru first started giving Indira Gandhi yoga lessons, until her assassination in 1984, Brahmachari was closely associated with her and several members of her family. This included her father, Prime Minister Nehru, who also took yoga lessons from Brahmachari and inaugurated the Vishwayatan Yogashram in 1959, and her son, Sanjay, with whom Brahmachari established several businesses that were later implicated in tax evasion and other kinds of financial scandals.[43] Brahmachari would come to be known as the Flying Swami for his love of airplanes and luxury, and his interactions with national and international elites.[44] Like Sanjay Gandhi, who died in 1980, Brahmachari would also die in a plane crash in 1994.

When the Vishwayatan Yoga Ashram became an organ of the state as the Central Research Institute for Yoga in 1976, it was during the time of Indira Gandhi's Emergency rule, when many other foundations of public life were being deinstitutionalized as part of a suspension of democratic and civil liberties. In our conversations with government officials during fieldwork, it became clear that the story of Brahmachari was a cautionary tale for them—a warning that the "guru model" of yoga instruction, as far as the yoga infrastructural state was concerned, was incongruent with the functioning of ministries in a secular liberal democracy. Yoga, they said, should not be associated with any individual but instead should be understood as the birthright of all Indians. Association with gurus risked the careful and consistent work done by government officials for decades around expressing yoga as an inheritance and right of Indian citizens in the fields of education, research, and public health.

This conceptualization of yoga as free public health and alternative medicine, or as an alternative *to* medicine, was deepened beginning in the 1990s. In 1995, the Department of Indian Systems of Medicine and Homeopathy was formed under the INC government led by Narasimha Rao. In 2003, under the BJP government led by Vajpayee, this department was renamed AYUSH, an acronym for Ayurveda, Yoga, Naturopathy, Unani, Siddha, and Homoeopathy. The acronym also spells a Sanskrit word, *āyuṣa*, that means "long-life" or "longevity." Over several decades, under the direction of governments of many partisan persuasions—the INC and its allies (1991–1995, 2004–2014), the left-of-center United Front coalition government (1995–1997), and the BJP and its allies (1998–2004)—AYUSH operated within the Ministry of Health and Family Welfare to carry out research and training in traditional Indian forms of medicine. In 2014, after the BJP returned to power with Narendra Modi at the helm, AYUSH was elevated to the status of a ministry, and in 2021, was renamed the Ministry of Ayush. The ministry would no longer be known by the acronym, AYUSH, but instead by the Sanskrit word *āyuṣa*. One official called it the "Ministry of Life," while Indian press reports often refer to the Ministry of Ayush as the "Ministry of Yoga," suggesting that yoga became its primary focus after 2014.[45] Subsequently, the Ministry of Ayush absorbed the Morarji Desai National Institute for Yoga, the epicenter for carrying out all activities associated with International Yoga Day every year.

The Department of AYUSH and later Ministry of Ayush served as government entities in charge of the kind of research previously done by independent organizations founded in the colonial period, such as the Yoga Institute and Kaivalyadham, both of which continue to undertake the scientific study of yoga. During fieldwork, we attended a conference on yoga hosted by the

Ministry of Ayush in New Delhi in which a lively debate occurred about whether the role of such conferences should be to promote "the authorization of yoga as science" or to reject the idea that "Indian science must be validated by the West as 'science' at all." They argued that if science was premised on rationality and observation, which is universal, then there is no "Western" science. Others felt that India's unique cultural modes of thought suggested an "Indian science" germane to the study of yoga. The Ministry of Ayush, therefore, supports both the study of yoga through the lens of science and a rearticulation of yoga as itself a scientific mode of inquiry, sometimes construed as unique to India.

Many other scholars discuss the elevation of the Ministry of Ayush and the creation of International Yoga Day, so we only briefly mention these events here. We agree that both are very significant, but we also suggest that they are not the only defining moments in the history of yoga's bureaucratic infrastructure. When scholars invoke the Ministry of Ayush, it is often to emphasize its post-2014 history, overlooking its preceding decades of existence. Just as the institution of yoga within Indian government schools is a project carried out under every major national government since independence in 1947, the establishment of AYUSH/Ayush and of yoga within a bureaucratic system is not the innovation of any single political party. All major political parties in power in New Delhi since independence have instituted or supported yoga within India's educational and health bureaucracies.

Yoga as a subject of state action and attention has more than seventy years of history that cannot be distilled into the last decade alone, which is where the bulk of yoga studies attention has been trained. The political uses of psychophysical yoga by the state are varied across this long postcolonial period and, as we have argued elsewhere, yoga is often bent to the political ideologies of those who wield it, part and parcel of political strategy. Our aim in making this point about the history of psychophysical yoga and the state is not meant to lessen the significance of or apologize for the pernicious politics of hate and violence enabled by religious fundamentalism in India. But any analysis of the contemporary intertwining of yoga and politics that does not recognize the longer history that we outline here remains incomplete.

Despite the many continuities from the 1950s onward that we engage above, we agree with other scholars who study the contemporary politics of yoga in India that significant changes have occurred since 2014, particularly in the ways that yoga's infrastructure bureaucracy has been deepened and further developed. The inauguration of International Yoga Day provided a new arena for psychophysical nationalism within India and further projected this as a mode of soft power onto a global stage. These changes are rightly read by scholars as framed by the politics of Hindu majoritarian nationalism.[46] What we have tried to demonstrate in this conclusion is that the history of bureaucratic structures that place yoga at the heart of the Indian state exist independently of any single political leader or political party. Instead, these structures operate within India's "steel frame," as its civil service was dubbed during the colonial era. We suggest that psychophysical yoga itself has been yoked by the Indian state over seven decades, harnessed by the main technique of state power, its modern bureaucracy. Encoded in our understanding of yoga as nonteleological and adaptable to any ideology, it can be deployed for different purposes by different actors over this time.

As in the longer history that we trace throughout this book, yoga has been bent to different ends, from war making and governance in the classical period to self-rule and sovereignty in more recent centuries. Yoga as political thought and action has a pliable, adaptive capacity. The bureaucratic infrastructure of psychophysical yoga in independent India from 1947 to the 2010s had the stated aims of revitalizing indigenous Indian physical culture and health practices, as we have suggested in this conclusion. Since 2014, the harnessing of psychophysical yoga by the Indian state has had the aim of consolidating a majoritarian politics organized around a purportedly authentic Indic, Hindu identity in order to project that image throughout India and abroad.

As authors, we realize that much of this book can be construed in ways unintended by us. Scholarship is always political, and as a book about yoga as political thought, the political runs through much of it. Over the last eight years, we have presented versions of this work in several venues, from small university seminars and intimate workshops to large keynote speeches and academic conferences, in the United States and internationally, and in all cases the reception of this work crosses political spectrums. We have been told, in well-meaning ways, that one can read in our work an implicit endorsement of Hindu right-wing appropriations of yoga as primarily Hindu, or at least we provide the material for such an appropriation by the Hindu right-wing and its ideologues. At the same time, we have been critiqued by Hindu right-wing ideologues and have received threatening and harassing communications.[47] Some have told us that we "hate Hindus" because the history we tell of yoga involves not just peace but also war and the world of politics. Others have simply told us that the yoga we describe does not reflect their practices, traditions, memories, or lineages, and so is not "authentic." Our intention has not been to offend anyone. This book is about a length of history and human expression that is not the sole possession of any political, religious, or cultural community.

Although most of this conclusion focuses on the intersection of the Indian state and psychophysical yoga, we end by returning yoga to the individual. As we suggest elsewhere, Orientalists argued that, in the "East," the individual is bypassed in favor of the collective, but in yoga, we find a preeminent technology of the self.[48] Across all three spheres of yoga that we identify in the introduction to this book—philosophical, psychophysical, and political—yoga is a tool in the hands of the individual, whether charioteer, king, poet, warrior, revolutionary, or everywoman. Yoga encodes political stratagems for going into battle and for the demands of governance that follow victory. It suggests routes to sovereign self-rule when faced with implacable obstacles, and it defines righteous action amid the grime of politics and the horror of war. In our account, yoga has as much to offer as a theory of political action as it does for the very different challenges of physical distress and a restless spirit. With all this in mind, we can modify our representation of the three spheres of yoga from the introduction to our book by locating within the three spheres the key texts and practices that we discuss throughout (figure C.2).

Yoga as philosophy—exemplified by the *Yoga Sūtras* and Sāṃkhya—comes to share space with yoga as politics in the *Mahābhārata*, the *Bhagavad Gītā*, and the modern use of *karma-yoga* in the nationalist period. Psychophysical practices like *haṭha yoga* and modern postural yoga intersect with yoga as politics through the Surya Namaskar at the hands of the Raja of Aundh. And yoga as politics also exists in isolation in texts such as the *Ṛg Veda* and the *Arthaśāstra*, where the other two spheres of yoga find no mention.

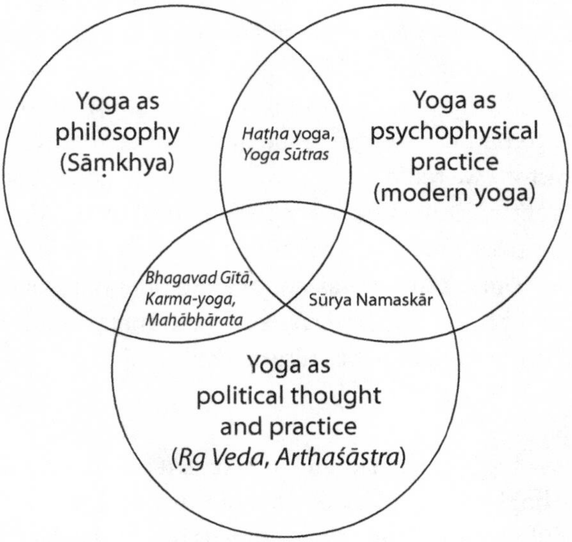

Figure C.2 Three spheres of yoga, updated

We might speculate about other relationships that these three spheres of yoga have to each other beyond the texts in which their meanings intersect. One representation of how these spheres of yoga might relate to each other is as a set of nested circles, much like the concentric *maṇḍala* theory. At the center sits the sovereign actor, for whom yoga is a means of controlling something, the basic articulation we propose about yoga as a political idea. The next ring might be psychophysical yoga, such as *haṭha* or modern yoga, a powerful means of controlling the body and mind. The outermost ring is a yogic philosophy of transcendence and freedom, which could be spiritual freedom or political freedom, or something in between.

Or, alternatively, the three spheres of yoga might relate to each other as a sequence. Yoga as philosophy addresses itself to the practitioner whose aim is spiritual freedom. It offers a technique to liberate the self from the mortal plane. But the task of preparing the mind and body for that ultimate pursuit falls to psychophysical yoga, which enables one's body to be powerful, to have force (*haṭha*) in the pursuit of one's aims and enables the mind's churning to cease. In turn, the pursuit of this psychophysical control requires a yogi to find a well-governed land with social and political stability. Yoga as politics may refer to the process of controlling one's opponents in a shared field of power to create the conditions for the other two kinds of yoga to flourish. As expressed by the anticolonial figures we study in this book, it is up to each of us to create a well-governed land if we do not already find ourselves living in one, even if this means challenging the premise that a given articulation of yoga is a way to this end, as Dr. Ambedkar did when he criticized the nationalist use of the *Bhagavad Gītā*.

Whether logically prior or central, both representations suggest that the social and political are also the proper domains for aspiring yogis. The warrior yogis that we find in the historical archives as well as the martial ascetics immortalized in fiction are not anomalous or exceptional figures. They are right at the heart of yoga in all its forms. We argue that every form of yoga is a yoga of power, a way to harness something, to apprehend it and control it, or a way to limit the force of another's power over oneself.

One implication of the history we trace is that the aspiring yogi must engage her sociopolitical context as much as she does her breath and body, mind and spirit. As we note in the interlude, key *haṭha* yoga texts prescribe a well-governed land for the practice of yoga. And perhaps a well-ordered yoga studio or aesthetically designed ashram is not a good enough stand-in for a well-governed society and polity, however one defines that ideal. The yogi dreams of a hut of her own in a peaceful well-governed land. Our hope is that yogis of all kinds in India and around the globe can forge virtuous, prosperous, and peaceful lands in which to live and practice, now and into the future.

Acknowledgments

THIS BOOK HAS BEEN nearly a decade in the works, and we have accumulated many debts that are a pleasure to acknowledge here.

For her unflagging support, patience, and astute advice, we thank Wendy Lochner at Columbia University Press (CUP). She believed this project would materialize in book form even during the years when we gave her little evidence for that belief. The editorial team at CUP has been wonderfully supportive. Our thanks to Kalie Hyatt, Leslie Kriesel, Julia Kushnirsky, and Elliott Cairns. We also would like to thank Sunny Khurana, Indiver Kumar Tyagi, and Marianne L'Abbate.

For assistance with several digitization projects related to this book, we thank Mohammed at SCI Weavers, Backstage Library Works, Perfect Image, Espen Bale at the British Film Institute, and Nick Gottschall at the University of Washington South Asia Center.

Some of the material that we present in our conclusion on yoga and the postcolonial Indian state is drawn from our essay "Legal Yoga," in *A History of Hindu Practice*, edited by Gavin Flood (Oxford: Oxford University Press), 404–424. We thank Gavin Flood and OUP for permission.

During field research, many individuals and institutions generously shared their views and materials with us. Our thanks to the excellent staff at the Shri Bhavani Museum and Library at Aundh, Kaivalyadam at Lonavala, the Yoga Institute at Santa Cruz, the Bhandarkar Oriental Research Institute, the Jayakar Library at Savitribai Phule Pune University, officials in the

Ministries of Education and Ayush in New Delhi, Justice B. N. Srikrishna, and the Pant and Madgulkar families in Pune. Our thanks to Sucheta Paranjape and Priti Ramamurthy for facilitating introductions to the Pant family, and to Milind Bedekar and Sanjay Upadhye for introducing us to the Madgulkar family. We're very grateful to Sagar Naik for his research assistance.

At the University of Washington, we are fortunate to be surrounded by generous and insightful colleagues and friends. Many of our colleagues in South Asia studies have heard us speak about this work, and several have offered valuable advice about it. Our thanks to Jameel Ahmed, Jayadev Athreya, Manish Chalana, Purnima Dhavan, Nick Gottschall, Radhika Govindrajan, Sudhir Mahadevan, Joe Marino, Heidi Pauwels, Priti Ramamurthy, Rich Salomon, Gowri Shankar, Kuldeep Singh, and Anand Yang. We'd like to thank Kuldeep Singh in particular for his expert design input on the cover.

The departments where we teach at the University of Washington—the Jackson School of International Studies and the Comparative History of Ideas—encourage the disciplinary trespassing that characterizes this book. We thank our colleagues for their intellectual company and friendship over the last decade and a half. We're particularly grateful for the advice and support of Dan Chirot, Sara Curran, Vanessa Freiji, Danny Hoffman, María Elena García, Judith Howard, Reşat Kasaba, Sabine Lang, Tony Lucero, Joel Migdal, Scott Radnitz, Chandan Reddy, and Cabeiri Robinson.

At the University of Washington, we thank Kathy Woodward and the Simpson Center for the Humanities for providing support and intellectual community. For research support, we are grateful to the College of Arts and Sciences, the South Asia Center, the Jackson School of International Studies, and the Henry M. Jackson Foundation. We're fortunate to have one of the best libraries in the world for the study of South Asia, and we appreciate the support of librarians Jessica Albano and Deepa Banerjee.

We thank the hosts, students, and audiences at several institutions and workshops where one or both of us have given talks about this work over the last eight years. Their insightful questions and critiques have sharpened immensely our arguments in this book. These include the Simpson Center for the Humanities at the University of Washington, the Centre for Studies in Religion and Society at the University of Victoria (British Columbia), Brandeis University's Soli Sorabjee Lecture Series (Boston), the University Seminar on South Asia hosted by Columbia University (New York), the V. M. Sirsikar Memorial Lecture at Savitribai Phule Pune University, the

Parekh Institute of Indian Thought at the Centre for the Study of Developing Societies (New Delhi), the Centre for Yoga Studies at the School of Oriental and African Studies (London), B. N. Pandey Memorial Lecture in the History of India at the University of Toronto, the Political Theologies and Development Workshop hosted by the Asia Research Institute at National University Singapore, the South Asia Graduate Student Conference at the University of California (Los Angeles), and the Politics of Religion at Home and Abroad Workshop (Chicago). We also shared our work with colleagues and audiences at the Western Conference of the Association for Asian Studies meeting hosted by El Colegio de México in Mexico City and the Annual Conference on South Asia at the University of Wisconsin, Madison.

We're indebted to many scholars for their engagement with the ideas of this book and advice on crucial points. We thank Janaki Bakhle, Carla Bellamy, Daniela Bevilacqua, Jason Birch, Guiseppe Bolotta, Cathy Boone, Neilesh Bose, Paul Bramadat, John Cort, Whitney Cox, Prachi Deshpande, Rajeshwari Deshpande, Rachel Dwyer, Christoph Emmrich, Michael Feener, Lars Martin Fosse, Philip Fountain, Farah Godrej, Jack Hawley, Nell Hawley, Elizabeth Shakman Hurd, Ayesha Irani, Andrea Jain, Will Kabat-Zinn, Shraddha Kumbhojkar, Steven Lindquist, Tim Lubin, Amanda Lucia, Angelika Malinar, Rachel McDermott, Christopher Jain Miller, Lisa Mitchell, Sagar Naik, Andrew Nicholson, Alok Oak, Rosalind O'Hanlon, Shailaja Paik, Sucheta Paranjape, Shruti Patel, Devdutt Pattanaik, William Pinch, Seth Powell, Hemant Rajopadhyaye, Srilata Raman, Ramnarayan Rawat, Yael Rice, Malini Roy, James Russell, Rich Salomon, Adheesh Sathaye, Patricia Sauthoff, Svati Shah, Ursula Sims-Williams, Harleen Singh, Shana Sippy, Michael Slouber, Caley Smith, Pushkar Sohoni, Winnifred Fallers Sullivan, and Audrey Truschke. Whitney Cox, Steven Lindquist, Hemant Rajopadhyaye, Andy Rotman, Richard Salomon, Adheesh Sathaye, and Caley Smith served generously as Sanskritists-on-call. Gayatri Chatterjee has remained a constant, brilliant interlocutor in this project and in all others. Shaman Hatley, Sucheta Paranjape, Steven Lindquist, Andy Rotman, and Jarrod Whitaker read portions of the book and gave crucial critique. We're deeply indebted to Joe Alter, Prathama Banerjee, Jim Mallinson, and Mark Singleton for reading the entire manuscript and offering critical insights.

In addition to the people we've mentioned already, dear friends have endured many conversations on the subjects of this book, including Paige Bartels, Camilo Borrero, Sonya Borrero, Jae Chung, Leah Clarkson, Naisargi Davé, Deepali Desai, Crispin Faber, Jurg Faber, Catherine Kamerling, Henry

Kamerling, Surabhi Kukke, Kevin Lalley, Nicole Mellow, Chad Naughton, Uzma Rizvi, Arie Thompson, Paige Trabulsi, Murtaza Vali, and Karl Wachter.

We are fortunate to have the warm and loving support of dear family and friends in India. In particular, we thank the Baiskars, the Paranjapes, the extended Gogte clan, and the Waghmares. In the United States, our family and friends, especially the Kale family, have tolerated this book's slow progression for almost a decade. Shobha Kale was with us when we first dreamed of this project over morning chai in 2015, and has spoken with us about it too many times to count over the years. Minal Kale and Vidula Kale read early versions of the introduction and offered valuable advice. William E. Novetzke and the Greene family have supported our endeavors over the years. We lost Mary E. Novetzke on December 16, 2019, her birthday. Christian's interest in yoga began when his mother gave him her copy of *The Autobiography of a Yogi* when he was a kid. She would have loved to know this book is in part a result of her eclectic, curious mind.

A book represents hours, days, and years spent in research and writing, which is time not spent doing other things. We end with an insufficient thanks to those "other things," namely, our extraordinary, beautiful, and irrepressible children, Sahil and Siyona. Sahil helped with the bibliography and notes, and Siyona with the book's graphics.

Finally, we thank our dog, Kahlo, for leading us on many hours of walks over the last four years. While he sniffed and barked, we discussed and debated much of this book.

Glossary

THE GLOSSARY CONTAINS non-English words from Sanskrit, Marathi, Hindi, Urdu, Pali, and Persian, as well as non-English words adopted in English. Since many of the words below exist across these languages, we do not cite each individual language. However, where a distinction of language is important, we mention this in the text or notes to the book.

ABHYĀS/ABHYĀSA: study.

AHIṂSĀ: noninjury.

ANĀSAKTI: unattachment.

ĀNVĪKṢIKĪ: to look toward; rational, empirical, critical inquiry; a mode of apprehension; associated with the political idea of yoga in the *Arthaśāstra*.

ĀPADDHARMA: duty or norms (*dharma*) in a time of difficulty (*āpad*).

ARTHA: meaning, aim, purpose, wealth, matters, business.

ĀSANA: posture, seat, abiding.

ĀTMA/ĀTMAN: soul, essence of individual being; self, as in *ātma-caritra*, self-deeds, autobiography.

AYOGA: not yoga; unharnessed, separated, undisciplined.

ĀYUṢA: duration of life, long life, longevity.

BAHUJAN: many people, the majority; in modern use, a term that often describes non-Brahman people, usually a community of people designated as belonging to the Other Backward Classes, as determined by the Indian state.

BHAKTI: sharing; a term for devotion to a deity, guru, or concept, both as a solitary practice and as a social practice (like pilgrimage, devotional performances, etc.).

BHAKTI-YOGA: the harnessing of *bhakti*, harnessed by means of *bhakti*; a term drawn from the *Bhagavad Gītā*.

BRAHMAN/BRAHMIN: *brāhmaṇa*; the self-described highest level of the *varṇa* class-caste typology; in the *Ṛg Veda*, a male priest who chants and performs sacrifices.

CARAKHĀ: a wheel, the spinning wheel used to spin cotton or jute into thread.

CASTE: from the Portuguese *casta*, race, lineage, tribe; in English, designating either or both *varṇa* and *jāti*, particularly as these exist in colonial and modern India.

DALIT: broken, torn, ground down; especially in Marathi and among particular groups, but throughout Indian languages, a term for people traditionally deemed "untouchable" in Hindu orthodox social thought and practice.

DAṆḌA: stick, rod, staff; by metonym, political power, authority, right to punish, potential for violence and/or force.

DAṆḌA-NAMASKĀR: a *namaskār* (see below) performed by making the body prone and stiff on the ground like a rod (*daṇḍa*); sometimes part of martial physical exercise and training, like a push-up; in Marathi, also used to describe the *sūrya-namaskār* and the *sāṣṭāṅga-namaskār*.

DAṆḌANĪTI: the right or moral (*nīti*) use of political power, violence, and/or force (*daṇḍa*).

DARŚANA: observation; a term for philosophy in Hinduism, such as Yoga and Sāṃkhya; a devotional way of viewing a deity.

DHAMMA: Pali, cognate with *dharma* in Sanskrit; in Buddhism, the teaching of the Buddha.

DHĀRAṆĀ: exercising concentration, meditation.

DHARMA: established, firm from *dhṛ*, to hold, bear, maintain, fix; morality, right, virtue, justice, doctrine, custom, social order, duty; in Hinduism, as in *Dharmaśāstra* (treatise on social and/or religious order), normative hierarchical social order around *varṇa* and gender prescriptions; in modern use, especially in English, the term more or less means religion.

DHĪ: thought.

DHYĀNA: meditation.

DṚṢṬI: sight; combined with yoga, "the control of sight" (*dṛṣṭi-yoga*).

FAKĪR: an ascetic of any religion (colonial period usage); now more commonly a Muslim ascetic; also rendered *faqīr*.

HAṬHA: force; firm determination and action; in combination with yoga, *haṭha yoga*, a tradition articulated in texts from approximately the twelfth century onward in Buddhism and Hinduism to name a kind of psychophysical practice that provides postures and positions (*āsana*), meditation techniques, breathing techniques, and other methods of mind-body practice; a key source for modern postural yoga.

JĀTI/JĀT: birth; the division of society by systems of endogamy and commensality into thousands of individual and hierarchical castes; in Marathi, a type or variant used in reference to particular species of plant and animal life.

JÑĀNA: knowledge, especially philosophical, religious, metaphysical knowledge; in *jñāna-yoga*, the harnessing of such knowledge for some aim, especially in the *Bhagavad Gītā*.

KĀMA: pleasure, affection, desire, love, sexual pleasure, as in *Kāmasūtra*.

KARMA: action, work, labor, activity, also the result of action, for example; in *karma-yoga*, especially in the *Mahābhārata* and *Bhagavad Gītā*, the harnessing of both action and the result of action, so acting without attachment to the fruits of action; in twentieth-century political contexts, self-less action in the name of nationalism.

KARMAYOGIN: the one who enacts *karma-yoga*; the title of a periodical edited and written by Aurobindo Ghose from 1909 to 1910.

KHĀDĪ: hand-spun cotton; in early twentieth century, a symbol of Indian self-rule and independence, especially associated with M. K. Gandhi.

KṢEMA: pacify, secure; peace, security, prosperity, a secure state. Derived from two almost identical roots (*kṣi*): "to possess" and "to destroy," which together, mean to possess and pacify by force.

KSHATRIYA: *kṣatriya*; a member of the sovereign, kingly class in Hinduism; in the *varṇa* typology, the second-highest type; sometimes glossed as "warrior caste"; *kṣatriya-dharma* refers to the duties prescribed in orthodox Hindu texts for members of these communities.

LOKĀYATA: extending from the world, worldly, materialistic, empirical; as "Lokāyata," a materialist, atheistic philosophy of classical India; in the *Arthaśāstra*, a method of apprehension through empirical observation that informs political strategy.

MALLKHĀṂB: From Sanskrit *malla-khāmbha*, wrestler (*malla*), post (*khāṃbha*), a kind of exercise and martial art involving a vertical wooden pole, often as a training exercise for wrestling and other martial arts, especially in Maharashtra.

MAṆḌALA: a circle or circular array; in the *Arthaśāstra*, a theory of "encircling" power around a king.

MANTRA: a thought instrument; some form of text and/or speech or vocalization meant to affect one's own mind, other people, or things.

MATA: thought, mind; opinion.

MOKṢA: freedom, liberation, release; a soteriological goal in much of Hinduism, Sikhism, and Jainism; in Buddhism as well, but rendered in Pali *mokkha*; more accurately, however, the goal of liberation in Buddhism is *nirvāṇa* and *nibbana* (Pali).

MOKṢADHARMA: the way of liberation/freedom; a name for a section of the Śānti Parvan (Book 12) of the *Mahābhārata* in which yoga is expressed as a philosophical means to liberation.

NAMASKĀRA/NAMASKĀR: making (*kāra*) a salute (*namas*); an act of honoring, saluting, respecting someone or something; sometimes done with joined palms pointing up and a slight bow; also done in other bodily ways, particularly through making the body prone before the thing being saluted or honored. See also *daṇḍa-namaskār*, *sāṣṭāṅga-namaskār*, and *sūrya-namaskār*.

NAMASTE: salute (*namas*) to you (*te*); a respectful phrase of greeting, common in modern Indian languages as well.

NAULĪ: a technique of *haṭha* and modern yoga that involves the auto-massage of abdominal muscles and organs.

NIRVĀṆA: blown out, extinguished, as in a candle's flame; ultimate soteriological goal of Buddhism; rendered *nibbana* in Pali.

NĪTI: leading; a term for policy, ethics, right conduct; political practice, proper governance, political wisdom.

PARVAN: a division of time, applied as division or section of the *Mahābhārata*, as in Śānti Parvan (Book Twelve).

PRĀṆĀYĀMA: the course or control (*yāma*) of breath (*prāṇa*); methods of breath control associated with psychophysical yoga.

PURĀṆA: ancient; classical Sanskrit works of past events, history, legends, myths, and so on.

RAHASYA: a secret matter; also, the essential point of that matter.

RĀJA: also *rājā* in Marathi, a king or ruler, as in the Raja of Aundh; also royal, kingly, political order, or rule, as in the British Raj.

RĀJA-DHARMA: a section of the Śānti Parvan in the *Mahābhārata* regarding kingly duties and strategies of governance.

RĀJARṢI: a king with the equanimity, self-control, and wisdom of a sage (*ṛṣi*).

ṚṢI: a sage in Hinduism; in particular, one of the titles given to authors of the Vedic texts, such as the *Ṛg Veda*.

ṚTA: art, truth, right, rite, especially in Vedic texts.

ŚAIVA: of Shiva; applied to anything related to the worship, theology, mythology, or philosophy associated with the Hindu deity, Shiva, particularly yoga and *tantra* practices.

ŚAMA: peace, tranquility, rest, from the verbal root (*śam*) meaning to pacify, ally, subdue, kill, extinguish, and conquer, as well as to become fatigued over such exertions.

SAMĀDHI: joining, combining, union, completion, accomplishment, absorption; intense application of the mind in concentration; a state of achieving an intense state of concentration; also, the tomb of a person who has achieved a permanent state of concentration.

SĀṂKHYA: rational enumeration, calculation, discrimination; the name of one of the classic schools of Hindu philosophy particularly related to Yoga as philosophy and Śaiva thought and practice.

SAṂNYĀSĪ: a person in Hinduism who renounces the world (*saṃnyāsa*).

SANT: a good person, especially used to refer to exceptional figures who are sacred in devotional or *bhakti* communities in India (a "saint"); also usually a poet or composer, often a "saint-poet."

ŚĀNTI: peace, tranquility; the time after war, as in the Śānti Parvan in the *Mahābhārata*.

SĀṢṬĀṄGA-NAMASKĀR: a *namaskār* done with (*sa*) eight (*aṣṭa*) limbs (*aṅga*); a prone prostration before a subject of honor, like a teacher, deity, the sun, and so on.

ŚĀSTRA: a Sanskrit treatise or body of literature on a given subject.

SATYĀGRAHA: holding on to truth; a concept developed by M. K. Gandhi to refer to his political thought and activities; a *satyāgrahī* is an adherent to this Gandhian concept.

SAVARṆA: with *varṇa*: a term that refers to people who, by virtue of caste/*jāti*, consider themselves within one of the four *varṇa* social categories; this excludes people considered "untouchable" in the normative Hindu *varṇa* typology.

SHUDRA: *śūdra*; the fourth type in the *varṇa* typology, a class associated with labor, especially agricultural labor; considered inferior to the first three classes and precluded from hearing the Vedic texts and from other Hindu ritual and textual worlds; this term is often glossed as "Bahujan" in contemporary language and associated with the Indian government category of Other Backward Classes.

ŚLOKA: a verse form in Sanskrit and other Indian languages, found, for example, in the *Ṛg Veda* and *Bhagavad Gītā*.

ŚOKA: sorrow.

SOMA: in Vedic texts, a drink consumed by the deity Indra before battle, and by priests and warriors; a primary object of one of the major sacrificial rites of the Vedic texts.

SŪKTA: well-said, a term for Vedic verse.

SŪRYA: the sun, as both astronomical object and Hindu deity.

SURYA NAMASKAR: *sūrya-namaskār*; a *namaskār* to the sun (as astronomical object and/or deity), performed also as a *sāṣṭāṅga-namaskār* and/or a *daṇḍa-namaskār*; a movement series considered foundational to modern yoga, popularized by the Raja of Aundh and others in the early twentieth century. See also *daṇḍa-namaskār*, *sāṣṭāṅga-namaskār*, and *sūrya-namaskār*.

SŪTRA: a thread; an aphoristic line or text on a given subject, as in *Yoga Sūtras* of Patanjali.

TANTRA: a loom, or the weave in a cloth; a term for a class of texts and practices (both often dialogic) considered to have metaphysical or mystical power.

UNTOUCHABLE: the English rendering of a set of terms such as *aspṛśya* ("not to be touched") or *cāṇḍāla*, or a gloss for a category of *jāti* considered in the category of the lowest or even outcaste members of the orthodox Hindu typology of social order; often considered a derogatory term by people subjected to this designation; the practice of untouchability is formally illegal in modern India and the eradication of this practice is the goal of many social and political movements.

VAISHYA: *vaiśya*; the third type of the orthodox Hindu *varṇa* typology, associated with business and merchant livelihoods.

VĀṆĪ: sound, voice, music, words; in *vāṇī-yoga*, indicating means of harnessing sound, such as the use of *mantra*.

VARṆA: appearance, color; a typology of socioreligious hierarchy in Hinduism, often applied to *jāti* groups; enumerated as Brahman, Kshatriya, Vaishya, Shudra, in that order, each considering itself superior to the one after; this typology has been highly contested and challenged over time, from Buddhism to contemporary social justice movements.

VEDA: knowledge, specifically of ritual; another name for the verses of the Vedic text.

VINYĀSA: movement, assemblage; an arrangement of movements as part of the modern practice of psychophysical yoga.

VIṢĀDA: despair, despondency; applied in particular to the despondency of Arjuna at the start of the *Bhagavad Gītā*; *viṣāda-yoga* refers to the title given to the first chapter of the *Bhagavad Gītā* that describes Arjuna's mental state, when he is controlled or yoked by despair; also a term used by Dr. B. R. Ambedkar to describe the Buddha's despair or quandary over whether to share his teachings, the *dhamma*, with humanity.

VYĀYĀMA/VYĀYĀM: exertion, effort, especially exercise of a physical kind; in the *Arthaśāstra*, refers to military exercises and various forms of military operations, such as mobilizing one's army; in Marathi, Hindi, and other Indian languages, refers also to martial arts; psychophysical yoga is often considered a mode of *vyāyām*.

YOGA: yoke, yoking; use, employment, control, and so on; a means of controlling something.

YOGĀBHYĀSA: the study of yoga.

YOGA-KṢEMA: as a *dvandva* (copulative) compound: war and peace, exertion and rest, settlement and acquisition; as a *tatpuruṣa* (determinative) compound: peace from war, rest from exertion, settlement after acquisition; in the *Arthaśāstra*, names the fundamental goal or activity of the state; in Buddhism, another term for *nirvāṇa*, the fundamental goal of Buddhism.

YOGA-PURUṢA: yoga-man; in the *Arthaśāstra*, a male spy master.

YOGAŚĀLA: a school for the study of yoga.

YOGĀSANA: a position or posture within psychophysical yoga.

YOGA-STRĪ: yoga-woman; in the *Arthaśāstra*, a female spy master.

YOGA SŪTRAS: *yoga-sūtra*; the text attributed to Patanjali (Patañjali); also called the *Pātañjalaya-Yoga-Śāstra*.

YOGEŚVARA: lord (*iśvara*) of yoga; a reference to Krishna in the *Bhagavad Gītā*.

YOGI, YOGĪ, YOGIN: masculine noun designating one who practices yoga.

YOGINĪ: feminine noun designating one who practices yoga.

Notes

Preface

1. In Kale and Novetzke 2020a, we consider this case and others in which yoga entered the U.S. legal domain alongside the history of yoga instruction in India's school system. We return to the subject of yoga as psychophysical practice in India's education and health bureaucracies in our conclusion.
2. We analyze this dispute alongside the larger debate about yoga as cultural appropriation in Kale and Novetzke 2021.

Introduction

1. The yoga and Sanskrit scholars James Mallinson and Mark Singleton provide this typology in their book, *Roots of Yoga*. In the introduction they distinguish between "yoga as practice," by which they mean the psychophysical yoga that is the subject of their book, and "Yoga as a doctrinal or philosophical system," which they do not discuss (Mallinson and Singleton 2017: xi). In *A History of Modern Yoga*, Elizabeth De Michelis likewise confines her discussion to psychophysical and philosophical systems of yoga, but provides further typologies within these spheres to differentiate between denominational, meditational, and postural yoga (De Michelis 2004).
2. We use the title *Yoga Sūtras* in this book because this is how the text is best known. However, a more accurate title would be the *Pātañjalayogaśāstra*, which would include both the *sūtras* and the commentary (*bhāṣya*).

3. The estimates on the date range of the *Ṛg Veda* vary. We follow the date range given by Jamison and Brereton in their translation, upon which we heavily rely. See Jamison and Brereton 2014: 5.
4. The estimates for this date range vary. We follow Brockington 1998: 26, and van Buitenen 1973: xxv.
5. There is considerable scholarly debate about dates of this text. Because the *Bhagavad Gītā* is part of the *Mahābhārata*, we do not give separate dates for the former. For example, Patton (2008: xxv) suggests that the full form of the *Bhagavad Gītā*, as we have it now, occurred around 200 BCE to 200 CE.
6. Olivelle (2013: 25–31) divides the text into three major phases: source materials (ca. 100 BCE to 100 CE), the original composition (ca. 50–125 CE), and the later recension (ca. 175–300 CE).
7. Monier-Williams, Leumann, and Cappeller 1899: 856–857.
8. See Figueira 2023: 67.
9. See Monier-Williams, Leumann, and Cappeller 1899: 856–858, and Mayrhofer 1986: 417. The word yoga as a "yoke" for a horse entered the Vedic lexicon already layered with meaning drawn from the shared martial culture of the Indo-Europeans (whoever they might have been). See Anthony 2007 and Doniger 1999. While the Sanskrit of the *Ṛg Veda* is an already established literary language by 1400 BCE, if not well before, the language finds genealogical siblings in other ancient Indo-European languages. These other languages include Avestan, the ancient Iranian language of the sacred scriptures of the Zoroastrian or Parsi religion (Avesta or the Avestan Gāthās), which are from a period very roughly coterminous with the *Ṛg Veda*, so perhaps the middle of the second millennium BCE. Also included in this language family are ancient Latin and Greek. All four languages—Sanskrit, Avestan, Latin, and Greek—share some common ancestor language that scholars reconstruct as "Proto-Indo-European," and this familial character is evident in the many similarities of vocabulary, roots, and grammar shared across these languages and their descendants, such as English, Hindi, Spanish, German, French, Russian, and Persian, among many others. Within this context, very central and important words tend to share phonological similarities, like the word for mother: *mata*, *madre*, *mutter*, *mère*, *mama*, and *mâdar*.
10. See Mallinson and Singleton 2017: 3–45 for a discussion of yoga as both action and result/goal, but within "the attainment of liberation or supernatural powers by means of prescribed psychophysical methods" (3).
11. The word can have the simple meaning of "union" as in a junction or point of contact. In theological contexts, such as those of Patañjalāya Yoga, Sāṃkhya Yoga, and Tantra, the word can convey an intimate unification with the divine (e.g., iśvara), or union between the human and divine, and so on. Here, yoga is both the striving for this unification and the completed state of it. For more on these meanings of yoga in psychophysical and theological worlds, see Mallinson and Singleton 2017.
12. Monier-Williams, Leumann, and Cappeller 1899: 1287. Some *haṭha* yoga techniques have effects on others, not just the *haṭha* yogi. See Mallinson and Singleton 2017: 359–394, for a survey of "yogic powers," many of which act outside

the yogi's body on others—such as "drawing people into one's power" (382). See also Birch 2011.

13. Thanks to one of our anonymous reviewers for suggesting that we sharpen and clarify our meaning here. We thank Shaman Hatley for suggesting a relationship here to the "yogic power" of *yogipratyakṣa* or "the perception of the yogi" which Mallinson and Singleton describe as a "means of acquiring authoritative knowledge" (2017: 359).
14. Foucault 1978.
15. Foucault 1970.
16. This idea is perhaps also shared with yoga as a philosophy, particularly in relationship to Sāṃkhya, which posits a closed system of elements, qualities, and forces that interact to evolve and devolve to various states of matter and mind.
17. See Alter 2000. Our thanks to an anonymous reviewer for this point.
18. For examples of dialectical thought in classical India, see the thought of figures like the Buddhist thinkers Nagarjuna (ca. third century CE) and Dharmakirti (seventh century CE), and the Hindu figures Shankara (ca. eighth century CE) and Udayana (tenth century CE). See Ganeri 2017.
19. For an early version of this argument, see Kale and Novetzke 2016.
20. Adorno 1992.
21. Homonyms often occur in heterogenous languages that borrow words from other languages, as is the case with English. Sanskrit is a homogenous, highly phonetic, and technically structured language; the word Sanskrit (*saṃskṛta*) means "perfected" and "completed." Homonyms pose a structural problem in Sanskrit, but they do sometimes exist. One example relevant for this book is the verbal root *kṣi*, which means both "to possess, rule over" and "reside undisturbed" (Monier-Williams, Leumann, and Cappeller 1899: 327 and Whitney 1885: 29), and yields the word *kṣema*, "giving rest or ease or security," a word apparently derived from the meaning of both roots, as we discuss in chapters 1 and 2, to rule over so as to have security. This kind of homonym is not uncommon among verbal roots in Sanskrit. However, in languages like Marathi and Hindi that borrow words from Sanskrit and other languages, one does find homonyms. For example, in Marathi, a word for "love," *kām*, is pronounced and written exactly as a word for "work," *kām*. The former is derived from the Sanskrit word *kāma* and the latter from the Sanskrit word *karma*. In Sanskrit, these two words are not homonyms, but in Marathi, they are. More examples could be given for other Indian languages. We thank Adheesh Sathaye for this example.
22. Ginu Kamani, "A New Position on the Kamasutra: On Sex, Sanskrit, and Fallibility of Richard Burton," *Mans World*, March 20, 2018, https://www.mansworldindia.com/currentedition/from-the-magazine/new-position-kamasutra/.
23. For more on this text, see Olivelle 2013, Singh 2017, McClish 2019. On its modern reception, see Banerjee 2012 and 2020.
24. See *Arthaśāstra* 6.2.4 and 7.1.1. See also Scharfe 1989: 206–207.
25. Singh 2017: 349.
26. Mouffe 2013. Chantal Mouffe applies these ideas about agonism to analyze modern liberal democracy and the politics of the European Union.

27. See "agonism, n.," *OED Online*, March 2023, Oxford University Press, https://www-oed-com.offcampus.lib.washington.edu/view/Entry/4095?redirectedFrom=agonism& (accessed May 30, 2023).
28. Bourdieu 1993.
29. See Schmitt 1976 [1932]: 33 and 2007 [1963]: passim. See de Ruiter 2012.
30. For studies of the neoliberal ends to which yoga is put, see Godrej 2022b. See also Jain 2020.
31. On yoga's entanglements with capitalism, see Jain 2015.
32. On the connection between yoga and fascist impulses, see Imy 2016: 320–343.
33. Krishnamacharya's *Yoga Makaranda* was written in Kannada in 1934.
34. This discussion draws on our previous work: Kale and Novetzke 2016; Kale and Novetzke 2020b: especially pages 43–44. While political theology does not feature prominently in this book, we believe the term is useful to think about multiple overlapping subjects and disciplinary perspectives.
35. As noted, we do not generally adopt the ideas of Carl Schmitt, not only because of his position within the National Socialist regime of Germany but also because of the irrelevance of his absolutist conceptualizations of ideas like sovereignty and the political to our project.
36. Schmitt's chapter on political theology opens by stating: "All significant concepts of the modern theory of the state are secularized theological concepts." See Schmitt 2005 [1922]: 36.
37. Banerjee 2020.
38. Foucault 2024 [1978]: 2, 156.
39. Many works center this subject, but see, for example, Moin 2012.
40. Kale and Novetzke (2020a), in particular, considers the judgment in the *Encinitas* case of 2015, where the judge argued rather paradoxically that yoga was "religious" and "not religious" at the same time.
41. Kale and Novetzke 2016, 2017, 2020a, 2020b, 2021.
42. Akers 2002; Behl and Doniger 2012a, 2012b; Behl, Weightman, and Pandey 2000; Birch et al. 2024; Bryant 2009; Chapple and Casey 2003; Dehejia 1986; Diamond and Aitken 2013; Diamond, Glynn, and Jasol 2008; Ernst 2016; Feuerstein 1980; Foxen and Kuberry 2021; Hatley 2007a, 2007b, 2013; Mallinson 2004, 2007, 2024; Mallinson and Singleton 2017; Mallinson and Szántó 2021; Samuel 2008; Sanderson 1988, 2009; Sarbacker 2021; and White 1996, 2000, 2003, 2009, 2011, 2014.
43. Bouillier in Neelsen 1992: 3–21; Gold in Lorenzen 1995: 120–132; Lorenzen 1978; Pinch 2006. C.f. Bouillier 2013: 164. A book with which we share our title—Julius Evola's *The Yoga of Power* [Lo Yoga della Potenza] written in 1925 in Italian—is not about politics but rather a history of *tantra* and Śakti forms of yoga. It is, however, a work deeply informed by Evola's fascist ideology (Urban 2006: 140–161).
44. Alter 2000, 2004; Bevilacqua 2018; Bevilacqua and Stuparich 2022; Singleton 2010.
45. Bucar 2022; De Michelis 2004; Foxen 2020; Syman 2010.
46. Lucia 2020.
47. Jain 2015, 2020.

48. Godrej 2022a, 2022b.
49. Black 2024; Gautam and Droogan 2018: 18–36; Gupta and Copeman 2019: 313–329; Lakshmi 2020; Sood 2018, 2023.
50. A notable recent exception is Banerjee 2020. Like Banerjee, we analyze the concept of *karma-yoga* and the writing and thought of Gandhi and Aurobindo; however, her deeper focus is on writers and thinkers from eastern India (Bankimchandra Chattopadhyay and Tagore, for example), while our book shifts to writers and political figures from western India like Tilak and the Raja of Aundh.
51. Even when ideas of yoga are central to political action, as with nationalist figures like Gandhi, much of the scholarship in U.S. academia bypasses the study of yoga in favor of studying other aspects of politics. For example, Rudolph and Rudolph (1967) examine the nature of Gandhi's political charisma, and Mantena (2012) examines Gandhi's political pragmatism. Where U.S. political scientists have explicitly engaged yoga, it is typically construed as psychophysical practice that has been instrumentalized by political actors and within political institutions. For example, Godrej (2022a, 2022b) looks at how psychophysical yoga has been embraced as a tool of discipline within U.S. prisons.
52. Banerjee 2020: 3.
53. Kapila 2021: 2.
54. Getachew and Mantena 2021: 362. The reference within this quote is to the subtitle of Partha Chatterjee's 2004 book, *Politics of the Governed*.
55. We recognize what Shameem Black has called a "clear danger . . . in looking into India's yogic histories" given the power of Hindu fundamentalism in recent decades, and that "[s]uch a project may seem all too close to textual practices where exclusionary visions of nationalism justify gendered, caste-based, and religious hierarchy" (Black 2024: 27).
56. For examples of Novetzke's work that deal with caste and gender inequality, see Novetzke 1993, 2008, 2011, and 2016. A forthcoming work is tentatively titled *Savitribai and Jotirao Phule* (Delhi: HarperCollins, expected 2026). For examples of Kale's work on socioeconomic and political inequalities, see Kale 2014, 2020; and Kale and Mazaheri 2019.
57. See Kale and Novetzke 2021.
58. Mallinson and Singleton 2017: xi.
59. We refrain from providing specific details in order to preserve the anonymity of our interview subjects.

1. Yoga as War and Peace in the *Ṛg Veda* and the *Mahābhārata*

1. For example, see Singleton 2010: 14, 180.
2. For example, a certain strain of Hindu fundamentalism claims that "everything is in the Vedas." We do not endorse this view. Although "yoga" is found in the *Ṛg Veda*, the word is not used to describe the psychophysical or philosophical

sort, as this chapter shows. For more on efforts to find these forms of yoga in the text, see note 4.

3. See, for example, Novetzke 2016.
4. We do not engage here the various debates about yoga as psychophysical practice or soteriological philosophy in the *Ṛg Veda*, but someone interested in this issue can see Werner 1977 and more recent discussions in Mallinson and Singleton 2017: xii–xiii. From our own reading of this text, there is no clear indication that "yoga" means anything like the psychophysical practices or soteriological philosophies that will later come to dominate the meaning of this term. We also avoid an engagement with the reading of the Indus Valley seals that seem to depict a person seated with legs crossed as indicative of psychophysical yogic practices. Until the Indus Valley script is deciphered, there is no compelling evidence to link a common way of sitting worldwide with a highly specific practice of yogic posture and meditation.
5. Mallinson and Singleton 2017: xiii.
6. The Indus Valley seals may present an older mode of communication, but no one yet is able to comprehend the seals' meaning. Some have argued that the seals represent a language (see Rao et al. 2009; Parpola 1994), while others have argued that the seals do not represent a language (Farmer, Sproat, and Witzel 2004).
7. Though historians will use the text to write histories of the period, the text does not purport to represent history, and as an archive it is neither interested in recording material "facts" nor is it in any way socially capacious in its scope. It pays little attention to general society, current affairs, or anything other than the sacrificial cosmic world and, self-reflexively, its own poetic nature.
8. A host of scholars have traced the martial emphases of the *Ṛg Veda*. Michael Witzel (1995) has used the ample data of the *Ṛg Veda* to write political and social histories of the Vedic period, arguing that a record of politics and kingship is replete in the *Ṛg Veda*. Jan Heesterman (1985, 1993) has traced the intersections of ritual and martial-political culture, hypothesizing that the origin of Vedic rites was a ritualized enactment of war meant to consecrate warriors and that its origin may have been war itself *as ritual*. Though this hypothesis has many challenges (see Whitaker 2011: 164–165), it points toward the martial origins and even compulsions that drove the creation of the *Ṛg Veda* text and its liturgies. Jarrod Whitaker illuminates the "masculine ideology" of the *Ṛg Veda* and how the text poetically and ritually constructs an ideal of martial masculinity. Whitaker traces an "androcentric martial ideology" expressed by the composers of the *Ṛg Veda* and in service to a dominant male martial culture that valorized the figure of the warrior as both a human and divine model (2011: 5, 161). This is particularly clear, as Whitaker says, in the ritualization and mythic origins of the *soma* sacrifice (2011: 5–10, 21). Whitaker suggests that the differentiation between "warrior" and "priest" may have been a later Vedic invention; in the earliest layers of the Vedic ritual world, they were likely one and the same, priests were also warriors, at least in the rhetoric of the text,

though perhaps not in whatever constituted the social world of this time (2011: 24, 29; see also Heesterman 1985, 1993). Steven Lindquist suggests that the portrayal of priests as warriors may have been an attempt by the authors of the text to further arrogate to themselves the power of their political benefactors and may not have any relationship to lived social reality. The text, Lindquist reminds us, is a literary one, not a work of history or social science, and so its ability to represent lived reality is questionable (Lindquist, personal communication 2019). This makes sense for the martial, mobile culture that is described in the *Ṛg Veda*, even if this culture did not constitute the whole, or even a dominant part of, lived social reality in this long period. The text then is one of social, religious, and political *poiesis*, a closed and circular system that makes a literary-liturgical-political world from words. We do not read the *Ṛg Veda* as a report on the conditions of life (political or mundane) in ancient India but rather as a powerful creative literary text, highly influential in the formation of many other discursive worlds, but still only a sliver of the past set amid a much occluded and lost history.

9. See Jamison and Brereton 2014: 38. See also Whitaker 2011.
10. See Jamison and Brereton for Indra as a warrior and the consumption of *soma* in relation to battle (2014: 68).
11. *Ṛg Veda*: 1.162; 1.163; 10.86 and see the royal consecration ritual in 10.121. See also Jamison and Brereton 2014: 32, 33–34. Other royal sacrifices can be found in Book Ten. Maharaja Jai Singh II of Jaipur performed an *aśvamedha* ritual for his coronation in 1741. Our analysis of the *Ṛg Veda* is based on Barend A. van Nooten and Gary B. Holland's edition (1994). Our translations are all drawn from Jamison and Brereton 2014, and we are guided by their excellent "introduction" and commentaries. We are grateful to Jamison and Brereton for their extraordinary work on and translation of the *Ṛg Veda*, without which our study would not be possible in this form, and on the digital text created by Karen Thomson and Jonathan Slocum at the University of Texas, Austin.
12. See Whitaker 2011.
13. See Whitaker 2011: 24, 29.
14. Each of the words given here ("art," "truth," "right," "rite") has an etymological connection to the word *ṛta*, and we chose them as our gloss because of this resonance in English. However, this list of English glosses for *ṛta* could be expanded. See Mahony 1998.
15. The word here is *samīka*, a fight, battle, or conflict.
16. Translation of *Ṛg Veda*: 4.24.3–6, 11 by Jamison and Brereton 2014: 597–598. See also Whitaker's translation (2011: 21).
17. Jamison and Brereton (2014: 14) argue that Book Four is one among the earliest "Family Books" composed within the *Ṛg Veda* corpus.
18. Ferrara 2020: 1–27. See her useful appendix noting all occurrences of yoga given by order of the age of the books of the *Ṛg Veda*. One may count twenty-two instances if one considers the reduplicated compound in *yógeyoge* in *Ṛg Veda*: 1.30.7 as two words rather than one, which would mean eight instances of the word meaning "harnessing a horse to a war chariot for battle" out of

twenty-two instances. A Paninian reading would render it as two separate but repeated words connoting repetition, which is its meaning here. We thank Rich Salomon for his advice on this point. The word index by Vishveshvaranand and Nityanand records nineteen occurrences of the word in some nominal form (1908: 339). In addition, "yoga" appears with prepositions six other times: *jiyog* ["conjoined" or "accompanying"] at *Ṛg Veda*: 1.136.6, 2.30.10, 6.28,3, 10.37.7; *prayoga* ["harnessing"] at *Ṛg Veda*: 10.7.5; *prāyoga* ["harnessed"] at *Ṛg Veda*: 10.106.2. It appears three more times as *yogiyā* ["harness strings"] at *Ṛg Veda*: 3.6.6., 7.70.4, 10.53.11.

19. *Ṛg Veda*: 1.34.9 (a donkey, not a horse, in this case but still yoked to a chariot); 8.67.8; 8.58.3; 10.39.12.
20. *Ṛg Veda*: 1.56.1, *Ṛg Veda*: 5.43.5.
21. *Ṛg Veda*: 2.8.1.
22. Other animals, such as cows—the other prized animal of the Vedic world—are sometimes tethered, harnessed, or otherwise controlled, and sometimes the root word *yuj* is used to describe this kind of restraint, but not the word yoga. In most cases, however, cows in the Vedas are kept in pens or herded rather than harnessed for their power. One possible exception is *Ṛg Veda*: 1.34.9, cited above, where the animal is a *rāsabha*, a donkey rather than a horse, though of the same *equus* genus. This is the only reference we can find to an animal other than a horse being subjected to yoga in the *Ṛg Veda*. Note that this statement does not hold true for yoga when it appears with a preposition (*jiyoga*, *prayoga*, *prāyoga*), but it does apply to the similar derivation, *yogiyā*, or "harnessing strings," which applies only to horses (see *Ṛg Veda*: 3.6.6, 7.70.4, 10.53.11), a curious note for those interested in explorations of the trace of psychophysical yoga in the *Ṛg Veda*. There is a well-known *śloka* in the *Ṛg Veda* (10.136) that describes the *keśin* or "Long-Haired One," a figure that was apparently an ascetic (*muni*). Many scholars looking for traces of psychophysical and meditative yoga point toward this figure and this verse to establish their existence in the Vedic period. However, the verse contains no mention of yoga (even though the word appears in the Tenth Book more than in any other book). *Ṛg Veda*: 3.6.6 contains a mention of "long-haired ones" but of the *equus* sort; however, these long-haired ones *are* described in relationship to yoga. Ferrara (2020, 14) points out that Guillame Ducœur has noted the "horse-like features employed in the description of the Keśin." This would mean that the only *keśin* in the *Ṛg Veda* associated with yoga is a horse not a human. Our thanks to Steven Lindquist for making this point.
23. See for example the *Kaṭha Upaniṣad* (ca. third century BCE), one of the earliest texts of philosophical and psychophysical yoga, where the metaphor of chariot, horses, sense, and self is integrated into this kind of yoga.
24. yóga; *Ṛg Veda*: 1.5.3; Jamison and Brereton 2014: 94. Our insertions are in brackets and bolding here and below. Note the resonance with the old English concept of agonism noted in our introduction, where it meant "the victor's prize in contest."
25. yóge-yoge; *Ṛg Veda*: 1.30.7; Jamison and Brereton 2014: 130.

26. yógam ā́ veda; *Ṛg Veda*: 10.114.9; Jamison and Brereton 2014: 1583. Regarding the "fallow bays" of Indra, these are female horses that are not pregnant. For comparison, see the use of yoga to refer to harnessing Indra's fallow bays to his chariot in *Ṛg Veda* 1.56.1, cited above. Our thanks to Whitney Cox for help on this text.
27. See Jamison and Brereton 2014: 24, for a discussion of the martial imagery used to describe poetry and ritual in the *Ṛg Veda*.
28. *Ṛg Veda*: 10.35.9 describes yoking the "pressing stones" (*grāvana*) used to extract Soma. See Jamison and Brereton 2014: 1433.
29. dhīnā́ṃ yógam; *Ṛg Veda*: 1.18.7; Jamison and Brereton 2014: 111.
30. matáyo áśvayogāḥ; *Ṛg Veda*: 1.186.7; Jamison and Brereton 2014: 391.
31. ṛtásya yóge; *Ṛg Veda*: 3.27.11; Jamison and Brereton 2014: 500. See also the use of *yogiyā* or "reins" in relationship to the yoking of thoughts (*Ṛg Veda*: 3.6.6).
32. ṛtásya yóge; *Ṛg Veda*: 10.30.11; Jamison and Brereton 2014: 1423.
33. The association between the word yoga and the yoking of thought perhaps transcends this Vedic context as well. It is also present in the Avestan Gathas, for example. Here is how Harvey, Lehmann, and Slocum translate *Yasna* 20, verse 10 of the *Avestan Gāthā*: at̰ asištā **yaojantē** | ā hušitōiš vaŋhāuš **manaŋhō**, translated as "And the swiftest [steeds] **will be yoked** to the dwelling place of Good **Mind**." See Harvey, Lehmann, and Slocum 2019.
34. For more, see Day 1982.
35. See Monier-Williams, Leumann, and Cappeller 1899: 938. For example, the word appears here four times in *Ṛg Veda*: 3.27: 1, 3, 8, and 11. The word *vāja* ("war prize") is extremely common in the *Ṛg Veda*. See Vishveshvaranand and Nityanand 1908: 371ff.
36. Mahony 1998: 3–4.
37. See Sharma 1977: 177–191.
38. The word appears most often as a *dvandva* ("copulative") compound (*yoga* and *kṣema*, "war and peace") in the *Ṛg Veda*, but even here and in later texts may be understood as a *tatpuruṣa* compound, a dependent determinative compound where one term modifies another (e.g., *kṣema* from *yoga*, "peace from war," "welfare from security", etc.). In our readings here and later, we find that the word often carries the meanings of both compound forms, open to multiple interpretations.
39. púṣyāt kṣéme abhí yóge bhavāti; *Ṛg Veda*: 5.37.5; Jamison and Brereton 2014: 704.
40. Our thanks to Caley Smith for this insight. While this text does not refer to yogis as such, we are reminded that William Pinch (2006: 103) writes of the seasonal nature of war and ascetic life in Mughal India when yogis and *sadhus* would join military groups after the harvest, alternating between asceticism/alms seeking and war, meaning that many yogis were also soldiers and spies simultaneously. Pinch notes of the eighteenth-century yogi that he was "many things at once . . . ascetic and archer, soldier and spy" (103). As a "yogi" here, the ascetic perhaps fulfilled both the "yoking" for war and for peaceful alms seeking. The relationship through yoga here to seasons of harvest and war is

perhaps also still present in contemporary India where a part-time *sadhu* is derogatorily called a *phasalī*, from *phasal* for "harvest," the *sādhu* who only joins after the harvest. Our thanks to Jim Mallinson for this phrase and point.

41. See Palihawadana 1968: 185–190.
42. pāhí kṣéma utá yóge váraṃ no; *Ṛg Veda*: 7.54.3; Jamison and Brereton 2014: 947.
43. śáṃ naḥ kṣéme śám u yóge no astu; *Ṛg Veda*: 7.86.8; Jamison and Brereton 2014: 992.
44. índraḥ kṣéme yóge háviya índraḥ; *Ṛg Veda*: 10.89.10; Jamison and Brereton 2014: 1537.
45. yogakṣemáṃ; *Ṛg Veda*: 10.166.5; Jamison and Brereton 2014: 1647. See the treatment of this verse in Neri and Pontillo 2019: 144. For more on frogs and poetry in the *Ṛg Veda* see Jamison 1991.
46. Ferrara 2020: 10. See also Monier-Williams, Leumann, and Cappeller 1899: 327, and Whitney 1885: 29, where they note that these two meanings are derived from two verbal roots, as opposed to two meanings derived from one verbal root as Ferrara suggests. However, Ferrara's point nonetheless stands that the word has these simultaneous meanings which we consider interrelated and interdependent. The root that yields "to possess, govern" appears to exist only explicitly here in the *Ṛg Veda*. We thank Jim Mallinson for this observation. It is interesting to speculate on the root meaning of *kṣema*. If it is derived from the roots of *kṣi*, it means at times to "possess" but also to "destroy," and so the meaning of "settlement" indicates perhaps the people one has had to "possess and destroy" to acquire and settle land, but it may also mean the destruction of what once stood on land, as in cultivation of land and its settlement and habitation. The word *kṣatriya* may bear a relationship to *kṣi* as well through *kṣatra*, "domination, wealth, power," and so a *kṣatriya* is one who dominates, is powerful, overwhelms and controls territory but also acquires, destroys, and settles territory, which is to say, governs. In the later two texts studied here, we will see that it is the *kṣatriya* who enacts both yoga and *kṣema*. The interrelated concepts of *kṣema* and *kṣatriya* seem apparently intertwined through yoga in the texts we study here, and perhaps in much wider scope as well. We thank Caley Smith for a discussion of this idea.
47. Ferrara 2020: 13. Here, Ferrara reads *yoga-kṣema* not as a *dvandva*, the way it is read by most translators, but as a *tatpuruṣa*. In this case, yoga modifies *kṣema* in an ablative sense, the *kṣema* derived from *yoga*. Ferrara's conclusion here is very similar to that of Neri and Pontillo 2019: 144ff. In the modern period, the word often simply means "welfare." See, for example, the "Yogakṣema Sabhas" or "Welfare Association," such as the Nambudiri Yogakṣema Sabha of 1908. See also the address by Finance Minister Sitharaman in 2022 and the slogan of the Life Insurance Corporation of India, noted in chapter 2.
48. See Neri and Pontillo 2019: 148ff on the history of this term, especially in Buddhism and Pali, where it becomes synonymous with *nirvāṇa/nibbāna*, the ultimate goal of Buddhist soteriology. They also argue that the term, especially in this context, is a *tatpuruṣa* meaning "security from bondage" or "rest from exertion."
49. Oguibénine 1984: 90, 92.

50. Oguibénine 1984: 93.
51. Oguibénine 1998: 233–236.
52. Ferrara 2020: 10 and 11.
53. The war is underway when Sanjaya (the narrator of the *Bhagavad Gītā*) tells the story of the *Bhagavad Gītā* because we know already that Bhishma is dying. However, the story Sanjaya tells returns to the start of the war.
54. The first translation of the *Bhagavad Gītā* occurs within the thirteenth-century text, the *Jñāneśvarī*, a commentary on the text written in Marathi and culturally located in Maharashtra, the main site for much of chapters 3 and 4. For more on the text, see Novetzke 2016.
55. For example, Tulsi Gabbard and Pramila Jayapal took their oaths with the *Bhagavad Gītā* as members of the U.S. House of Representatives in 2013 and 2017, respectively, and Rishi Sunak took his oath as the prime minister of the United Kingdom on the *Bhagavad Gītā* in October 2022. See Richard Davis (2015) for more on the life of the *Bhagavad Gītā*.
56. See Mallinson and Singleton 2017: xiii; Brockington 2003; Fitzgerald 2012.
57. Fitzgerald 2012: 46.
58. Sāṃkhya refers to a dualistic philosophy based on the enumeration of elements and cosmic forces and is often associated with philosophical and psychophysical yoga. For Sāmkhya in the epics, see Schreiner 1999; Brockington 2003; Fitzgerald 2012: 49ff.
59. See *Kaṭha Upaniṣad*: 3:11, for an extended engagement with chariots and horses as metaphors for the mind, self, senses, and so on. See Mallinson and Singleton 2017 for the most extensive engagement with texts on streams of yoga within philosophy and especially psychophysical practice.
60. Notable exceptions are the work of Alexis Sanderson (2009) on the Śaiva Age; Benoytosh Bhattacharyya (1964) and Patton Burchett (2019) on the Tantric Age; and Ronald Davidson (2002) where yoga and allied forms like *tantra* are explored in relationship to kingship and political power. Although we could not find the word yoga in reference to the concept of *janapada*—a political territorial division in Vedic ancient and classical Sanskrit texts—our theorization of yoga occasioned this comment from an astute reader, Andy Rotman, who noted that we are "positing a certain political relationship of subjugation/domestication where both parties thrive but the hierarchy remains . . . it's almost vassalization . . . this corresponds in some ways to the early *janapadas* and the ways they annexed each other" (Rotman, personal communication 2023). It is beyond the scope of this work to track this relationship, but Rotman's insight is provocative. We thank Rotman for this and for his reading of this chapter and the next.
61. The frequency of the term yoga in Book Three, the Forest Book, appears primarily to concern yoga as superhuman power. For example, this book recalls the details of Kunti's "immaculate conception" of Karna through the sun God Surya (*Mahābhārata* 3.308) as a kind of yoga. See the translation by Johnson (2005: 257): "the Sun . . . entered her by yoga, and gave her a child . . . But the Sun did not defile her."

62. We consider Book Eleven, "The Book of Women," to be the story of the formal conclusion of the war as well as the last iteration in the genre of war narrative that characterizes the preceding books. As the title of the following book, Book Twelve—"Peace"—suggests, the context of Book Eleven is not yet one of peace. Hostilities still simmer and violence still threatens: Dhritarashtra briefly tries to kill Bhima and the Pandavas pursue a fleeing Ashvatthaman. Book Eleven describes what comes at war's end: the meeting of surviving adversaries, the funerary rites and lamentations, especially the reflection on the war's effect by the women who have lost their warrior kin. This suggests that this book holds the formal conclusion of the war, the ending of hostilities, and a shift to a time of treaty, even if it is not a book that narrates actual battle. Book Eleven continues to reflect on the battles of the recent past, while Book Twelve looks to governance in the future post-war world. We thank Nell Hawley for discussing this point with us.
63. See Malinar 2007.
64. See Modi 1950: 88ff. Our thanks to Angelika Malinar for this reference.
65. *Bhagavad Gītā*: 18.75. For the meaning of *yogeśvara* as "lord/master/sovereign of war strategy," see Mehendale 1995.
66. See Malinar 2007.
67. See *Bhagavad Gītā*: 6.10–18.
68. For example, see *Bhagavad Gītā*: 2.47–50, 3.7, 4.1–3, 5.1–2, 5.11.
69. *Bhagavad Gītā*: 6.1–3.
70. See *Bhagavad Gītā*: 6.5–8, 15.11.
71. See *Bhagavad Gītā*: 5.21, 6.29, 8.27, 9.28.
72. *Bhagavad Gītā*: 4.42: *yogam ātiṣṭha uttiṣṭha bhārata.*
73. Mehendale 1995.
74. *Bhagavad Gītā*: 11.4, 11.9.
75. Mehendale 1995: 26–27. This is perhaps a reference to yoga as cosmic philosophy or Sāṃkhya.
76. *Bhagavad Gītā*: 18.76.
77. Mehendale 1995: 26.
78. Mehendale 1995: 29.
79. Mehendale 1995: 40ff. We thank Sucheta Paranjape for this reference and for her astute reading of this chapter.
80. *Mahābhārata*: 6.13.5.
81. Fitzgerald 2004: 140–141. We say the *Bhagavad Gītā* precedes Book Twelve knowing that, in the sometimes complicated chronology and narrative of the epic, the telling of the *Bhagavad Gītā* in Book Six is itself preceded by the account that Bhishma has been felled, and so the *Bhagavad Gītā* as told follows Bhishma's demise, but the conversation that the *Bhagavad Gītā* records does precede Bhishma's death.
82. For the continuation of the subjects and narrative context of Book Twelve into Book Thirteen, see Fitzgerald 2012: 142–143. Much of the concept of "donation" here involves alms and gifts to Brahman men.
83. See, for example, Fitzgerald 2012; Brockington 2003.
84. Fitzgerald 2004: 81–82, 92. Note that Fitzgerald argues that Book Twelve and the management of Yudhishthira's *śoka* or sorrow through compelling

him not to renounce kingship, politics, and war but to learn the moral rules (*dharma*) of governing is a refutation of the Buddhistic kingly model of Ashoka (2004: 114ff, 135ff). Consider also Dr. B. R. Ambedkar's argument that the *Bhagavad Gītā* is also a refutation of Buddhism. See Ambedkar 2014 [1927] and chapter 3 of this book.

85. See *Mahābhārata*: 12.66.33, 12.156.5–10. For a study of the *Āpaddharmaparvan*, see Bowles 2007.
86. *Mahābhārata*: 12.47.34–9, 12.50.32–33. See also *Mahābhārata*: 12.26.3–4, where Vyasa is described as *yogavid*, one who knows yoga, a common statement about sagacious people like him. This is probably Yoga philosophy of some kind.
87. *Mahābhārata*: 12.47.65–68.
88. A common meaning is to do something properly, to do it "by yoga," as in *Mahābhārata*: 12.113.17.
89. *Mahābhārata*: 12.104.32. We thank Sucheta Paranjape for pointing out this use of yoga to us.
90. *Mahābhārata*: 12.106.23–24.
91. For example, *Mahābhārata*: 12.25.24, 29; 12.59.42, 48, 51, 73.
92. *Mahābhārata*: 12.101.9–10, 12.103.26.
93. *Mahābhārata*: 12.68.36.
94. *Mahābhārata*: 12.136, 13, 12.138.51.
95. *Mahābhārata*: 12.120.18.
96. *Mahābhārata*: 12.161.21.
97. *Mahābhārata*: 12.72.16.
98. *Mahābhārata*: 12.97.12.
99. *Mahābhārata*: 12.72.9.
100. *Mahābhārata*: 12.63.29.
101. See James Fitzgerald's translation of this line as "all disciplines of yoga meditation are declared on the basis of the Lawful Deeds of the king" (Fitzgerald 2004: 324).
102. *Mahābhārata*: 12.128.10. We thank Richard Salomon, Jim Mallinson, Andy Rotman, and Caley Smith for help with this translation, although any fault of this translation is the authors' alone.
103. See *Mahābhārata*: 5.36.55, 5.123.23, 5.127.5, 1.60.43, 1.75.9, 1.87.16, 2.63.17, 3.281.102, 5.38.38.
104. The title of Book Five is *ud-yoga*, "gearing-up" for war. The Udyoga Book details preparations for war on both sides, as well as efforts to avert war by diplomatic negotiation. Here, *yoga-kṣema* is discussed as the ability to acquire and hold property securely; the possibility for prosperity; a secure state that can ensure prosperity, safety, and the means for profit; coming to define a state of stability ensured by force; the aftermath of war; and the state of peace and prosperity that is hoped will follow war. For examples, see *Mahābhārata*: 5.36.55, 5.38.38, 5.123.23, 5.127.5.
105. *Mahābhārata*: 6.24.45; *Bhagavad Gītā*: 2.45.
106. See Patton 2008: 28. See also the discussion of this passage and the other in the *Bhagavad Gītā* that contains this word in the work of Neri and Pontillo (2019: 144ff, 148), where they translate the term as "rest from exertion." See a parallel text in Book Fourteen (The Horse Sacrifice) within the *Anugītā* or

selective summary of the *Bhagavad Gītā. Mahābhārata*: 14.46.43: "[One should be] beyond duality, beyond worship, and also beyond self-serving rituals; beyond self-centeredness, beyond ego, and also beyond *yoga-kṣema*."

107. *karmaṇyevādhikāraste mā phaleṣu kadācana* (*Bhagavad Gītā*: 2.47; *Mahābhārata:* 6.26.47). This concept of action without attachment to the fruits of action is a key idea in the *Bhagavad Gītā* and will be essential for its political interpretation in the modern period. Angelika Malinar has noted that this book exemplifies an engagement with *buddhi yoga*, or the faculty of "discrimination," that allows one to be detached from the fruits of actions (2007: 69ff). Renouncing the fruit of actions is also a concept that will be refuted in the *Arthaśāstra*, as we will see in chapter 2.

108. *Bhagavad Gītā*: 9.22; *Mahābhārata*: 6.33.22. See Fosse 2007: 89. Alex Cherniak (2008: 239) in his rendering of the sixth book of the *Mahābhārata* for the Clay Sanskrit Library Series, leaves "yoga" untranslated but preserves the *dvandva* compound: "I bestow yoga and security upon the people who are always diligent, attending to me and thinking of no one else." See a similar passage and sentiment in Book Twelve (*Mahābhārata*: 12.336.67).

109. Neri and Pontillo refer to this "something material, toward which wise men have to become indifferent" (2019: 152). The mundane materiality indicated by *yoga-kṣema* perhaps marks the transition of this term from the Vedic and more simple meaning of "war and peace" or "acquisition and settlement" to the idea of "stable material well-being and wealth."

110. Neri and Pontillo describe how *yoga-kṣema* or *yogakkhema* cross the lines of Buddhism and Hinduism, and in both cases, refer to the "Summum Bonum," the highest good imagined in each tradition, but in different ways. In Buddhist Pali texts like the *Suttapiṭaka*, *yogakkhema* indicates *nibbāna* (*nirvāṇa*) (2019: 153). However, in Hindu texts, they argue the word has both a spiritual and a "secular" or mundane meaning (2019: 147), including "venturing out to conquer new land" (2019: 142) in the *Taittirīya-upaniṣad* and in the *Bhagavad Gītā* representing the "kingly programme" that "provides [a king's] subjects with all they need" (2019: 146). They conclude that, in the *Bhagavad Gītā*, the meaning of *yoga-kṣema* is "inherited [from] the old Vedic secular meaning" as a *dvandva* compound even as it evolved, perhaps in dialogue with Buddhism, into a *tatpuruṣa* compound meaning "rest from exertion" (2019: 154).

111. The one reference to *yoga-kṣema* in the *mokṣadharma* section is strikingly like the mention of the term in the *Bhagavad Gītā*: 9.22: Hari (Vishnu, Krishna) will provide *yoga-kṣema* to those who are devoted to him. In this instance, however, it is not *bhakti* that is the instrument of devotion but rather those who follow the *mokṣadharma*, the teachings of this portion of Book Twelve.

112. *Mahābhārata*: 12.17.7. We thank Hemant Rajopadhyaye for his help reading these several references to *yoga-kṣema* in Book Twelve. The text is a little enigmatic about who is being addressed by Yudhishthira. The flow of the text suggests that it is his brother, Bhima, but Fitzgerald argues that Bhima may be the audience for Yudhishthira's musings about renunciation. Yudhishthira is referring to himself, speaking to himself in the second person in a kind of soliloquy. See Fitzgerald 2012: 200, 694.

113. *Mahābhārata*: 12.70.9.
114. *Mahābhārata*: 12.70.20.
115. *Mahābhārata*: 12.70.20.
116. Bhishma's instruction to Yudhishthira, which continues into Book Thirteen, contains four references to *yoga-kṣema*. However, this section is quite specifically about giving donations (*dāna*) to Brahmans. The consistent justification for this system of patronage rests on the claims repeated throughout this text that Brahmans, not kings, preserve *yoga-kṣema* in a kingdom (*Mahābhārata*: 13.5.30 and *Mahābhārata*: 13.60.18), that the king's wealth and power (*artha*) is the possession of the Brahman, who is the foundation of *yoga-kṣema* (*Mahābhārata*: 13.61.37). A king who does not recognize this dependence on Brahmans for "prosperity" by giving donations of land to Brahmans rules over a kingdom without *yoga-kṣema* (*Mahābhārata*: 13.61.39); only those kings who grant land to Brahmans will see *yoga-kṣema* preserved in their kingdom (*Mahābhārata*: 13.61.41). The exaggerated emphasis on the superiority of Brahmans and hence their entitlement to gifts perhaps sets this book apart from the others on lessons for a king. In any case, here, *yoga-kṣema* is clearly indicative of a state of security and prosperity enforced through the king's actions.
117. *Mahābhārata*: 12.72.11.
118. *Mahābhārata*: 12.73.22.
119. *Mahābhārata*: 12.139.9.
120. *Mahābhārata*: 12.75.1.
121. *Mahābhārata*: 12.87.24.
122. *Mahābhārata*: 12.76.30.
123. *Mahābhārata*: 12.88.11.
124. *Mahābhārata*: 12.88.33.
125. Our formulation builds off the insights and translations of Neri and Pontillo 2019.
126. See, for example, *Mahābhārata*: 12.88.33: cattle traders, who may wander beyond and work outside the physical boundaries of the state, should be warned of foreign dangers.
127. Fitzgerald 2004: 315–316; *Mahābhārata*: 12.80.16–18. Words inserted in brackets are our additions.

2. Yoga as Political Strategy in the *Arthaśāstra*

1. Government of India 2022: 21. Gloss of *yoga-kṣema* is in the original. See *Mahābhārata*: 12.72.11.
2. Chikermane 2022. See the retort from Mallikarjun Kharge (2022), who invoked characters from the epic, in particular, Ekalavya, a "low caste" (Shudra, tribal, perhaps Dalit) figure: "As I understand, this budget is for Arjun and Dronacharya and not for Ekalavya. There is nothing for the poor in this budget."
3. Ramanujan 1999.

4. The Sanskrit phrase seems to read, "I bring welfare."
5. "'Striking Success' Among State Undertakings," *Times of India*, December 27, 1963, 7.
6. For *śāstra* as "theory" and *prayoga* as "practice," see Pollock 1985: 499–519. In the *Arthaśāstra*, *prayoga* does mean "a practical activity," but it does not seem to convey a special meaning set in conversation with the idea of *śāstra*. Yoga, however, as we note here, does have a specialized practical meaning.
7. The *Arthaśāstra* is often sold in bookstores or categorized in libraries under other rubrics, such as "management" and "business," to appeal to modern audiences.
8. Mallinson and Singleton, for example, do not include the *Arthaśāstra* in their timeline of texts important for understanding yoga and mention the text only once, in relationship to female ascetics (see Mallinson and Singleton 2017: 54). David Gordon White (2009) does engage with the text in his book, *Sinister Yogis*, and we comment on that engagement here, but his search is for the yogis and yoga of the psychophysical kind and not for yoga as political thought. We know of no major scholarly treatment of yoga as a political concept in the *Arthaśāstra*.
9. For a sense of this canon, see Mallinson and Singleton 2017. For some of the problems of relying on premodern canons for modern practice, see Singleton 2010, especially the introduction.
10. The *Arthaśāstra*'s first line praises two figures—Śukra and Bṛhaspati—who are considered the origin or authors of two texts in the same genre as the *Arthaśāstra*: the *Śukranīti* and the *Bṛhaspati Sūtra*. We briefly examined these texts for our study. However, these texts were composed much later than the *Arthaśāstra*. The *Bṛhaspati Sūtra* is perhaps from somewhere between the sixth century and the thirteenth century CE (see Thomas and Datta 1921: 8), and the *Śukranīti* may be as early as the sixteenth century or as recent as the nineteenth century CE (see Gopal 1962). For this reason, neither text was ideal for our purposes. However, they are still quite interesting. The *Bṛhaspati Sūtra*, for example, uses the word yoga to mean "employment," especially of people, that is, a "job" (e.g., *Bṛhaspati Sūtra*: 1.77, 179, 2.52 in Thomas and Datta 1921). The text evinces an awareness of Sāṃkhya as philosophy (e.g., 3.35). It also refers to performing a mode of honoring a master (*svāmi*) as a *daṇḍa-namaskāra*, but there's no sense in which this is a form of exercise (*vyāyāma*) or psychophysical yoga. Otherwise, the word yoga does not indicate psychophysical or philosophical practice in this text. In contrast, the *Śukranīti* refers to yoga as both philosophy (4.3.55–59) and psychophysical practice (4.3.114–115; 4.4.147–151; 4.4.161–162), and the text cites *yogaśāstra* (4.3.100–101). See Oppert 1882 for the Sanskrit text of the *Śukranīti*. If this is a nineteenth-century text, as Gopal (1962) argues, it perhaps reflects the intersection of these two spheres of yoga with a treatise on "political science" (*nītiśāstra*) in this time.
11. These links between the epic and the *Arthaśāstra* perhaps move back and forth through time given that both texts are produced over centuries. Neri and Pontillo (2019), for example, argue that the commentarial tradition of interpreting *yoga-kṣema* in the *Bhagavad Gītā* verse 9.22, noted above, "plausibly depend[ed] on the late kingly *Arthaśāstra* ideal" (153).

12. McClish and Olivelle (2012) place the text between 100 BCE and 100 CE. Thomas Trautmann (1968: 314) sets the date for its final form as late as 250 CE. The *Arthaśāstra* is probably based on a text McClish refers to as the *Daṇḍanīti*—"the administration of punishment" (2019: 7)—which likely dates to the first century BCE. A figure calling himself "Kautilya" may have edited and emended the *Daṇḍanīti* in the third century CE, McClish argues, producing essentially the text we have today (2019: 152ff). As noted earlier, Olivelle (2013: 25–31) divides the text into three major phases involving the sources of the text (ca. 100 BCE to 100 CE), the original composition (ca. 50–125 CE), and the later recension (ca. 175–300 CE).
13. Olivelle 2013: 8.
14. For more on this, see Olivelle 2013: 33, 37–38 and Lubin 2015: 241. Our thanks to Tim Lubin for pointing this out to us.
15. For modern commentary of the text, see Banerjee 2020, especially chapter 2.
16. See McClish (2019), especially for the rise of Brahmanical influence he traces between this text's prototype, the *Daṇḍanīti*, and the final *Arthaśāstra*.
17. A figure that we discuss in chapter 4, the Raja of Aundh, recalls in his Marathi autobiography that he studied the *Arthaśāstra* in college at Deccan College in the late nineteenth century, a decade or so before the text's "rediscovery" in 1905 by Shamasastry. He may mean "political science" here, but he sets it besides the *Mahābhārata*, suggesting an engagement with actual texts rather than genres. See Pant 1946a: 118–119, 450, 616; Pant 1946b: 10, 363–364, 469, 519, 523. See also Banerjee 2012: 28 for more on the text before Shamasastry's publication.
18. Ramaswamy 1935: 11–12, 51–52. Cited in Misra 2016: 310.
19. See Spellman 1964, Trautmann 1968, and Trautmann and Das 2012.
20. Strand 2021: 72–87.
21. Misra (2016) argues that the main political fault lines in twentieth-century India are not between Gandhi's rejection of industrial modernity and Nehru's westernized views; rather, they are between those who took a pragmatic, realpolitik view of politics and those who viewed politics as a domain primarily for moral endeavor, a view shared by Gandhi and Nehru. The latter group rejected the *Arthaśāstra* for lacking a moral core, as Misra demonstrates through her reading of Nehru's *Discovery of India*, among other texts.
22. One can mark this transition in the work of Thomas Trautmann, whose 1968 dissertation was a philological and historical study of the *Arthaśāstra*, reprised in 2012 (with Gurcharan Das) as "The Science of Wealth" and published in a series about "The Story of Indian Business" (Trautmann 1968; Trautmann and Das 2012).
23. Misra 2016: 331–333.
24. Misra (2016: 333–334, 335–336) also points out that several politicians over the last several decades—and especially finance ministers—have quoted passages from the *Arthaśāstra*. Two examples from different points on the political spectrum are Congress politician Pranab Mukherjee and Bharatiya Janata Party politician Arun Shourie.
25. In addition to scholarship on how the *Arthaśāstra* can guide business strategy, management schools in India have plumbed the text to offer crash courses

in Indic resources for business professionals. As one example, the Indian Institute of Management in Calcutta offers a four-day executive education program called "Mastering Strategy: Insights from Indic Arthashastra Traditions." Accessed June 7, 2023 at https://www.iimcal.ac.in/sites/default/files/pdfs/IIMC-MDP_MS_Nov-11-15-2024_FINAL_0.pdf.

26. Davies 2013: 49–66.
27. Boesche 2005: 157–172.
28. See Gowen 1929; Sil 1985: 101–142; Boesche 2010: 253–276; Gray 2014: 635–657.
29. Weber 2004 [1917]: 87–88.
30. Gray 2014: 638–641. What Gray means by "political theology" appears to be the Brahmanism that underwrites the last recension of the text, as well as references to Hindu texts, such as the Vedas, and other orthodox Hindu concepts. These distinctions of religion or "non-religion" are highly heuristic when applied to India around 300 CE. This lack of a clear distinction between politics and religion also means that it is not likely that a concept would move in some measurable way from a theological context to a political one, following the classic formation of the idea of political theology by Carl Schmitt, as the two categories would not exist in the same way. It is also not our opinion that Brahmanism or Brahmanical thought and practice constitute a realm distinct from politics. Brahmanical patriarchy has always been political as much as it is religious, a fundamental ideology premised on gender, property, and power. For an astute study of some of these questions of religion and politics as distinct or intertwined in the *Arthaśāstra*, see McClish 2019.
31. Spellman 1964; Bisht 2019: 55.
32. Singh 2017: 359. In this section, she is reading the definition of *yoga-kṣema* at the start of book 6, chapter 2, that we engage below. We have inserted Sanskrit terms in brackets.
33. Banerjee 2020: 45 and Banerjee 2012.
34. For example, Singh does address the word yoga in a footnote, commenting on its appearance in the text alongside *sāṃkhya* and *lokāyata* as one among "various philosophical schools" (2017: 557n12).
35. One place where yoga does seem to indicate "war," as we saw in the *Rg Veda*, is with the word modified by the preposition *abhi* as in *abhiyoga* (e.g., *Arthaśāstra*: 5.37.5), which sometimes means a "lawsuit" or a legal dispute (e.g., *Arthaśāstra*: 2.8.30; 2.16.13; 3.11.33, 38, 41), but most of the time *abhiyoga* indicates an "attack" or "assault" or "to set upon," as in a battle (e.g., *Arthaśāstra*: 4.5.16; 5.1.22; 7.5.32; 7.8.8; 7.13.1, 11–16, 38, 41; 8.4.16; 10.2.17).
36. *Arthaśāstra*: 1.19.32, 4.3.11.
37. *Arthaśāstra*: 4.4.14.
38. *Arthaśāstra*: 4.4.19, 7.14.44.
39. *Arthaśāstra*: 5.2.45, 13.2.38.
40. *Arthaśāstra*: 4.3.23, 9.1.15, 10.6.48.
41. White 2009: 22, 26. See also Shearer 2020: 63–64; Samuel 2008: 237.
42. See *Arthaśāstra*: 4.5.1–18, 1.11.
43. See *Arthaśāstra*: 1.11.4–8, where the text suggests the best spies to pose as ascetics are former, now "apostate" (*udāsthita*), ascetics.

44. *Arthaśāstra*: 1.19.32.
45. White (2009) cites *Arthaśāstra*: 5.6.21–22 (260), 1.11.13–20, and 1.12.22 (298). Of these, *Arthaśāstra*: 5.6.21–22 does not seem to refer to ascetics.
46. *Arthaśāstra*: 1.11.13–20.
47. *Arthaśāstra*: 4.5.1–18. See *Arthaśāstra*: 1.11.1 for *bhikṣukī*.
48. *Arthaśāstra*: 1.19.32, 4.3.11, 4.3.40.
49. *Arthaśāstra*: 5.6.48.
50. *Arthaśāstra*: 13.2.1.
51. See also Shearer 2020: 63–64; Samuel 2008: 237.
52. Many other terms exist for secret agents in the *Arthaśāstra*, such as *praṇidhi* and *apasarpa*, and so on.
53. *Arthaśāstra*: 1.11.1. In addition to *bhikṣukī*, one finds other female figures, such as *muṇḍā* ("female shaven-head ascetic") and *parivrājikā* ("female wandering ascetic").
54. *Arthaśāstra*: 1.11.4–8.
55. *Arthaśāstra*: 1.11.9–12.
56. *Arthaśāstra*: 1.11.13–20.
57. Some *haṭha* yoga texts also seem aware of such phony ascetics. For example, in the *Dattātreyayogaśāstra* (ca. 1100–1300 CE) one reads, "It is a well-known fact that men who wear religious garb but undertake no religious practices deceive people by talking of yoga for purposes of lust and gluttony" (Mallinson and Singleton 2017: 61).
58. *Arthaśāstra*: 4.5.1–18.
59. For example, *Arthaśāstra*: 1.19.32.
60. *Arthaśāstra*: 1.19.32, 4.3.11, 4.3.40.
61. *Arthaśāstra*: 4.3.11, 4.3.40, 4.3.44.
62. For the powers of psychophysical yoga, see Mallinson and Singleton 2017: 359ff.
63. See also the *Harivaṃśa* 96.13–15, cited in White (2009: 259n74) where the word *yoga-puruṣa* is similarly used.
64. See *Arthaśāstra*: 1.21.29.
65. See *Arthaśāstra* 1.11 for an entire chapter of the *Arthaśāstra* devoted to this figure and the use of secret agents.
66. *Arthaśāstra*: 13.4.41.
67. *Arthaśāstra*: 9.3.26–34.
68. *Arthaśāstra*: 12.1.26.
69. *Arthaśāstra*: 5.2.32.
70. *Arthaśāstra*: 5.6.35.
71. *Arthaśāstra*: 11.1.42.
72. *Arthaśāstra*: 1.1.14. See Monier-Williams, Leumann, and Cappeller 1899: 466.
73. *Arthaśāstra*: 1.1.15.
74. *Arthaśāstra*: 7.17.42, 7.17.60, so named after the Hindu deity of water.
75. *Arthaśāstra*: 1.16.34, 7.6.41, 9.3.18, 12.4.29, 12.5.2, 13.2.36–37, 14.3.88.
76. *Arthaśāstra*, for example, 1.18.10, 5.1.54, 7.3.6 12.2.8, 13.2.50.
77. Olivelle 2013: 273.

78. Kangle 1972: 317.
79. Shamasastry 1929 [1915]: 291.
80. Singh 2017: 359.
81. Rangarajan 1992: 546.
82. McClish 2019: 163. See *Arthaśāstra*: 1.4.3; 1.5.2; 1.7.1.
83. *Arthaśāstra*: 1.4.3–4.
84. McClish in his study and textual genealogy of the *Arthaśāstra*, links the concept of *daṇḍanīti* with *yoga-kṣema* through the *Arthaśāstra* source text that he names the *Daṇḍanīti*. See McClish 2019: 163ff.
85. Olivelle 2013: 69.
86. *Arthaśāstra*: 1.5.2.
87. *Arthaśāstra*: 7.5.26. Recall the two instances of *yoga-kṣema* in the *Bhagavad Gītā*, which also prescribes that, while *yoga-kṣema* must be the goal of the warrior-king, he should pursue it without attachment (*Bhagavad Gītā* 2.45) or through devotion to Krishna (*Bhagavad Gītā* 9.22) rather than through attachment to the fruits of his actions, that is, to *yoga-kṣema* itself.
88. *Arthaśāstra*: 7.14.18.
89. *Arthaśāstra*: 7.15.12.
90. *Arthaśāstra*: 13.1.12.
91. *Arthaśāstra*: 1.15.13.
92. *Arthaśāstra*: 3.11.3.
93. *Arthaśāstra*: 8.1.23, 8.4.9.
94. *Arthaśāstra*: 8.2.7.
95. *Arthaśāstra*: 1.13.7–8.
96. *Arthaśāstra*: 6.2.11.
97. Olivelle 2013: 10. Olivelle specifically refers to *Arthaśāstra*: 6.1.1 as laying out the "blueprint for structuring the text."
98. *Arthaśāstra*: 6.2.1–3.
99. Olivelle 2013: 273. This passage has received much attention from scholars and translators because its meaning is not entirely clear. In the notes to his translation of the *Arthaśāstra*, Olivelle (2013: 657) says of the passage above that "the translation of the compound *yogakṣema* poses several problems." Olivelle notes that the term usually means "security or security measures" and mentions the Vedic use as well, which he states is "prominent" in the *Arthaśāstra* (657), suggesting that the sense of war or conflict—what he calls "the trek . . . in search of wealth"—in the Vedic text is still implied in yoga's meaning here (657). However, Olivelle prefers the most literal translation of *vyāyāma* as "exertion" and *śama* as "rest" in his edition (273). Shamasastry (1929 [1915]: 291) appears to move closer to an interpretation that invokes war in his translation, where he reads *śama* and *vyāyāma* as "peace" and "industry," and yoga and *kṣema* as "acquisition (of property)" and "security." Kangle (1972: 317) seems to follow Shamasastry's reading of all terms but prefers "activity" for *vyāyāma*. Rangarajan (1992: 546), a political economist, provides an interpretive translation more suited for modern international relations, seeing *śama* as "nonintervention" and *vyāyāma* as "overt action," implying military action. He also takes

yoga to mean "acquiring new territory," and *kṣema* is rendered as "ensuring the security of the state within existing boundaries" (Rangarajan 1992: 546).

100. See Tambiah 1985, particularly chapter 7.
101. Singh 2017: 309.
102. As Upinder Singh summarizes, the six measures are "peace/treaty (*sandhi*), war/initiating hostilities (*vigraha*), staying quiet (*āsana*), initiating a military march (*yāna*), seeking shelter (*saṃśraya*), and the dual policy of peace or treaty with one king and war against another (*dvaidhībhāva*)" (Singh 2017: 349).
103. *Arthaśāstra*: 6.2.4, 7.1.1.
104. Scharfe 1989: 206–207.
105. See Upinder Singh's discussion of the *maṇḍala* theory (Singh 2017: 308–311).
106. This one exception occurs in *Arthaśāstra*: 2.36.12 in a section on rules for governing a city and for surveilling the movement of people at night. The passage seems to indicate that there is a designated *kṣemarātri*, a "secure night [time]," when, as Olivelle notes, "free movement is permitted" (Olivelle 2013: 580). We believe the implication is that increased security is in place so that the usual surveillance methods (householders reporting to the superintendent the coming and going of guests, for example) is suspended. It sounds like an ancient version of a block party.
107. Ferrara 2020: 10. Also note again Monier-Williams, Leumann, and Cappeller 1899: 327, and Whitney 1885: 29, for the opinion that these two meanings are derived from two verbal roots, not one. The root that yields "to possess, govern" appears to exist explicitly only in the *Ṛg Veda*, but the implicit meaning seems to endure here as well.
108. As noted above, Olivelle understands the terms *vyāyāma* and *śama* to mean "exertion" and "rest" (2013: 273). Kangle prefers "activity" and "peace," (1972: 317) whereas Shamasastry translates them as "industry" and "peace" (1929: 365). Rangarajan prefers "overt action" and "non-intervention" (1987: 546).
109. *Arthaśāstra*: 7.17.1–2.
110. *Arthaśāstra*: 1.11.21, 9.3.35–36, 13.5.17.
111. Monier-Williams, Leumann, and Cappeller 1899: 1053.
112. In modern Indian languages like Marathi and Hindi, the word *vyāyām* means "exercise" but also, especially in Hindi, "martial arts." The *Śukranīti* also appears to consider *vyāyāma* a component of martial arts (see Benoy 1913: 218) as well as the movement of soldiers (Benoy 1913: 230, 253).
113. *Arthaśāstra*: 2.31.6, 2.31.18.
114. *Arthaśāstra*: 8.3.46.
115. *Arthaśāstra*: 2.1.30, 8.4.5.
116. *Arthaśāstra*: 7.12.18, 8.4.20.
117. *Arthaśāstra*: 1.16.29, 2.33.8, 7.13.30, 8.5.7, 9.1.39, 9.2.5, 10.4.16.
118. Olivelle 2013: 273.
119. The text describes the internal construction of the state in terms of barons and ministers; essential properties to be defended, like agricultural land and forts; the arrangement of primary departments like the treasury and the army.

120. *Arthaśāstra* 6.2 is often cited as one source for the ancient adage: "the enemy of my enemy is my friend."
121. Kajari Kamal (2022: 4), in her study of the *Arthaśāstra*, writes that "*yogakṣema* enjoins the ruler to secure the survival of the state including through resort to war (*daṇḍa*). The right use of coercive state power is the central question of Kautilyan statecraft."
122. Our thanks to Andy Rotman, Jim Mallinson, Joseph Marino, and Rich Salomon for advice on this passage.
123. See Malamoud 2003.
124. Weber 2004 [1917]: 33.
125. See, for example, *Bhagavad Gītā*: 2.47; chapter 3 of this book.
126. See Ruben 1926: 355ff, cited in Kangle 1965: 100. The passage Ruben cites is discussed below in this chapter.
127. See *Arthaśāstra*: 1.6.4–12; 8.3.41, 43.
128. See Olivelle 2013: 66–67.
129. *Arthaśāstra*: 1.2.10.
130. For example, see Singh 2017: 557n12; Chowdhury 2020: 175–178; Bisht 2019: 19–20. It is not clear how Kangle (1972: 6) takes yoga here because he simply refers to it as one among "the oldest philosophical systems of India." Shamasastry (1929 [1915]) and Rangarajan (1992) make no comment in their notes. Several scholars have identified this reference to yoga as pointing toward some other philosophical system, such as Nyāya or Vaiśeṣika. For example, McClish and Olivelle (2012: 4n1) suggest that "in this context [Yoga] probably refers to the system of logic, later known as Nyaya, rather than to the well-known system of mental training." See also Olivelle 2013: 468; Chousalkar 1981: 55–76; Chousalkar 2018; Chattopadhyay 1976: 249–250. Kamal (2022: 3) refers to yoga here as "Vaisesika." Dasgupta et al. (1969: 227) mentions this passage but assumes it is part of technical methods of "Yoga concentration" and not explicitly that of Patanjali. Elsewhere in their work, however, Dasgupta et al. (1969: 277) seem to think that all examples of *ānvīkṣikī* are references to Nyāya. Bilimoria and Mohanty (2018: 98) also appear to read *ānvīkṣikī* as Nyāya. This is noteworthy given Nyāya refers to modes of epistemology, including logic, inference, and empiricism—modes of apprehension. These ideas comport with a concept of political strategy based on gathering proper empirical information.
131. See McClish and Olivelle 2012: xx; Trautmann 1968: 314. See Mital (2000) for an argument for preserving the traditional date of composition around the fourth century BCE.
132. See Ruben 1926: 355ff, cited in Kangle 1965: 100.
133. James Fitzgerald (2012: 49–51) comments on Yoga and Sāṃkhya as a pair in the context of the *Mahābhārata*. See also Malinar 2007; Schreiner 1999.
134. Figures from the *Mahābhārata* (and the *Rāmāyaṇa*) are mentioned in the text; however, we could find no mention of the *Bhagavad Gītā* or Krishna, although Arjuna is mentioned (*Arthaśāstra* 1.6.5ff).
135. These are usually enumerated as desire (*kāma*), anger (*krodha*), greed (*lobha*), delusion (*moha*), arrogance (*mada*), and jealousy (*mātsarya*).

136. *Arthaśāstra*: 1.7.1.
137. For example, see *Bhagavad Gītā* 3.37 and 16.4; Patanjali's *Yoga Sūtras*: 2.34, in Bryant 2009: 263ff.
138. See Singh 2017: 127, 142.
139. *Arthaśāstra*: 1.5.16.
140. It is worth noting that the more common term for a school of philosophy, *darśana*, does not appear in relation to these ideas, although both words carry the same connotation of "sight," a way to see something, a point of view.
141. *Arthaśāstra*: 1.2.1. The word is also described as a "specialized form of Vedic knowledge" (*Arthaśāstra*: 1.2.3) and appears in the *Arthaśāstra* only in the first five chapters of the first book.
142. *Arthaśāstra*: 1.5.7–8.
143. *Arthaśāstra*: 1.2.12; Olivelle 2013: 67.
144. *Arthaśāstra*: 1.4.3.
145. Olivelle 2013: 467. Note that Olivelle refers to the three terms as indicating philosophical systems, although he equates "Yoga" with "Nyāya" rather that Patanjali's *Yoga Sūtras* (468).
146. Potter 1977: 20.
147. Kangle 1972: 100, also see Kangle 1972: 99–100, 130.
148. Gupta 2004: 2.
149. Bhattacharya 2012: 134–135.
150. Ganeri 2017: 9.
151. For example, *Arthaśāstra*: 1.5.7.
152. For example, *Arthaśāstra*: 2.7.2.
153. *Arthaśāstra*: 1.4.3.
154. *Arthaśāstra*: 1.4.4.
155. *Arthaśāstra*: 1.2.5, 1.4.5, 5.4.1, 15.1.30.
156. See Pollock 1985. See also Edgerton 1965 [1924], who refers to *sāṃkhya* as "theory" and yoga as "practice" in his translation, as cited in Malinar 2007: 70n29.

Interlude

1. Sanderson 2009. See also the long history of *tantra* traced from the sixth century CE to the present as part of the British Museum exhibit "Tantra: Enlightenment to Revolution" curated by Imma Ramos, https://www.britishmuseum.org/exhibitions/tantra-enlightenment-revolution#explore-tantra. For a succinct engagement with *tantra* with mention of its relationship to yoga, see Hatley 2020. See also Goodall et al. 2020.
2. Sanderson 2009: 253.
3. Quote from Burchett 2019: 29ff. See Bhattacharyya 1964.
4. Davidson 2002: 4. This politicization is apparent in the deep influence within Tibet of Tantric Buddhism and its traditional leaders, who starting in the seventh century CE are also practitioners of the yoga of Tantric Tibetan Buddhism.

We thank Shaman Hatley for this reference and an astute reading of the interlude.

5. We thank Shaman Hatley for making this point.
6. Birch 2011.
7. See Mallinson and Singleton 2017: 46ff.
8. Mallinson and Szántó 2021: 3–4. As the authors put it, in addition to being the earliest text focused on physical yoga, "it introduces many practices and principles fundamental to the yoga method often categorised in subsequent Sanskrit texts as haṭha" (Mallinson and Szántó 2021: 3). It is noteworthy that the *Amṛtasiddhi* is a text composed in and with reference to a Buddhist context.
9. Mallinson and Szántó 2021: 87 (Sanskrit text, section 19, verse 5) and 139 (English translation).
10. Mallinson and Szántó 2021: 42 (Sanskrit text, section 1, verse 3) and 108 (English translation). See also Mallinson and Szántó 2021: 84 (Sanskrit text, section 17, verse 2) and 137 (English translation), and 103 (Sanskrit text, section 36, verse 5) and 150 (English translation).
11. Birch et al. 2024: section 1, verses 12–14.
12. Mallinson and Singleton 2017: 62.
13. The idea that yoga should be practiced in ideal and comfortable conditions is not necessarily the norm across all communities that practice yoga, especially ascetical ones. For example, in Maharashtra, the ascetical yogic community of the thirteenth century, the Mahanubhavs, are instructed by their guru, Chakradhar, to "stay in places where you know no one and no one knows you . . . throw away your life at the foot of a tree at the end of the land." As Anne Feldhaus points out, this yogic-ascetic community seemed to search out discomfort and precarity as the preconditions of their practice; they rejected the yogi's hut and the well-governed land. See Feldhaus 1983: 200. See also a discussion of the essence of these passages in Feldhaus 2003: 183ff. For a discussion of the Mahanubhavs, vernacularization, and political power, see Novetzke 2016: 185–186. Note that in the passages of *haṭha* yoga cited above, and in other texts, the *haṭha* yogi should choose a stable polity but practice at its periphery rather than at its center. From the sample of texts cited by Mallinson and Singleton (2017), one can read that the yogi should "avoid all company" (58), practice yoga "on the top of a mountain or at the foot of a tree . . . [in] empty mountain caves, temples or empty houses" (59), "in a hidden . . . sheltered [spot]" (60), "not . . . in . . . a city or near people," but in "a secluded location" (61) that is nonetheless contained within a well-governed stable kingdom.
14. On Al-Biruni's translations into Arabic, see Verdon 2024.
15. Verdon 2024: 4.
16. See Ernst 1996, 2003, 2005, and Ernst and D'Silva 2024.
17. See Behl and Doniger 2012a, 2012b; Behl, Weightman, and Pandey 2000.
18. Hatley 2007b: 353–354.
19. Irani 2021.
20. See Diamond and Aitken 2013; Diamond, Glynn, and Jasol 2008; Parikh 2015.
21. See Truschke 2016.
22. Truschke 2020: 116.

23. Truschke 2020: 118.
24. Pinch 2006.
25. Bevilacqua and Stuparich 2022. See also Bevilacqua 2018. The current chief minister of India's most populous state, Uttar Pradesh, is a Nātha yogi. See Marrewa-Karwoski 2017.
26. See Burchett 2019; Novetzke 2008, 2016.
27. As Deshpande 2007 describes, in the late nineteenth and early twentieth centuries, Ramdas's legacy became a site where questions of region, religion, and caste were debated and contested among scholars and political activists. We discuss Ramdas's links to early forms of the Surya Namaskar in chapter 4.
28. See Dasgupta 1982; Bhattacharya 2012.

3. Yoga as Revolution in Anticolonial Nationalism

1. White 2009 titles his book after these "sinister" figures.
2. As examples from the press, see "Editorial: Article 3," *Times of India*, March 9, 1891, 3; E. A. W., "The Occult in India: Ghosts and Ghost Doctors," *Times of India*, July 7, 1909, 5; "Yogi Who Used to Swallow Poisons: Fatal Demonstration, Delay in Taking Yoga Exercises," *Times of India*, March 29, 1932, 8; "Swallowing Head of Live Viper, Bombay Performance," *Times of India*, March 16, 1932, 7. For scholarship on this subject, see Pinch 1996.
3. Churchill and James 1974: 4985. The term *fakīr* in Churchill's English parlance would have been interchangeable with the word "yogi." For the elision between *fakīr* and *yogi* in the English public sphere of the early twentieth century, as well as a register of the fear of sedition attached to these terms, see Colby and Williams 1918: 343–344.
4. Davis 2018: 63.
5. Mill 1826: 351–356. Mill's scathing description of yogis begins: "But the excess to which religion depraves moral sentiments in Hindus is most remarkably exemplified in the supreme, the ineffable merit which they ascribe to the saint who makes penance his trade." Negative views of yoga circulated outside the English-language sphere as well, as with Hegel, who believed the practice of yoga epitomized the moribund nature of India and its spirit. See Figueira 2023: 62. See also Rathore and Mohapatra 2017.
6. On Emerson, Thoreau, and Whitman's varied engagements with the *Bhagavad Gītā*, see Figueira 2023, chapter 4. On Thoreau's broader engagement with Indic ideas, including his self-fashioning as a yogi, see Davis 2018.
7. De Michelis 2004.
8. Singleton 2010.
9. See Notovitch 1894. See Kersten 1986 for a recent iteration of this old idea. For a scholarly treatment of this legend, see Joseph 2012.
10. The small group of nationalists we consider in this chapter is meant to be indicative rather than exhaustive. Many other nationalists read the *Bhagavad Gītā* in relation to the unfolding dynamics of anti-imperialist politics, including

Subhas Chandra Bose, Vivekananda, V. D. Savarkar, Vinoba Bhave, and Periyar, and may also have engaged with the text's ideas of yoga. See Gowda 2011 on nationalists' engagements with the *Bhagavad Gītā*, which has chapters on many of the thinkers we discuss as well as essays on Bankimchandra Chattopadhyay, Vinoba Bhave, and Vivekananda. On V. D. Savarkar's engagement with the *Bhagavad Gītā* and *karma-yoga*, see Chaturvedi 2013 and Bakhle 2024. Savarkar's tendencies toward atheism and the critique of Hindu practices he deemed divisive (like caste and cow protection) meant he used the *Bhagavad Gītā* in complicated ways but never centered it within his political ideology. See Bakhle 2024 for a rather startling passage in Savarkar's Marathi writing where he argues that to decenter the worship of the cow by orthodox Hindus one might just worship all useful animals, like a donkey, and he sarcastically proposes the creation of a "donkey Gita" (202–203).

11. See Lorenzen 1978, Pinch 2006, and Bhattacharya 2012.
12. Chattopadhyay's 1882 text is criticized for its retelling of the Saṃnyāsī Rebellion in a way that rendered Muslims no longer partners in the resistance but corrupt local rulers and the reason for the decline of Hindu society. In other words, Chattopadhyay is often criticized for *excluding* Muslims from the heroic aspects of this narrative, an extension of excluding Muslims from the history of yoga. For a detailed reading of the place of *karma-yoga* in *Anandamath* as well as in other novels by Chattopadhyay, see Banerjee 2020.
13. On how colonial-era laws inadvertently made the religious the vehicle for the political, see Pinney 2009.
14. For more on this subject, see Davis 2015 and Ganachari 1995.
15. Chakrabarty and Majumdar 2013: 340–1; Chaturvedi 2013.
16. Savarkar also began his engagements with the *Bhagavad Gītā* while in prison in the Andamans, though he wrote from memory because his text had been confiscated, along with his glasses. In his memoirs, he writes that the act of confiscating his *Bhagavad Gītā* struck his fellow prisoners as unusually cruel, suggesting this was not the norm. The text and his glasses were eventually returned to him. Savarkar also lists many religious texts contained in the prison's library. See Chaturvedi 2013: 159–160. Chaturvedi notes that Savarkar says that he relied on the *Bhagavad Gītā* in particular "to educate fellow prisoners about politics and religion." However, as we note above, neither the text nor terms like *karma-yoga* ever seem to form a core source for his political philosophy. For a comprehensive view of Savarkar's thought, especially as expressed in Marathi, see Bakhle 2024.
17. On Lajpat Rai's relationship to Hindu nationalist politics and Hindu orthodoxy, see Bhargav 2022 and 2023.
18. Lajpat Rai 1908b: 153–158.
19. Lajpat Rai 1908b: 163.
20. On this point, see Sinha 2013: 25–47.
21. *Freeman's Journal and Daily Commercial Advertiser* (Dublin, Ireland), Saturday, December 9, 1899. Quoted in Sinha 2013: 37.
22. It is worth noting that Edwin Arnold held the titles of "Knight Commander of the Most Eminent Order of the Indian Empire" and "Companion of the Most

Exalted Order of the Star of India." Annie Besant, on the other hand, held no imperial titles and was an activist and leader for Irish and Indian home rule.

23. Lajpat Rai 1908a: 1–2.
24. Lajpat Rai 1908a: 55.
25. Lajpat Rai 1908a: 56. Sanskrit *devanāgarī* in original.
26. See the *Bhagavad Gītā* 5.1–2, as well as Lajpat Rai (1908a, 49ff) on this passage.
27. One finds multiple renderings of his name in English. In *Karmayogin* his name appears most frequently as "Aurobindo Ghose," but at times as "Aurobindo" and at others as "Babu Aurobindo" and "Babu Aurobindo Ghose." We follow the now common convention of referring to him as "Aurobindo" throughout. However, he is listed as "Ghose" in our bibliography and citations.
28. Heehs 2008: 142. See also Bose 2010: 123.
29. As a counterpoint, see Peter Heehs's notes regarding Aurobindo's consistent practice of yoga in various forms, especially its psychophysical and meditative forms, even during his highly political period (Heehs 1993: 72, 125–126, 136, 183, 233–234).
30. Ghose 2013: 43.
31. Ghose 2013: 2.
32. The source for the translation is Patton 2008: 44.
33. See, for example, Sartori 2013, which takes up Aurobindo's ideas about the *Bhagavad Gītā* after 1910, when Aurobindo "focused his attention on his spiritual practice, becoming the renowned 'Yogi of Pondicherry' " (320). Gowda 2011 similarly focuses his analysis on Aurobindo's later work on the *Bhagavad Gītā*, leaving out his writings in *Karmayogin*.
34. "Publisher's Note" in Ghose 1997 [1909–1910]: ii.
35. Several works exist on Aurobindo's political thought, for example Southard 1980: 353–376, Varma 1976, and Marwah 2024. The essay by Marwah is one of the few that deals explicitly with Ghose's writings in *Bande Mataram*, *Karmayogin*, and *Arya*, though he does not explore Ghose's engagement with yoga or the *Bhagavad Gītā*.
36. Ghose 1997 [1909–1910]: 9, 10.
37. See, for example, Ghose 1997 [1909–1910]: 24, 26.
38. Ghose 1997 [1909–1910]: 27.
39. Ghose 1997 [1909–1910]: 21.
40. Ghose 1997 [1909–1910]: 25.
41. Ghose 1997 [1909–1910]: 24.
42. Ghose 1997 [1909–1910]: 53.
43. Ghose 1997 [1909–1910]: 136.
44. Ghose 1997 [1909–1910]: 27–28.
45. Ghose 1997 [1909–1910]: 28.
46. For this concept of the "self" in this field of political thought, especially in relationship to Gandhi, see Chakrabarty and Majumdar 2013: 346.
47. Ghose 1997 [1909–1910]: 53.
48. Ghose 1997 [1909–1910]: 53.
49. Ghose 1997 [1909–1910]: 25.
50. Ghose 1997 [1909–1910]: 61–62.

51. Ghose 1997 [1909–1910]: 65.
52. Ghose 1997 [1909–1910]: 461.
53. Sartori 2013: 48–65.
54. Ghose, cited in Sartori 2013: 61.
55. Sartori (2013: 56) proposes that one can understand Aurobindo's *Essays on the Gita* published in 1916–1918 after his departure from Calcutta, as a "sophisticated and self-conscious articulation of the theological underpinnings of the Swadeshist vision at their most fundamental." Rather than seeing Aurobindo as first a political actor and later a spiritual one, we can think of him as a flexible thinker who approached the problem of the political from different vantages over time.
56. Sarkar 1973: 494.
57. Sarkar (1973: 485) also notes that "[b]ut for the vow on the Gita during initiation, there was in fact little of religion in the revolutionary society as founded by Aurobindo and his emissaries in 1902—and Aurobindo states that he started yoga regularly only from about 1904." Sarkar appears to sequester yoga within the realm of "religion," whereas we argue that yoga as religion *and* politics (and philosophy and psychophysical practice) existed not in contradistinction but in synthesis with one another. On Aurobindo, yoga, and religion, see also Heehs 1993.
58. See Ghosh 2017 for an examination of such political activity among *bhadralok* or "gentlemanly" society in Bengal in the first half of the twentieth century.
59. "Delhi Conspiracy Case: Counsel's Address to the Court," *Times of India*, May 2, 1914, 6; "The Delhi Trial; Approver in the Box; 10,000 Revolutionaries," *Times of India*, June 2, 1914, 7; "Delhi Sedition Case; Effect of Reading Books," *Times of India*, April 2, 1914, 7.
60. "Delhi Conspiracy Case; Counsel's Address to the Court," *Times of India*, May 2, 1914, 6.
61. "The Delhi Trial; Approver in the Box; 10,000 Revolutionaries," *Times of India*, June 2, 1914, 7.
62. "Rajabazar Case; Counsel's Address," *Times of India*, May 12, 1914, 5; "Rajabazar Bomb Case; Address for the Crown," *Times of India*, May 14, 1914, 8.
63. "Letter from the Government of Bengal, no. 1366-P.D., dated the—July 1914, submitting a copy of the judgment in the Raja Bazar Bomb Case in Simla Records 2, 1915. Authors: The Hon'ble Sir Asutosh Mookerjee, Kt. CSI, and The Hon'ble Thomas William Richardson, ICS. Government of India, Home Department, Political-A, Proceedings, September 1915, No. 310 (9–33)," 52. Hereafter "Letter from the Government of Bengal 1914."
64. "Rajabazar Bomb Case; Further Evidence," *Times of India*, May 4, 1914, 7; "Rajabazar Bomb Case; Address for the Crown," *Times of India*, May 14, 1914, 8.
65. Letter from the Government of Bengal 1914: 19.
66. "Rajabazar Bomb Case; Address for the Crown," *Times of India*, May 14, 1914, 8.
67. "Rajabazar Bomb Case. Assessors' Verdict of Not Guilty," *Times of India*, May 26, 1914, 8.
68. "Rajabazar Bomb Case. Assessors' Verdict of Not Guilty," *Times of India*, May 26, 1914, 8.
69. Letter from the Government of Bengal 1914: 19.

70. Letter from the Government of Bengal 1914: 53.
71. They were "Deśāce Durdaiva," "The Misfortune of the Country" (May 12, 1908); "Bombagolyāce Rahasya," "The Secret of the Bomb" (June 2, 1908); "He Upaya Ṭikāū Nāhī," "This Solution Is Not Sustainable" (June 9, 1908); and "Bombagolyācā Kharā Artha," "The Real Meaning of the Bomb" (June 26, 1908). For these citations see Kelkar 1908.
72. Kelkar 1908, 350 (p. 3 in appendix "Exhibits"). See also Tilak's statement in one of his articles against the bombing (Kelkar 1908: 355, p. 8 in appendix "Exhibits").
73. See Mukherjee 2020; Sadhukhan 2021.
74. Kelkar 1908: 254–255. For a similar engagement with the semiotics of the bomb in colonial India published just after Tilak's trial, see Pal 1909.
75. For the centrality of *mantra* to many forms of yoga, especially *haṭha*, see Mallinson and Singleton 2017, chapter 7.
76. Kelkar 1908: 368 (p. 21 of appendix "Exhibits").
77. For more on how the British come to view the *Bhagavad Gītā* as incendiary, see Ganachari 1995.
78. In this chapter, we focus on where Tilak draws from ideas of yoga specifically. For recent, more extensive engagements with Tilak's political thought, see Kapila 2021 and Oak 2022.
79. The English translation was published in two volumes in 1935 and 1936. The first volume begins with words of praise from a handful of "prominent personalities," who comment either on the importance of the *Bhagavad Gītā* itself or on Tilak's significance as a political thinker. See Tilak 1935: xi–xxiii. Some of these were the usual suspects—Vivekananda, Annie Besant, Aurobindo, Gandhi. This portion of the second volume, published in 1936, begins with praise from the Raja of Aundh (Tilak 1936: xxxiii–xxxiv), who is the focus of our next chapter. Rather than translate Tilak's text, we rely on the translation overseen by Tilak's sons, which represents a kind of "authoritative" version of his text in English. Where we engage with the Marathi, we rely on Tilak 1924a and 1924b.
80. For a lengthier discussion of the several interpretations of the *Bhagavad Gītā* that Tilak believes to be erroneous, like those by Sankara and Ramanuja, and the Marathi commentary by Jnaneshwar, see Figueira 2023, chapter 5, and Oak 2022.
81. Tilak 1935: xliv.
82. Tilak 1935: xxvi–xxvii.
83. Tilak 1935: 80–81. Tilak equates *pravṛtti* or "advancing forward" with *karma-yoga*, so both terms are rendered as "Energism" in English translation.
84. Tilak 1935: 16–17, 34, 37, 39.
85. Tilak 1935: 16, 35–37.
86. Tilak 1935: 66ff, 76ff.
87. Tilak consistently holds out the possibility of violence when other means fail. See, for example, his challenge to the concept of *ahimsā*: Tilak 1935: 44ff.
88. Tilak 1935: 76ff.
89. Tilak 1935: 79.
90. Tilak 1935: 80.

91. Tilak 1935: 77, 79.
92. Tilak 1935: 80.
93. Tilak 1935: 81.
94. Tilak 1935: 16.
95. Tilak 1935: 78.
96. Tilak 1935: 607.
97. Tilak 1922: 245–246. This was part of a speech he gave titled "Karma and Swaraj"; no date for the speech is given.
98. Tilak 1922: 245–246.
99. Tilak 1935: xxvii.
100. Renan and Giglioli 2018 [1882].
101. Noteworthy examples include Alter 1996 and 2000, Chakrabarty and Majumdar 2013, Devji 2012, Davis 2015, Skaria 2016, and McLain 2019.
102. Kale and Novetzke 2020b.
103. Duara 2015, 228. For more on the varied inspirations of Gandhi's politics, see Rudolph and Rudolph 2006.
104. Gandhi first mentions Patanjali in 1908 (Gandhi 1999: Vol. 9: 222) and continues to refer to him throughout his writings (see Gandhi 1999: Vol. 95: 190). He often refers to Patanjali as a moral philosopher (e.g., Gandhi 1999: Vol. 10: 475).
105. See Gandhi 1999: Vol. 36: 256.
106. See Gandhi 1999: Vol. 17: 34.
107. See Gandhi 1999: Vol. 24: 111.
108. The translation into Gujarati would appear in 1929. Gandhi's commentary, a series of public talks, began appearing in 1926 and included his "Anāsakti-yoga" introductory essay in 1930. See Gandhi 1999: Vol. 46: 164ff.
109. As a note of historical interest, we might also point out that many Indian nationalists found common ground with German nationalism along the lines of the old adage "the enemy of my enemy is my friend," itself an expression of how the *maṇḍala* theory envisions the field of political relations (and the *Arthaśāstra* is its possible source). Gandhi wrote two letters to Hitler, in July 23, 1939 and December 24, 1940, and though he called Hitler a "friend" and spoke warmly of Mussolini, Gandhi urged both men to avoid war. See Gandhi 1999: Vol. 76: 156ff and Vol. 79: 453ff.
110. Gandhi 1999: Vol. 37: 97, 99. Elsewhere Gandhi refers to *bhakti yoga* also as "the sovereign yoga" (Gandhi 1999: Vol. 55: 54).
111. Chatterjee 2004.
112. Chakrabarty and Majumdar 2013: 338.
113. Scott 2016.
114. Scott 2016: 209.
115. Chakrabarty and Majumdar 2013.
116. Chakrabarty and Majumdar 2013: 80–81.
117. Chakrabarty and Majumdar 2013: 80.
118. Note that B. R. Ambedkar articulates a similar position, that Gandhi's nonviolence existed because of violence elsewhere, writing "Gandhi's nonviolence

also is violence in a way." Cited in Kumar 2015: 147 as drawn from Ambedkar's "Amravati Address" (84–88), originally published in *Bahishkrit Bharat* on November 25, 1927.

119. Alter 2000: 28.
120. Monier-Williams, Leumann, and Cappeller 1899: 125.
121. Tilak 1935: 68.
122. Besant 1905: preface.
123. Roy 2013.
124. Roy 2013 provides details of the various incentives that were offered to recruit Indian peasants to the army, including signing bonuses, bonuses after a tour of duty, promises of canal-irrigated lands, and pensions. These incentives had to be expanded when the twentieth century's global wars required a larger Indian army force.
125. See Ambedkar in Moon 2014: 23–98.
126. Ghose 1997 [1909–1910]: 27–28.
127. See Kumar 2015: 147.
128. Figueira 2023:183; and Ambedkar in Narke and Moon 2014: 357.
129. Kumar 2015: 147.
130. Narke and Moon 2014: 363.
131. Narke and Moon 2014: 361.
132. Narke and Moon 2014: 362. It is interesting to note that, although Ambedkar does not engage with Gandhi's commentary, he refers to this sense of nonattachment to the fruits of caste-based actions as "*Anasakti*" in the text (Narke and Moon 2014: 362), a term more closely related to Gandhi's commentary than that of Tilak.
133. Narke and Moon 2014: 363.
134. Narke and Moon 2014: 360.
135. Narke and Moon 2014: 363.
136. For a thorough examination of the competing views of Tilak, Gandhi, and Ambedkar around the *Bhagavad Gītā* and Ambedkar's critique of *karma-yoga*, see Kumar 2015 and Figueira 2023.
137. The word *dhamma* is the Pali rendering of the Sanskrit *dharma*.
138. See Ambedkar 1957: 111ff.
139. For example, two of the earliest and best-known translations of the *Bhagavad Gītā* into English in this time both use this title system. Wilkins titles the chapter "The Grief of Ărjŏŏn," (1785: 27), and Arnold ends each book with its title, in this case "*Entitled 'Arjun-Vishâd,' Or 'The Book of the Distress of Arjuna'*" (1914 [1885]: 6). This convention continues in many translations of the text.
140. Ambedkar 1957: 111.
141. See Kumar 2015 for a discussion of this idea and its tension between Gandhi and Ambedkar as two differing proponents of this concept.
142. Ambedkar 1957: 111.
143. We thank Andy Rotman and Rich Salomon for advice on this point.
144. Ambedkar 1957: 113.

4. Yoga as Sovereignty in Princely India

1. On the heterogeneity of twentieth century sovereignty, including "subimperial states" and other "minor states," see Beverley 2020: 409–411.
2. Some scholars argue that Princely States were the sites of the worst feudal impulses and often aided colonial power, particularly so in eastern India. See, for example, Pati 2005. For examples of scholarship about how more positive indigenous visions for politics and governance were being imagined and enacted, particularly among Princely States in western and southern India, see Bhagawan 2003, Ikegame 2013, Nair 2011, Pillai 2023, and Sagar 2022.
3. Rothermund 1983: 15.
4. The opening sentences of each year's administration report of Aundh states this simply but directly: "The State does not pay any tribute to the Paramount Power or to any other State" (*Annual Administration Report of the Aundh State*, various years).
5. A full history of the fortunes of Aundh's rulers, from the time of Shivaji onward, is given in Rothermund 1983, which remains one of the few scholarly English-language books about Aundh.
6. Quoted in Rothermund 1983: 17.
7. "Satara Conspiracy Case," *Times of India*, September 21, 1910; "Aundh Conspiracy Case," *Times of India*, October 6, 1910; "Aundh Conspiracy Case," *Times of India*, October 7, 1910.
8. "Alleged Conspiracy," *Times of India*, March 6, 1911.
9. The opening pages of Sukthankar et al. 1966 (II), which is the Prologomena to the critical edition, reads: "At a meeting of the General Body of the Institute, held on July 6, 1918, Shrimant Balasaheb Pant Pratinidhi, Chief (now Ruler) of Aundh—the liberal and enthusiastic patron of diverse projects calculated to stimulate research, advance knowledge, and enhance Indian prestige—the president elect on the occasion, easily persuaded by a band of young and hopeful Sanskritists who had returned to India after completing their philological training abroad, with their heads full of new ideas, urged upon the audience the need of preparing a Critical and Illustrated Edition of the Mahābhārata, offering to contribute, personally, a lakh of rupees, by annual grants, towards the expenses of producing the edition."
10. In some images that we have found of the Raja, he wears a sacred thread; in others, such as the film we discuss in this chapter, he appears without it.
11. For the theory of the "brahmin double," see Novetzke 2011. The Raja was not averse to chastising and even condemning his fellow Brahmans and Brahmanical orthodoxy. For example, his illustrated book on Ellora recounts in detail his journey from Aundh to the archaeological site. On the way, the Raja and his large travel party stop in Ahmednagar to see the fort, visit the high school to urge students to practice Surya Namaskars, and address the Nagar Brahman Sabha. Of the last, the Raja writes: "It is said that the Brahman is the spiritual guide of all other Varnas. But the Hindus of Nagar are in such a hopeless

condition to-day that in a place like Nagar which has so large an element of the Brahman population, there are about 12,000 Hindu converts to Christianity. This is, in a way, a disgrace to Brahmans and to the Brahman Sabha. We told the members of the Sabha to think of the situation dispassionately" (Pant 1929 [1928]: 20).

12. Singleton 2010: 14. Mallinson and Singleton 2017 note that perhaps the first mention of the Surya Namaskar in a *haṭha* text is not until the mid-nineteenth century, although the signature "downward dog" (*gajāsana*, *adhomukhaśvanāsana*) does appear in a text a century earlier (95).
13. For Ramdas's philosophy of politics, see his text, *Dāsbodh*, in particular chap. 11, sec. 5 (Bhat 1915: 268ff).
14. See, for example, *Dāsbodh* 16.2.22 (Bhat 1915: 351): *sūryās namaskār*. Here, the word *sūrya* receives a dative caste ending (*-ās*) meaning, "to the sun," so the translation would be "salutation to the sun," which is grammatically shortened to a *tatpuruṣa* compound, *sūryanamaskār* in Marathi and other Indian languages.
15. Ramdas appeared to describe the Surya Namaskar as a form of yoga and as synonymous with the *sāṣṭāṅga namaskār*. In Book Four, chapter 6 of the *Dāsbodh*, in a section on "devotional honoring" (*vandanabhakti*), Ramdas describes how to perform various kinds of *namaskār* to various worshipful things like gods and revered teachers (Bhat 1915: 89ff). Ramdas writes, "One should worship the sun" (*sūryāsi karāveṃ namaskār*) (Bhat 1915: 89 [4.6.3]) and the kind of *namaskār* one should do to these highest of honorable things is called *sāṣṭāṅga* (Bhat 1915: 89 [4.6.4]), the "eight-limb prostration," which suggests that this *namaskār* to the sun is synonymous with the *sāṣṭāṅga namaskār*. In Book Sixteen, chapter 2, Ramdas refers to the *namaskār* being done to *sūrya*, as a form of yoga, when he writes of the practice and others in this chapter: "All the innumerable yogas and ideas about what one should do at the rising of the sun cannot be counted" (Bhat 1915: 350 [16.2.6]). He concludes this section, as noted above, by advising the reader to offer a "salute to the sun" or *sūryās namaskār* (Bhat 1915: 351 [16.2.22]). Nowhere did we read a more direct declaration of the Surya Namaskar as a yoga, but we think these associations are suggestive.
16. See Sarkar 1930: 11; O'Hanlon 2007: 511; Sarbacker 2023: 315; Singleton, 2010: 205. Note that the *daṇḍa* here may mean both "stick" and its common colloquial metonymic meaning of "martial power," as we saw in the *Arthaśāstra*. In other words, a martial exercise fit for soldiers and royal figures.
17. Mujumdar 1950: xxiii.
18. Singleton 2010: 102.
19. See, for example, Alter 2004: 23; Singleton 2010: 124, 180; Goldberg 2016: 184.
20. Pant 1946b: 367–369.
21. Pant 1969 [1922]: 16. The version that we obtained is held in the Bhandarkar Oriental Research Institute, filed under the subject names Nyāya, yoga, Tantra, and Vedānta.
22. The Raja says he stopped doing all other exercises, such as Sandow, in 1908. See Pant 1946b: 381. Perhaps he incorporated things he learned from Sandow into his Surya Namaskar practice, as Mark Singleton has argued (2016: 177), but

his own statements on his practice suggest that, rather than incorporate, he rejected these Western physical culture methods entirely and that his Surya Namaskar is not, from his point of view, a mixture of Western physical culture and Indian exercise or yoga methods. In this way, he is much like Yogendra, as Singleton notes (2010: 118), who also rejected these figures. Singleton's discussion of the Raja does not note that the Raja explicitly rejected these systems, as Yogendra did. And while the Raja does say, as Singleton notes (2010: 124), that he studied Sandow and other methods for "fully ten years," the Raja is specifically referring to the decade before 1908. After that point, the Raja says that he no longer practiced such methods.

23. Pant 1946b: 226, 370.
24. Pant 1946b: 375–376. In our interview with the Pant family, several of the Raja's descendants shared with us parts of an old, torn book with the title *Sāṣṭāṅga Namaskār* and an image of the Raja standing in *namaskār*, which is also found in all his other books. In addition to his name, two other names are given as authors—Ananta Lakshmi Mahajani and Savitribai Lakshmi Mahajani. There is no date or publication information remaining, but we suspect it is a collection of the Marathi articles the Raja wrote around 1920 and published by the publisher of *Purushartha*.
25. This is the date given in the preface to the Hindi version of the book (Pant 1939: 3). In the second edition of the English-language *Surya Namaskars*, the Raja says that the date is 1924 (Pant 1929 [1928]: i).
26. Pant 1939: 3.
27. By 1929 at least, word of the Raja's Surya Namaskar practice had reached Gandhi, who wrote a letter to K. V. Swami that year congratulating him for curing his own leprosy through the Surya Namaskar taught by the Raja. This was a detail that K. V. Swami wanted Gandhi to advertise widely for the benefit of others. See Gandhi 1999: Vol. 47: 244, 244n1.
28. Pant 1940: i.
29. Pant 1939: 3.
30. While the *Yoga Makaranda* does not contain special sections for women in particular, Krishnamacharya (2006 [1934]: 28) clearly states that yoga is for all people, men and women, and people of all castes, and specifically refutes the idea that yoga practice is only for men.
31. Compare this with the guru-oriented practices that form modern yoga lineages.
32. This is a guess on our part based on the earliest references we can find to the film. For example, *The Annual Administration Report of the Aundh State for the Year 1928–1929* records that the "Namaskar Cinema Film was shown by the Chief-saheb in the Parsee High School, Panchgani" (41). From around the same time, the second edition of the English *Surya Namaskars*, published in 1929, notes the film being "exhibited in towns, cities, colleges, etc." (Pant 1929 [1928]: iv).
33. For a discussion of what constitutes *vinyāsa*, see Singleton 2010: 184ff. It is noteworthy that this film was made a decade before films depicting Krishnamacharya and his students were made.

34. For the practice of *naulī* in *haṭha* yoga, see Mallinson and Singleton 2017: 49–50, 71–79.
35. See the following point in the film: 7:04.
36. "'Surya Namaskars'–The Secret of Health," *News Chronicle*, July 6, 1936, 7; "The Yoga Way to Fitness for Men, Slimness for Women," *The Daily Mirror*, July 25, 1936, 17.
37. Louise Morgan, "Surya Namaskars: A Rajah's 10-Point Way to Health," *News Chronicle*, July 30, 1936, 5; Louise Morgan, "Surya Namaskars No. 2," *News Chronicle*, August 6, 1936, 5; Louise Morgan, "Surya Namaskars—3," *News Chronicle*, August 13, 1936, 5; Louise Morgan, "Louise Morgan Gives the Final Lesson in Surya Namaskars," *News Chronicle*, August 20, 1936, 5.
38. Most of *The Ten-Point Way to Health* is either quoted verbatim or paraphrased from the *Surya Namaskars* book. However, two chapters do appear to be expanded versions of Morgan's articles: chapter 4 on breathing and chapter 5—arguably the core of the book—on the proper execution of the ten postures of the Surya Namaskar. Whatever the method of collaboration, the entire text is attributed to the Raja alone, with the exception of the introduction, which was written by Morgan.
39. Pant 1940: i.
40. The title is perhaps drawn from the original Marathi collection of the Raja's essays published around 1920 and noted above.
41. Atre 2009 [1933]: 10.
42. Atre 2009 [1933]: 41. We have discussed above yoga in Ramdas's thought and practice. For more on Jnandev, see Novetzke 2016: 117 and Kiehnle 1998.
43. See Novetzke 2011, 2016.
44. This is a theme from the Raja's *Ātmacaritra* and from his son's recollections (as in an *Unusual Raja*), where both recall how they rejected, avoided, and ridiculed their own father's attempts to teach them the Surya Namaskar.
45. "The Yoga Way to Fitness for Men, Slimness for Women," *Daily Mirror*, July 25, 1936, 17.
46. Pant and Morgan 1938: 44.
47. Pant and Pant 1970: title page.
48. Pant and Pant 1970: 8, 36ff.
49. See, by comparison, Singleton's discussion of the points of view of figures like Yogendra in 1928 or Krishnamacharya in the mid-1930s, who appeared to view the Surya Namaskar as outside the fold of yoga (Singleton 2010: 180–181).
50. Goldberg 2016:184.
51. Singleton 2010: 180; Mallinson and Singleton 2017: 482–483n27.
52. Singleton 2010: 124. See also Singleton 2016: 176–177.
53. Cited in Mallinson and Singleton 2017: 95.
54. Singleton 2010: 180. Singleton also notes this position on the Surya Namaskar and yoga by Yogendra, of the famous Yoga Institute in Santa Cruz, Mumbai, in 1928.
55. See, for example, Birch and Singleton's essay (2019) on a text that may have had the name, the *Haṭhābhyāsapaddhati*, and circulated within the martial

princely contexts of Mysore and the Maratha Confederacy in the nineteenth century (6ff). The "notebook" (*bāḍa*) that contains this text, and may have been an aid in yoga instruction, is in the collection of the Bharat Itihas Samshodhak Mandal in Pune and so likely part of the collection of V. K. Rajwade, a prominent Marathi historian whose primary interest was Maratha political history. The presence of this text on yoga in his collection suggests that he preserved it because he saw it as part of the history of Maratha political power. As Birch and Singleton make clear, the *Haṭhābhyāsapaddhati* may have been the source for some of the "more unusual *āsanas*" in the Kannada text *Vyāyāmadīpike* of 1896 (47), a text also described as containing "wrestling exercises," and therefore also a text of martial arts (57). Krishnamacharya's *vinyāsa* method itself "derived from techniques from wrestling traditions" (59). As the authors write, the similarities between these two texts suggest that "the *āsanas* and exercises [*vyāyāma*] common to both were part of a wider tradition of yoga that included conditioning exercises of a 'gymnastic' nature." (48). Our proposal is that these two concepts are deeply intertwined in the kinds of martial political culture in which both recensions of the *Haṭhābhyāsapaddhati* exists: the Princely State of Mysore and the Maratha Princely States. Following on Birch and Singleton's observation that "yoga's association with exercise (*vyāyāma*) was well established by the time of the *Haṭhābhyāsapaddhati*'s composition," we point out in chapter 2 the much older association already in place between yoga and *vyāyāma* in the third century CE (48). This is *vyāyāma* in a more expansive sense, but the association is clearly present.

56. Pant 1969 [1922]: 11–12; Pant 1939: 26–27.
57. Pant 1929 [1928]: 35. In *The Ten-Point Way to Health*, the section on vision is not present and the section on speech is found in chapter 11, "Health Through Speech" (Pant and Morgan 1938: 81–87).
58. This is a reference to *Bhagavad Gītā* 6.13 and it also appears in the Hindi and also in the English *Surya Namaskars*. Here is the Raja's translation of this verse from *Surya Namaskars*: "(One should sit) holding the back, neck and head erect, immovably steady, looking fixedly at the point of the nose, without looking around" (Pant 1929 [1928]: 35).
59. See Mallinson and Singleton 2017: 59.
60. Pant 1939: 26.
61. Pant 1969 [1922]: 12.
62. Pant 1946b: 381. As noted above, this can also mean "by the method of the Surya Namaskar," but neither meaning precludes the other because yoga is a method. This is the case with the following iterations of yoga in Marathi as well. The polyvalence of this term in Indian languages exceeds that of the term in English, and these uses reflect this much wider scope of meaning.
63. Pant 1969 [1922]: 13–14, 16. These are all described in the *Surya Namaskars* English text as well, but without the use of "yoga" or even "application" in most cases (Pant 1929 [1928]: 49–54).
64. For example, see Pant 1969 [1922]: 8–9; Pant 1939. See also Pant 1946b: 519, 523, 469.
65. Pant 1969 [1922]: 16.

66. Pant 1946b: 131–132. The reference to the Surya Namaskar is clearly implied through "proper exercise," or *yogya vyāyām*, which is the way the Raja commonly refers to the Surya Namaskar in his work. The reference is to the *Bhagavad Gītā*: 6.17.
67. Patton 2008: 74.
68. This differential in semantic range is not confined to texts of the 1920s and 1930s. Consider the two plaques—one in Hindi and one in English—that describe the Surya Namaskar sculpture to visitors in New Delhi's Indira Gandhi International Airport. In Hindi, the word yoga appears three times to describe the Surya Namaskar (the word *vyāyām* appears twice). In English, the word yoga does not even appear once, but rather we read only of "yogic postures." Even in 2011, in relationship to a sculpture created because of the highly popular worldwide practice of yoga, the use of this word differed significantly between these two languages. We thank Radhika Govindrajan for discussing these two passages and sharing her insights.
69. The library extends well beyond these topics as well, with a full collection of books and periodicals on physical culture, diet, nutrition, and health. Titles on asthma, rheumatism, and digestive troubles sit alongside the 1937 edition of K. V. Iyer's book, titled *Surya Namaskar*, given to him "with best compliments from" the author himself. His interests extended as well to history, philosophy, and literature, and all these subjects are represented in his library collection.
70. He refers to five texts: "Patanjali, Yajnavalkya, Vasistha, Hata-Yoga-Pradipica, Amrita-Bindu-Upanishad" as offering instruction about "deep breathing." This reference is in both the English version (Pant 1940:160) and *The Ten-Point Way to Health* (Pant and Morgan 1938: 98–99).
71. See Pant 1929 [1928]: 39.
72. See Pant 1932: 144. The Raja also references *mudrā* in his glossary as "any pose in yoga with psychological significance" (149).
73. Letter to H. G. O. Blake in 1849, cited in Davis 2018: 56.
74. For example, Gan 2013.
75. It is noted by Morgan in her introduction that the Raja gives the royalties for his books to educational charities in Aundh (Pant and Morgan 1938: 16).
76. Oman 1903: 51n2.
77. The original appeared in the *Sunday Referee* (London) on January 3, 1937, under the title "An Old Raja and His Fad." This was reprinted under the title "Tyranny of Fashion," *Truth* (London), January 6, 1937, 11.
78. These associations also existed in Marathi, Hindi, and other Indian languages, including Sanskrit, but in those languages, as opposed to English, the word yoga had a far broader range.
79. Our account of political and administrative reforms is drawn from various years of *The Annual Administration Report of the Aundh State*, the report on the *Administration of Justice in Aundh State, 1940–1941*, as well as Rothermund 1983. Aundh was not alone in embracing aspects of representative government. These were evident in several other Deccan and non-Deccan states, although it would be difficult to say in general whether these were genuine attempts at democratization or more cynical measures taken by royal houses trying to keep their subjects mollified and the British off their backs.

80. *The Annual Administration Report of the Aundh State for the Year 1923–1924.*
81. *Administration of Justice in Aundh State, 1940–1941*: 2.
82. Gandhi 1999: Vol. 79: 91.
83. *The Annual Administration Report of the Aundh State for the Year 1940–1941.*
84. Rothermund 1983 and Pant 1989 include the phrase "Aundh Experiment" in the titles of their books. The earliest use that we've found, however, seems to be as the title of a newspaper article published at the time of the Raja's initial proclamation: "Aundh Experiment," *Times of India*, November 5, 1938.
85. Following Indian independence, Apa Pant had a forty-year long diplomatic career and authored a number of books about Aundh, his father, and his own career experiences, many of which we rely on in our research for this book.
86. Rothermund 1983: xi.
87. Much of the information we present here about Maurice Frydman draws from two biographical essays written by Apa Pant and published in Sri Ramanasram's quarterly journal, *The Mountain Path*: Pant 1991a and Pant 1991b.
88. Pant 1991a: 35.
89. Nisargadatta and Frydman 1992 [1973]: 367, 451.
90. Nisargadatta and Frydman 1992 [1973]: 473.
91. Letter to S. D. Satavalekar, October 5, 1938, in Gandhi 1999: Vol. 74: 86.
92. Letter to Amrit Kaur, November 30, 1938, in Gandhi 1999: Vol. 74: 262.
93. Pant 1989: 36–39.
94. "Aundh Constitution," in *Harijan*, January 14, 1939, in Gandhi 1999: Vol. 74: 408–409.
95. It is worth noting that Gandhi played almost no role in the drafting of India's constitution, a project overseen by Dr. B. R. Ambedkar, as noted in chapter 3.
96. Rothermund 1983: 52. Note that Gandhi also called the *carakhā* and spinning a form of yoga. See chapter 3 and Kale and Novetzke 2020b.
97. Pant 1989: 75.
98. The budgets that we examined from the 1890s include no line item for education spending, which might have existed entirely in local schools like *pāṭhaṣāḷā*, which in turn were traditionally reserved for boys from elite castes.
99. *The Annual Administration Report of the Aundh State for the Year 1935–1936*: 45. A substantial section of each year's annual report is devoted to detailing the state's progress in education.
100. Rothermund 1983: 52.
101. *The Annual Administration Report of the Aundh State*, 1922–1923 and various years.
102. "A Progressive State: Visit to Aundh Chief Saheb's Original Administration," *Times of India*, January 15, 1926.
103. Our brief analysis of Aundh's public finances focuses on the state's support for education. There is more to be said about Aundh finances, including more critical observations about high tax rates, dissatisfaction among members of the Aundh Assembly about the Raja's spending on cultural initiatives, and Aundh's perennial budget deficits (see Pant 1989).
104. The Raja's speech is quoted in *The Annual Administration Report of the Aundh State for the Year 1927–1928*: 37.

105. *The Annual Administration Report of the Aundh State for the Year 1935–1936*: 46.
106. Pant 1946b: 428–429.
107. In 1933, Gandhi published in *Harijan* a report written by S. D. Satavlekar, an artist and Vedic-Ayurvedic scholar under the patronage of the Raja. Satavlekar was also a scholar of yoga as classical Indic medicine. Satavlekar's assessment of the Raja's efforts in 1933 suggest that the Aundh government attempted to end certain aspects of caste discrimination against "Untouchables," such as allowing universal unrestricted temple entry and access to water in exchange for commitments to give up consuming the meat of dead animals and to bathe regularly. On the former, the members of deemed "Untouchable" communities in Aundh were "indifferent as regards temple-entry"; pointed out that bathing required water, to which they were not allowed access; and said that the eating of dead animals was the only means of sustenance allowed by the systems of caste in place. The Raja appears to address each issue in turn but is unable to resolve the issue of "carrion" because the dominant non-Brahman caste, the report says, believed the Dalit community to be poisoning cattle on purpose. Satavlekar suggests that caste conflict in Aundh is primarily between Maratha castes and Dalit castes, and internal to Dalit castes: "Temples visited by the Harijans are boycotted for the most part by non-Brahmins . . . [t]he Mahar among . . . [Dalits] regards himself as superior to the five Mangs . . . [w]hen they sit down to feed in my house, they decline to sit in the same row." See Gandhi 1999: Vol. 60: 152–155. One should note that this assessment by Gandhi, whether factual or not, conforms to his elite caste patriarchal ideas about Dalit castes, labor, and cleanliness. See, for example, Joel Lee 2021: 121ff, or Gandhi's essay, "The Ideal Bhangi," in *Harijan*, November 28, 1936, in Gandhi 1999: Vol. 70: 126–128.
108. "Karve's College: Advice to Women," *Times of India*, January 8, 1925, 8.
109. "Education of Women, Physical Culture: India's Most Urgent Problem," *Times of* India, October 26, 1926, 10.
110. Pant 1940: 1.
111. Pant 1940: 71–72. The references to figures in the quotation are in sequence: a Chitpavan Brahman general (*senapatī*) of the Peshwa who died in 1818 in a battle against the British East India Company forces, a reference to the Raja's own ancestors, a Maratha ruler of Ujjain in the late eighteenth century, a Maratha general who led successful campaigns to expand Maratha rule in northern India. Notably such passages from *Surya Namaskar* are missing in *The Ten-Point Way to Health*. Our sense is that, more than toning down religious content (as Sarbacker [2023] has noted), the Raja tones down political content in the latter publication.
112. *The Annual Administration Report of the Aundh State for the Year 1927–1928*: 5, and various years.
113. "Physical Culture at Poona," *Times of India*, April 2, 1930, 13.
114. *The Annual Administration Report of the Aundh State for the Year 1933–1934*: 42.
115. " 'Surya Namaskar' in Schools," *Times of India*, February 21, 1934, 6.
116. "Compulsory Physical Training: Poona Colleges' Experiment," *Times of India*, November 15, 1927, 12.

117. *The Annual Administration Report of the Aundh State for the Year 1932–1933*: 4; *The Annual Administration Report of the Aundh State for the Year 1935–1936*: 3.
118. "Physical Culture in Mysore: Special Training Classes," *Times of India*, June 19, 1929, 7.
119. Singleton 2010: 179.
120. Goldberg 2016.
121. Birch and Singleton 2019. The text has no title, but the authors surmise the title may have been *Haṭhābhyāsapaddhati*. They speculate the date of the text to be the eighteenth century, but the two extant copies they consult are from the nineteenth century—one from Mysore and one from Pune.
122. We do not argue that Krishnamacharya's practices are derivative of the Raja's Surya Namaskar. Krishnamacharya's system is distinct from the Raja's Surya Namaskar. We also do not argue that the Raja's Surya Namaskar is the source of the whole of modern yoga. We are only interested in this moment of intersection around the Surya Namaskar at the cusp of the explosion of modern yoga across the globe, a process in which both the Raja and Krishnamacharya are key figures. We thank Mark Singleton for making this point.
123. Singleton 2010: 8.
124. Birch and Singleton (2019), drawing on their study of the *Haṭhābhyāsapaddhati* (ca. eighteenth century to nineteenth century), suggest they may see in and around this text the influence and presence of "Indian martial arts and wrestling" and "a yogic adaptation of some military training methods . . . widespread throughout South Asia before India was demilitarized by the British" (65). We argue that this "influence and presence" is a result of the genealogy of this strand of yoga that comes from and through the martial cultures of the Princely States.
125. Manjapra 2012: 60.
126. As Manjapra 2014: 146 puts it, "Both German and Indian economics in the nineteenth and twentieth centuries were responding to the ideology of laissez-faire universalism associated with Adam Smith—the ideology that directed British liberal imperialism."
127. Gerschenkron 1962.
128. Quoted in Manjapra 2014: 148.
129. *The Annual Administration Report of the Aundh State for the Year 1937–1938*: 21–23.
130. *The Annual Administration Report of the Aundh State for the Year 1942–1943*: 18.
131. According to the Memorandum of Association of Kirloskar Brothers, Limited, filed in 1920, the Raja of Aundh's capital contribution equaled that of Laxman Kirloskar and he served as one of the company's seven initial directors. Government of India National Archives. Kirloskar Brothers & Shivaji Works, 1936, PP_000000010085, Roll_00012_File_No_75, PA_Microfilm_Digitized Private Papers of M. R. Jayakar.
132. *The Annual Administration Report of the Aundh State for the Year 1937–1938*: 20–21.
133. "Aundh State: Industrial Progress," *Times of India*, September 14, 1923, A7.
134. "Aundh State: Industrial Development," *Times of India*, December 1, 1922, A4.
135. Our translation from the original Marathi. See Madgulkar 2021 [1963]: 123.

136. This is both recorded in the annual administration reports and recollected by his son Appa Pant in a foreword for Rothermund 1983: xvi.
137. Pant 1991b: 126.
138. Tupe 2000: 248.
139. We could find no scholarship on Swatantrapur itself, although Rothermund (1983: 50–51) refers to it by name, as does Apa Pant in several of his books. There also was no mention of Swatantrapur in any of the Aundh annual administration reports that we consulted, which included most reports from 1909–1910 until 1942–1943. Although the prison was established in 1939, it became functional only in 1944.
140. Pant 1989: 85.
141. For example, without mentioning either Aundh or its Raja, one recent news story tells that the open prison was established in "pre-independent India as an experiment influenced by Mahatma Gandhi's 'self-rule' principle and his philosophy of love and compassion." Debasish Panigrahi, "Swatantrapur Vasahat: Life Inside a Prison Without Walls," *Hindustan Times*, August 22, 2016.
142. In recent scholarship on open prisons in India (Senapaty 2023; Goyal 2021), there is no discussion of Aundh or Swatantrapur, although Goyal notes that it served as inspiration for the film by V. Shantaram. We spell the film's title in English as it is spelled in English in most of its advertising posters.
143. Madgulkar 2021 [1963]. One chapter, entitled "Aundh's Raja," recalls Madgulkar's childhood memories in Aundh, all of which deepens the view that we have from other sources of the Raja as a humane ruler and Aundh as a tiny but remarkable polity. Among the topics Madgulkar writes about are the Raja's attentiveness to the Surya Namaskar practice on his annual tours of Aundh, his opposition to untouchability (Madgulkar 2021 [1963]: 12), and how the author personally benefitted from the Raja's educational investments (128).
144. Our thanks to Anand Madgulkar, G. D. Madgulkar's son, who shared with us these details about Madgulkar's initial plans to write about Swatantrapur in an interview held in Pune at the Madgulkar family home, Panchavati.
145. Alter 2000: 103.
146. Kapila 2021: 6.
147. Quoted in Alter 2000: 93–94.

Conclusion: Yoga Infrastructure in India's Bureaucracy

1. One important exception is the ethnographic work of Bevilacqua 2018. See also Bevilacqua and Stuparich 2022.
2. See Jain 2020, especially chapter 5; Black 2024.
3. Kale and Novetzke 2020a. We thank Gavin Flood and Oxford University Press for permission to use some material from this publication here.
4. See Alter 2004; Singleton 2010.

5. "School for Training Yoga Teachers: Santa Cruz Institute Recognized by Govt," *Times of India*, July 13, 1958, 3; "Training in Yoga for Teachers: Camp at Lonavala," *Times of India*, March 26, 1959, 3.
6. "Training of Yoga Teachers: Govt. Grant for Institute," *Times of India*, May 24, 1959, 13.
7. Bharat Sevak Samaj (National Development Agency), n.d., "Know About Bharat Sevak Samaj," http://www.bssve.in/knowaboutbss.asp.
8. "Practise Yogic Exercises: Premier's Advice to Youth," *Times of India*, August 27, 1956, 3.
9. Responding to a question in parliament, Secretary to the Education Minister Mohan Das said that the center was prepared to give advice and grants to the states to promote yoga, but the implementation of yoga would be left to the state governments' education ministries: "Propagation of Yoga: Centre Prepared to Give Grants," *Times of India*, September 21, 1954, 11.
10. "National Policy on Education, 1986" sec. 8.21: 30.
11. Aggarwal 2002: 28.
12. Four stamps were issued in 1991. In 2016, the Indian government, under Narendra Modi, issued a set of twelve stamps, this time depicting the Surya Namaskar sequence. India was not alone in public commemorations of yoga. In 2011, the Chinese government issued a set of eight stamps portraying famous yoga guru B. K. S. Iyengar performing *āsanas*, released in conjunction with the China-India Yoga Summit held in Guangzhou in June 2011, which Iyengar attended. This occurred during the rule of Congress leader Manmohan Singh, the same year in which the Surya Namaskar sculpture was erected in Indira Gandhi International Airport.
13. National Curriculum Frameworks 1988: 31.
14. National Curriculum Frameworks 1988: 31.
15. National Curriculum Frameworks 2000: 48–9, 73–4, 87, 93.
16. National Curriculum Frameworks 2000: 13.
17. National Curriculum Frameworks 2000: 13–14. Newton refers to Isaac Newton (1642–1727), the English astronomer, scientist, and mathematician; Aryabhatta refers to an Indian mathematician, astronomer, and scientist who is said to have lived about 500 CE.
18. National Curriculum Frameworks 2000: 54.
19. See, for example, Truschke 2016 on Sanskrit in Mughal India.
20. Kale and Novetzke 2020a.
21. "Yoga Secular Practice, Says Ramdev," *Times of India*, June, 20, 2016, online edition; "Yoga Is 'Carrier of India's Spiritual Tradition': Yogi Adityanath," *Deccan Herald*, June 21, 2020, online edition; "Yoga Has No Religion, Can Become a Binding Force for World: PM Modi," *Business Standard*, June 22, 2018, online edition.
22. National Curriculum Framework 2000: 87.
23. Permanent Mission of India to the UN, 2014, "Statement by H. E. Narendra Modi, Prime Minister of India at the General Debate of the 69th Session of the United Nations General Assembly on September 27, 2014." Government of India, https://pminewyork.gov.in/IndiaatUNGA?id=NjUy.

24. "SC to Hear Plea on Making Yoga Compulsory at School, 2016," *The Hindu*, November 4, 2016, updated December 20, 2016, online edition, http://www.thehindu.com/news/national/SC-to-hear-plea-on-making-yoga-compulsory-at-school/article16436611.ece.
25. For example, see the introduction of a yoga textbook by the National Council of Educational Research and Training in 2015; and Akshaya Mikul, 2014, "NCERT Books a Yoga Day Date for Students," *Times of India*, updated June 8, 2015, online edition, http://timesofindia.indiatimes.com/india/NCERT-books-a-yoga-day-date-for-students/articleshow/47592916.cms?, accessed June 14, 2017. For another example, see National Council of Educational Research and Training, 2010, "Scheme on Quality Improvement in Schools: Component of Introduction of Yoga in Schools." This government policy document addresses the fact that the need for yoga teacher training expressed in the 1986 National Policy on Education and reiterated in the 2005 National Curriculum Framework had yet to materialize by 2010.
26. Interview with NCERT official, New Delhi.
27. National Education Policy 2016: 101.
28. Kale and Novetzke 2020a.
29. National Education Policy 2020: 4, 16.
30. National Education Policy 2020: 39, 53.
31. National Education Policy 2020: 50.
32. National Education Policy 2020: 55.
33. National Curriculum Framework 2023.
34. National Curriculum Framework 2023: 42, 47, 55, 387, 389, 392, 408, 413, 490, 541.
35. National Curriculum Framework 2023: 76, 390.
36. National Curriculum Framework 2023: 258, 483–484.
37. National Curriculum Framework 2023: 389, 480. For more on *mallakhāṃba* and yoga, see McCartney 2023.
38. In an interview, an official associated with the Ministry of Ayush mentioned the relationship between yoga and martial arts, especially *kalarīppāyaṭṭu*.
39. For example, during the COVID-19 pandemic, the Ministry of Ayush released a document detailing a "yoga protocol" for the mitigation of COVID-19 symptoms that emphasized Ayurvedic treatments but also included an extensive list of yoga *āsanas* and breathing techniques. See "National Clinical Management Protocol Based on Ayurveda and Yoga for Management of COVID-19," Ministry of Ayush, Government of India, no date.
40. Desai had previously served in the cabinet of Indira Gandhi, but once the Congress Party split in 1969, Desai joined the opposing flank. In the elections held after the Emergency period, Desai led the Janata Party in opposition to Indira Gandhi's faction of Congress and won, serving as prime minister from 1977 to 1979.
41. *Haṭhapradīpikā*, chapter 3, verses 94–95. See Mallinson et al. 2024, online.
42. According to Frank's (2002) biographical account of Indira Gandhi, Brahmachari first enters her orbit in 1958, when he arrives in Delhi impoverished, after accusations of sexual impropriety had forced him to leave Kashmir. Ten

years earlier, in 1950, however, India's Films Division produced an eighteen-minute English-language film, *Sukshma Vyayam: A Better Way to Health*, that features Dhirendra Brahmachari, with three other male yogis, performing a variety of *prāṇayāma* practices and *haṭha* yoga poses. In the next decades, the Films Division would make only a few additional films about yoga (in 1972 and 1998) until 2015, when a cluster of films was produced in rapid succession (2015, 2016, 2016, 2017), demonstrating the greater weight given to yoga after the Bharatiya Janata Party's (BJP) return to power in 2014.

43. Frank 2002. The Nehru-Gandhi family members weren't the only followers of Brahmachari. Many others at the highest echelons of Indian politics were also adherents of Brahmachari, including Morarji Desai, Lal Bahadur Shastri, Jayaprakash Narayan, and Rajendra Prasad. Brahmachari was not the only influential yogic figure. Nemichand Jain, aka, Chandraswami, was also closely associated with several political figures, including former Indian Prime Minister V. P. Narasimha Rao. For more on him and Brahmachari, see Jaffrelot in Copeman and Ikegama 2012: 85ff.
44. "Dhirendra Brahmachari, Yoga Master, 1970," *New York Times*, June 10, 1994.
45. See "From Toilet to Loneliness: The Most Weird [*sic*] Ministries Across the World," *Economic Times*, January 24, 2018. The article lists unusual government departments across the world. India's "Ministry of Yoga" is deemed the second weirdest in this article just after the United Kingdom's "Ministry of Loneliness."
46. See, for example, McCartney 2019; Puri 2019; Jain 2020; Lakshmi 2020; Miller 2020; Black 2024; Sood 2023.
47. See South Asia Scholar Activist Collective, 2023, *Hindutva Harassment Field Manual*, New York, https://www.hindutvaharassmentfieldmanual.org.
48. Kale and Novetzke 2016.

Bibliography

Primary Sources

Akers, Brian. 2002. *The Hatha Yoga Pradipika*. Woodstock, NY: YogaVidya.

Ambedkar, B. R. 1957. *The Buddha and His Dhamma*. Mumbai: Siddharth College Publications.

Ambedkar, B. R. 2014 [1927]. "Essays on the Bhagwat Gita: Philosophic Defense of Counter-Revolution: Krishna and His Gita." In *Dr. Babasaheb Ambedkar Writings and Speeches*, Vol. 3. Edited by Hari Narke and Vasant Moon, 357–380. Mumbai: Government of Maharashtra.

Arthaśāstra = Kangle 1969.

Arnold, Edwin. 1914 [1885]. *The Song Celestial or Bhagavad-Gîtâ*. London: Kegan Paul, Trench, Trübner.

Belvalkar, Shripad Krishna, ed. 1968. *The Bhagavadgītā: Being Reprint of Relevant Parts of the Bhīṣmaparvan from B. O. R. Institutes Edition of the Mahābhārata*. Second repr. Poona: Bhandarkar Oriental Research Institute.

Besant, Annie, and Bhagavan Das. 1905. *The Bhagavad-Gîtâ*. London: Theosophical Publishing Society.

Bhagavadgītā = Belvalkar 1968.

Bhat, Achyut Chitaman, ed. 1915. *Śrīsamarth Rāmadāsasvāmī-viracit Śrīdāsbodh*. Pune: Bhaṭ āṇi Manḍaḷī.

Birch, Jason, Mitsuyo Demoto, Jürgen Hanneder, Nils Liersch, and James Mallinson, eds. 2024. *Haṭhapradīpikā*. http://hathapradipika.online.

Bryant, Edwin. 2009. *The Yoga Sūtras of Patañjali: A New Edition, Translation, and Commentary with Insights from the Traditional Commentators*. E-book. New York: North Point.

Dāsbodh = Bhat 1915.

Gandhi, Mohandas Karamchand. 1999. *The Collected Works of Mahatma Gandhi* [Electronic Book]. Vols. 1–98. Delhi: Publications Division, Ministry of Information and Broadcasting, Government of India.

Ghose, Aurobindo. 1997 [1909–1910]. *Complete Works of Sri Aurobindo.* Vol. 8. Pondicherry: Sri Aurobindo Ashram Trust.

Ghose, Aurobindo. 2002 [1880–1908]. *Bande Mataram: Political Writings and Speeches.* Vol. 6–7. Pondicherry: Sri Aurobindo Ashram Trust.

Ghose, Aurobindo. 2013 [1906–1910]. *Tales of Prison Life* v2@2013. E-book. Pondicherry: Sri Aurobindo Institute of Culture.

Haṭhapradīpikā = Birch et al. 2024.

Jamison, Stephanie W., and Joel P. Brereton. 2014. *The Rigveda: The Earliest Religious Poetry of India.* New York: Oxford University Press.

Kangle, R. P., ed. 1969. *The Kauṭilīya Arthaśāstra: A Critical Edition with Glossary.* Part I. 2nd ed. Bombay: University of Bombay.

Kelkar, N. C., ed. 1908. *The Full & Authentic Report of the Tilak Trial.* Bombay: The Indu-Prakash Steam.

Krishnamacharya, T. 2006. *Yoga Makaranda or Yoga Saram (The Essence of Yoga) First Part.* Translated by C. M. V. Krishnamacharya and S. Ranganathadesikacharya. Madurai: Madurai C. M. V. Press. Original Kannada ed. in 1934. Original Tamil ed. in 1938.

Madgulkar, Gajanan Digambar. 2021 [1963]. *Mantaralele Divas* [*Magical Days*]. Aurangabad: Saket Prakashan.

Mahābhārata = Sukthankar et al. 1966.

Mallinson, James. 2004. *The Gheraṇḍa Saṁhitā: The Original Sanskrit and an English Translation.* Woodstock, NY: YogaVidya.

Mallinson, James. 2007. *The Śiva Saṁhitā: A Critical Edition and an English Translation.* Translated by James Mallinson. Woodstock, NY: YogaVidya.

Mallinson, James. 2024. *The Dattātreyayogaśāstra.* Collection Indologie 153. Haṭha Yoga Series 5. Pondicherry, India: Intitut Français de Pondichéry.

Mallinson, James, and Péter-Dániel Szántó. 2021. *The Amṛtasiddhi; and, Amṛtasiddhimūla: The Earliest Texts of the Haṭhayoga Tradition.* Pondicherry, India: Intitut Français de Pondichéry.

Moon, Vasant, ed. 2014. *Dr. Babasaheb Ambedkar Writings and Speeches Vol. I.* New Delhi: Government of India.

Morgan, Louise. 1936. "Surya Namaskars: A Rajah's 10-Point Way to Health." *News Chronicle.* July 30, 5.

Morgan, Louise. 1936. "Surya Namaskars No. 2." *News Chronicle.* August 6, 5.

Morgan, Louise. 1936. "Surya Namaskars—3." *News Chronicle.* August 13, 5.

Morgan, Louise. 1936. "Louise Morgan Gives the Final Lesson in Surya Namaskars." *News Chronicle.* August 20, 5.

Mujumdar, Dattatraya Chintaman. 1950. *Encyclopedia of Indian Physical Culture; A Comprehensive Survey of the Physical Education in India, Profusely Illustrating Various Activities of Physical Culture, Games, Exercises, Etc., as Handed over to Us from Our Fore-Fathers and Practised in India.* Baroda: Good Companions.

Narke, Hari, and Vasant Moon. 2014. *Dr. Babasaheb Ambedkar Writings and Speeches.* Vol. 3. 2nd ed. New Delhi: Government of India.

Nisargadatta, Maharaj, and Maurice Frydman. 1992 [1973]. *I Am That*. Durham, NC: Acorn.

Olivelle, Patrick. 2013. *King, Governance, and Law in Ancient India: Kautilya's Arthashastra: A New Annotated Translation*. New York: Oxford University Press.

Oppert, Gustav, ed. 1882. *Śukranītisāra*. Madras: Government Press.

Pal, Bipin Chandra. 1909. "The Etiology of the Bomb in Bengal." *Swaraj* (London). June 16.

Panigrahi, Debasish. 2016. "Swatantrapur Vasahat: Life Inside a Prison Without Walls." *Hindustan Times*. August 22.

Pant, Apa. 1989. *An Unusual Raja: Mahatma Gandhi and the Aundh Experiment*. Hyderabad: Sangam.

Pant, Apa B. 1991a. "Maurice Frydman: An Early Devotee." *Mountain Path* 28 (1–2): 31–36.

Pant, Apa B. 1991b. "Maurice Frdyman." *Mountain Path* 28 (3–4): 125–128.

Pant, Apa, and Bhawanrao Srinivasrao Pant. 1970. *Surya Namaskars, an Ancient Indian Exercise*. Bombay: Orient Longmans.

Pant, Bhawanrao Srinivasarao. 1929 [1928]. *Surya Namaskars*. English, 2nd ed. Aundh: R. K. Kirloskar.

Pant, Bhawanrao Srinivasrao. 1932. *Ajanta: A Handbook of Ajanta Caves Descriptive of the Paintings and Sculptures Therein*. Bombay: D. B. Taraporevala.

Pant, Bhawanrao Srinivasarao. 1939. *Sūrya-Namaskār*. Hindi. N.p.: n.p.

Pant, Bhawanrao Srinivasarao. 1940. *Surya Namaskars*. 5th ed. English. Aundh: Aundh State Press.

Pant, Bhawanrao Srinivasarao. 1946a. *Ātmacaritra: Khaṇḍa Pahilā*. Vol. 1. Marathi. Aundha: Da. Ga. Kulakarṇī.

Pant, Bhawanrao Srinivasarao. 1946b. *Ātmacaritra: Khaṇḍa Dusarā*. Vol. 2. Marathi. Aundha: Da. Ga. Kulakarṇī.

Pant, Bhawanrao Srinivasrao. 1969 [1922]. *Sūryanamaskār*. 9th ed. Marathi. Pune: Vyāyāmaviṣayak Eka Prakāśan.

Pant, Bhawanrao Srinivasrao, and Ramchandra Dattatraya Ranade. 1929. *Ellora: A Handbook of Verul (Ellora Caves)*. Bombay: D. B. Taraporevala.

Pant, Bhawanrao Srinivasrao, and Louise Morgan. 1938. *The Ten-Point Way to Health: Surya Namaskars*. London: Dent.

Rai, Lala Lajpat. 1908a. *The Message of the Bhagawad Gita*. N.p.: Indian Press.

Rai, Lala Lajpat. 1908b. *The Story of My Deportation, by Lala Lajpat Rai*. Pakistan: Jaawantrai, M.A.

Ṛg Veda = van Nooten and Holland 1994.

Sarkar, Jadunath, ed. 1930. *Selections from the Peshwa Daftar*. Bombay: Central Government Press.

Sukthankar, Vishnu S. et al., eds. 1966 [1933–1966]. *The Mahābhārata: For the First Time Critically Edited*. 19 vols., Bhandarkar Oriental Research Institute.

Tadpatrikar, Shriniwas Narayan. 1935. *Shri Bhavanrao Silver Jubilee Volume: A Publication of the Universal Appreciation of Twenty-Five Years' Most Progressive and Successful Rule of Shrimant Bhavanrao Alias Balasaheb Pandit Pratinidhi, Ruler of Aundh*. Aundh: Silver Jubilee Committee.

Thomas, F. W., and Bhagavad Datta, eds. and trans. 1921. *Brihaspati Sutra or The Science of Politics According to the School of Brhihaspati*. Lahore: Moti Lal Banarsi Dass.

Tilak, Bal Gangadhar. 1922. *Bal Gangadhar Tilak, His Writings and Speeches*. India: Ganesh.
Tilak, Bal Gangadhar. 1924a [1915]. *Rahasya-Vivecan arthāt Gītece karmayogapar Nirūpaṇ*. Part I. Marathi. Mumbai: New Art.
Tilak, Bal Gangadhar. 1924b [1915]. *Śrīmadbhagavadgītārahasya*. Part II. Marathi. Mumbai: New Art.
Tilak, Bal Gangadhar. 1935. *Śrī Bhagavadgītā-Rahaysa or Karma-Yoga-Śāstra*. Vol. 1. Translated by Bhalchandra Sitaram Sukthankar. Pune: Vaibhav.
Tilak, Bal Gangadhar. 1936. *Śrī Bhagavadgītā-Rahaysa or Karma-Yoga-Śāstra*. Vol. 2. Translated by Bhalchandra Sitaram Sukthankar. Bombay: Vaibhav.
van Nooten, Barend A., and Gary B. Holland. 1994. *Rig Veda: A Metrically Restored Text with an Introduction and Notes*. Cambridge, MA: Department of Sanskrit and Indian Studies, Harvard University.
Wilkins, Charles. 1785. *The Bhagvat-Geeta, or Dialogues of Kreeshna and Arjoon*. London: C. Nourse.
Yoga Sūtras = Bryant 2009.

Government Documents

Administration of Justice in Aundh State. Various years.
Annual Administration Report of the Aundh State. Various years.
Government of India. 2010. National Council of Educational Research and Training. "Scheme on Quality Improvement in Schools: Component of Introduction of Yoga in Schools."
Government of India. 2014. Permanent Mission of India to the UN.
Government of India. 2022. Budget 2022–2023 Speech of Nirmala Sitharaman Minister of Finance. February 1.
Government of India. 2023. Budget 2023–2024.
Government of India. N.d. Ministry of Ayush. "National Clinical Management Protocol Based on Ayurveda and Yoga for Management of COVID-19."
Government of India. National Curriculum Framework for School Education. Various years.
Government of India. National Education Policy/National Policy on Education. Various years.

Archives and Libraries

Bhandarkar Oriental Research Institute
British Library
Government of India, National Archives
Jayakar Library at Savitribai Phule Pune University
Shri Bhavani Museum and Library, Aundh

Newspapers and Periodicals

Business Standard (New Delhi)
Deccan Herald (Bangalore)
Economic Times (Mumbai)
The Hindu (Chennai)
Hindustan Times (New Delhi)
Karmayogin (Calcutta)
Kesari (Pune)
Maratha (Pune)
New York Times (New York)
News Chronicle (London)
Sunday Referee (London)
Times of India (Mumbai/Bombay)

Films and Plays

Atre, P. K. 2009 [1933]. *Sāṣṭāṅga Namaskār*. Pune: Paracure Prakashan Mandir.

Do Ankhen Barah Haath. 1957. Directed by V. Shantaram. Mumbai: Rajkamal Studios. Black and white, Hindi.

Hindoo Fakir. 1902. Directed by Thomas Edison. West Orange, NJ: Edison Manufacturing Company. Black and white, silent short.

[No title]. Film featuring Krishnamachrya. 1938. No producer given. Black and white, silent short.

Sukshma Vyayam: A Better Way to Health. 1950. Directed by N. S. Thapa. Mumbai: Films Division, Government of India. Black and white, short film, English.

Surya Namaskar. 1928. Aundh: Bhawanrao Srinivasarao Pant. Black and white, silent short (catalogued in the British Film Institute as 1935).

Secondary Sources

Adorno, Theodor W. 1992. *Negative Dialectics*. New York: Continuum.

Aggarwal, D. 2002. *History and Development of Elementary Education in India*. New Delhi: Sarup.

Alter, Joseph S. 1996. "Gandhi's Body, Gandhi's Truth: Nonviolence and the Biomoral Imperative of Public Health." *Journal of Asian Studies* 55 (2): 301–322.

Alter, Joseph S. 2000. *Gandhi's Body: Sex, Diet, and the Politics of Nationalism*. Philadelphia: University of Pennsylvania Press.

Alter, Joseph S. 2004. *Yoga in Modern India: The Body Between Science and Philosophy*. Princeton, NJ: Princeton University Press.

Anthony, David W. 2007. *The Horse, the Wheel, and Language: How Bronze-Age Riders from the Eurasian Steppes Shaped the Modern World*. Princeton, NJ: Princeton University Press.

Bakhle, Janaki. 2024. *Savarkar and the Making of Hindutva*. Princeton, NJ: Princeton University Press.

Banerjee, Prathama. 2012. "Chanakya/Kautilya: History, Philosophy, Theater and the Twentieth-Century Political." *History of the Present (Champaign, IL)* 2 (1): 24–51.

Banerjee, Prathama. 2020. *Elementary Aspects of the Political: Histories from the Global South*. Durham, NC: Duke University Press.

Behl, Aditya, and Wendy Doniger. 2012a. *Love's Subtle Magic: An Indian Islamic Literary Tradition, 1379–1545*. New York: Oxford University Press.

Behl, Aditya, and Wendy Doniger. 2012b. *The Magic Doe: Qutban Suhravardi's Mirigavati*. New York: Oxford University Press.

Behl, Aditya, S. C. R. Weightman, and Shyam Manohar Pandey. 2000. *Madhumālatī: An Indian Sufi Romance*. Oxford: Oxford University Press.

Benoy, Kumar. 1913. *Sukra-Niti-Sara: The Sacred Books of the Hindus Volume XIII, Parts I & II*. Allahabad: Panini Office.

Beverley, Eric Lewis. 2020. "Introduction: Rethinking Sovereignty, Colonial Empires, and Nation-States in South Asia and Beyond." *Comparative Studies of South Asia, Africa, and the Middle East* 40 (3): 407–420.

Bevilacqua, Daniela. 2018. *Modern Hindu Traditionalism in Contemporary India: The Śrī Maṭh and the Jagadguru Rāmānandācārya in the Evolution of the Rāmānandī Sampradāya*. Abingdon, UK: Routledge.

Bevilacqua, Daniela, and Eloisa Stuparich, eds. 2022. *The Power of the Nāth Yogīs*. Amsterdam: Amsterdam University Press.

Bhagawan, Manu. 2003. *Sovereign Spheres: Princes, Education, and Empire in Colonial India*. New York: Oxford University Press.

Bhargav, Vania Vaidehi. 2022. "A Hindu Champion of Pan-Islamism: Lajpat Rai and the Khilafat Movement." *Journal of Asian Studies* 81 (4): 689–705.

Bhargav, Vania Vaidehi. 2023. "The Hinduism and Hindu Nationalism of Lala Lajpat Rai." *Religions (Basel, Switzerland)* 14 (6): 744–763.

Bhattacharya, Ananda. 2012. "Reconsidering the Sannyasi Rebellion." *Social Scientist (New Delhi)* 40 (3/4): 81–100.

Bhattacharyya, Benoytosh. 1964. *An Introduction to Buddhist Esoterism*. 2nd ed. Varanasi: Chowkhamba Sanskrit Series Office.

Bilimoria, Purusottama, and J. N. Mohanty, eds. 2018. *History of Indian Philosophy*. Abingdon, UK: Routledge.

Birch, Jason. 2011. "The Meaning of Haṭha in Early Haṭhayoga." *Journal of the American Oriental Society* 131 (4): 527–554.

Birch, Jason, and Mark Singleton. 2019. "The Yoga of the *Haṭhābhyāsapaddhati*: Haṭhayoga on the Cusp of Modernity." *Journal of Yoga Studies* 2: 3–70.

Bisht, Medha. 2019. *Kautilya's Arthaśāstra: Philosophy of Strategy*. Abingdon, UK: Routledge.

Black, Shameem. 2024. *Flexible India: Yoga's Cultural and Political Tensions*. New York: Columbia University Press.

Boesche, Roger. 2005. "Han Feizi's Legalism Versus Kautilya's Arthashastra." *Asian Philosophy* 15 (2): 157–172.

Boesche, Roger. 2010. "Moderate Machiavelli? Contrasting The Prince with the Arthashastra of Kautilya." *Critical Horizons: Journal of Social & Critical Theory* 3 (2): 252–276.

Bose, Sugato. 2010. "The Spirit and Form of an Ethical Polity: A Meditation on Aurobindo's Thought." In *An Intellectual History of India*. Edited by Shruti Kapila, 117–132. Cambridge: Cambridge University Press.

Bouillier, Véronique. 2013. "Religion Compass: A Survey of Current Researches on India's Nāth Yogīs." *Religion Compass* 7 (5): 157–168.

Bourdieu, Pierre. 1993. *The Field of Cultural Production: Essays on Art and Literature*. New York: Columbia University Press.

Bowles, Adam. 2007. *Dharma, Disorder, and the Political in Ancient India: The Āpaddharmaparvan of the Mahābhārata*. Leiden: Brill.

Brockington, John L. 1998. *The Sanskrit Epics*. Leiden: Brill.

Brockington, John L. 2003. "Yoga in the Mahabharata." In *Yoga: The Indian Tradition*. Edited by Ian Whicher and David Carpenter, 13–24. London: Routledge.

Bucar, Elizabeth M. 2022. *Stealing My Religion: Not Just Any Cultural Appropriation*. Cambridge, MA: Harvard University Press.

Burchett, Patton. 2019. *A Genealogy of Devotion: Bhakti, Tantra, Yoga, and Sufism in North India*. New York: Columbia University Press.

Chakrabarty, Dipesh, and Rochona Majumdar. 2013. "Gandhi's Gītā And Politics as Such." In *Political Thought in Action: The Bhagavad Gita and Modern India*. Edited by Shruti Kapila and Faisal Devji, 66–87. Cambridge: Cambridge University Press.

Chapple, Christopher Key, and John Thomas Casey. 2003. *Reconciling Yogas: Haribhadra's Collection of Views on Yoga*. Albany: State University of New York Press.

Chatterjee, Partha. 2004. *The Politics of the Governed: Reflections on Popular Politics in Most of the World*. New York: Columbia University Press.

Chattopadhyay, Bankimchandra. 2005 [1882]. *Anandamath, or The Sacred Brotherhood*. Translated by Julius J. Lipner. London: Oxford University Press.

Chattopadhyay, Bankimchandra, and Chittaranjan Bandyopadhyay. 1983. *Ānanda Maṭha: Racanāra Preraṇā o Pariṇāma, Ta̱tsaha Baṅkimacandrera Ānanda Maṭhera Prathama Saṃskaraṇera Phaṭokapi*. Kalikātā: Ānanda.

Chattopadhyaya, Debiprasad. 1976. *What Is Living and What Is Dead in Indian Philosophy*. New Delhi: People's Publishing House.

Chaturvedi, Vinayak. 2013. "Rethinking Knowledge with Action: V. D. Savarkar, the Bhagavad Gita, and Histories of Warfare." In *Political Thought in Action: The Bhagavad Gita and Modern India*. Edited by Shruti Kapila and Faisal Devji, 155–176. Cambridge: Cambridge University Press.

Cherniak, Alex. 2008. *Mahabharata. Book Six, Bhishma*. Vol. 1. New York: New York University Press.

Chikermane, Guatam. 2022. "Anchored in Bharat, Budget 2022 Exudes Confidence, Powers India's Growth." Observer Research Foundation. February 1. https://www.orfonline.org/expert-speak/anchored-in-bharat-budget-2022-exudes-confidence/.

Chousalkar, Ashok. 1981. "Political Philosophy of the Arthashastra Tradition." *Indian Journal of Political Science* 42 (1): 54–66.

Chousalkar, Ashok S. 2004. "Methodology of Kautilya's Arthashastra." *Indian Journal of Political Science* 65 (1): 55–76.

Chousalkar, Ashok S. 2018. *Revisiting the Political Thought of Ancient India: Pre-Kautilyan Arthashastra Tradition*. New Delhi: Sage.

Chowdhury, K. R. 2020. "Anvikshiki in Arthashastra." *International Journal of Sanskrit Research* 6 (2): 175–178.

Churchill, Winston S., and R. R. James, eds. 1974. *Winston S. Churchill: His Complete Speeches, 1897–1963*. Vol. 5. New York: Chelsea House.

Colby, Frank Moore, and Talcott Williams. 1918. *The New International Encyclopedia*. 2nd ed. Vol. 8. New York: Dodd, Mead.

Copeman, Jacob, and Aya Ikegame, eds. 2012. *The Guru in South Asia: New Interdisciplinary Perspectives*. London: Routledge.

Dasgupta, Atis. 1982. "The Fakir and Sannyasi Rebellion." *Social Scientist (New Delhi)* 10 (1): 44–55.

Dasgupta, Surendranath, R. R. Agarwal, and S. K. Jain. 1969. *History of Indian Philosophy*. Allahabad: Kitab Mahal.

Davidson, Ronald M. 2002. *Indian Esoteric Buddhism: A Social History of the Tantric Movement*. New York: Columbia University Press.

Davies, Philip H. J. 2013. "The Original Surveillance State: Kautilya's Arthashastra and Government by Espionage in Classical India." In *Intelligence Elsewhere*. Edited by Philip H. J. Davies and Kristian C. Gustafson, 49–66. Washington, DC: Georgetown University Press.

Davis, Richard H. 2015. *The Bhagavad Gita: A Biography*. Princeton, NJ: Princeton University Press.

Davis, Richard H. 2018. "Henry David Thoreau, Yogi." *Common Knowledge* 24 (1): 56–89.

Day, Terence P. 1982. *The Conception of Punishment in Early Indian Literature*. Waterloo, Ontario: Wilfrid Laurier University Press.

Dehejia, Vidya. 1986. *Yoginī, Cult and Temples: A Tantric Tradition*. New Delhi: National Museum.

De Michelis, Elizabeth. 2004. *A History of Modern Yoga: Patañjali and Western Esotericism*. 1st paperback ed. London: Continuum.

de Ruiter, Adrienne. 2012. "The Political Character of Absolute Enmity: On Carl Schmitt's The Concept of the Political and Theory of the Partisan." *Archiv Für Rechts-Und Sozialphilosophie* 98 (1): 52–66.

Deshpande, Prachi. 2007. *Creative Pasts: Historical Memory and Identity in Western India, 1700–1960*. New York: Columbia University Press.

Devji, Faisal. 2012. *The Impossible Man: Gandhi and the Temptation of Violence*. Cambridge, MA: Harvard University Press.

Diamond, Debra, and Molly Emma Aitken. 2013. *Yoga: The Art of Transformation*. Washington, DC: Smithsonian Institution.

Diamond, Debra, Catherine Ann Glynn, and Karni Singh Jasol. 2008. *Garden & Cosmos: The Royal Paintings of Jodhpur*. Washington, DC: Smithsonian Institution.

Doniger, W. 1999. "Presidential Address: 'I Have Scinde': Flogging a Dead (White Male Orientalist) Horse." *Journal of Asian Studies* 58 (4): 940–960.

Duara, Prasenjit. 2015. *The Crisis of Global Modernity: Asian Traditions and a Sustainable Future*. Cambridge: Cambridge University Press.

Edgerton, Franklin. 1965 [1924]. *The Panchatantra*. London: G. Allen and Unwin.

Ernst, Carl. 1996. "Sufism and Yoga According to Muhammad Ghawth." *Sufi* 29: 9–13.

Ernst, Carl. 2003. "The Islamization of Yoga in the Amrtakunda Translations." *Journal of the Royal Asiatic Society*, 3rd ser., 13 (2): 199–226.

Ernst, Carl. 2005. "Situating Sufism and Yoga." *Journal of the Royal Asiatic Society* 15 (1): 15–43.

Ernst, Carl W. 2016. *Refractions of Islam in India: Situating Sufism and Yoga*. New Delhi: Sage.

Ernst, Carl W., and Patrick D'Silva. 2024. *Breathtaking Revelations: The Science of Breath from the 'Fifty Kamarupa Verses' to Hazrat Inayat Khan*. Jackson, MI: Omega.

Evola, Julius. 1992 [1925]. *The Yoga of Power: Tantra, Shakti, and the Secret Way*. Translated by Guido Stucco. Rochester, VT: Inner Traditions.

Farmer, Steve, Richard Sproat, and Michael Witzel. 2004. "The Collapse of the Indus-Script Thesis: The Myth of a Literate Harappan Civilization." *Electronic Journal of Vedic Studies* 11 (2): 19–58.

Feldhaus, Anne. 1983. *The Religious System of the Mahanubhava Sect: The Mahanubhava Sutrapatha*. New Delhi: Manohar.

Feldhaus, Anne. 2003. *Connected Places*. New York: Palgrave Macmillan.

Ferrara, Marianna. 2020. "Rest After War: Yóga in the Ṛgveda and Its Scholarly Understanding in the Nineteenth and Twentieth Centuries." *Mythos (Palermo)* 14 (1): 209–238.

Feuerstein, Georg. 1980. *The Philosophy of Classical Yoga*. Manchester: Manchester University Press.

Figueira, Dorothy M. 2023. *The Afterlives of the Bhagavad Gita: Readings in Translation*. Oxford: Oxford University Press.

Fitzgerald, James L. 2004. *The Mahābhārata. Vol. 7, Book 11, the Book of Women. Book 12, the Book of Peace, Part One*. Chicago: University of Chicago Press.

Fitzgerald, James L. 2012. "A Prescription for *Yoga* and Power in the *Mahābhārata*." In *Yoga in Practice*. Edited by David Gordon White, 43–57. Princeton, NJ: Princeton University Press.

Fosse, Lars Martin. 1997. *The Crux of Chronology in Sanskrit Literature: Statistics and Indology: A Study of Method*. Oslo: Scandinavian University Press.

Fosse, Lars Martin. 2007. *The Bhagavad Gita. Original Sanskrit and an English Translation*. Woodstock, NY: YogaVidya.

Foucault, Michel. 1970. *The Order of Things: An Archaeology of the Human Sciences*. New York: Pantheon.

Foucault, Michel. 1978. *The History of Sexuality, Volume 1: An Introduction*. Translated by R. Hurley. New York: Pantheon.

Foucault, Michel. 2024 [1978]. *The Japan Lectures: A Transnational Critical Encounter*. London: Routledge.

Foxen, Anya P. 2020. *Inhaling Spirit: Harmonialism, Orientalism, and the Western Roots of Modern Yoga*. Oxford: Oxford University Press.

Foxen, Anya P., and Christa Kuberry. 2021. *Is This Yoga? Concepts, Histories, and the Complexities of Modern Practice*. Abingdon, UK: Routledge.

Frank, Katherine. 2002. *Indira: The Life of Indira Nehru Gandhi*. Boston: Houghton Mifflin.

Gan, Vicky. 2013. "Early Films (Including One by Thomas Edison) Made Yoga Look Like Magic." *Smithsonian Magazine*. November 18. https://www.smithsonianmag

.com/smithsonian-institution/early-films-including-one-by-thomas-edison-made-yoga-look-like-magic-180947717/.

Ganachari, Aravind. 1995. "British Official View of 'Bhagwat Gita' as 'Text-Book for the Mental Training of Revolutionary Recruits.'" *Proceedings of the Indian History Congress* 56: 601–610.

Ganeri, Jonardon, ed. 2017. *The Oxford Handbook of Indian Philosophy*. Oxford: Oxford University Press.

Gautam, Aavriti, and Julian Droogan. 2018. "Yoga Soft Power: How Flexible Is the Posture?" *Journal of International Communication* 24 (1): 18–36.

Gerschenkron, Alexander. 1962. *Economic Backwardness in Historical Perspective: A Book of Essays*. Cambridge, MA: Belknap Press of Harvard University Press.

Getachew, Adom, and Karuna Mantena. 2021. "Anticolonialism and the Decolonization of Political Theory." *Critical Times (Berkeley, CA)* 4 (3): 359–388.

Ghosh, Durba. 2017. *Gentlemanly Terrorists: Political Violence and the Colonial State in India, 1919–1947*. Cambridge: Cambridge University Press.

Godrej, Farah. 2022a. *Freedom Inside? Yoga and Meditation in the Carceral State*. New York: Oxford University Press.

Godrej, Farah. 2022b. "Yoga, Meditation, and Neoliberal Penality: Compliance or Resistance?" *Political Research Quarterly* 75 (1): 47–60.

Goldberg, Elliott. 2016. *The Path of Modern Yoga: The History of an Embodied Spiritual Practice*. Rochester, VT: Inner Traditions.

Goodall, Dominic, Shaman Hatley, Harunaga Isaacson, and Srilata Raman. 2020. *Śaivism and the Tantric Traditions: Essays in Honour of Alexis G. J. S. Sanderson*. Leiden: Brill.

Gopal, Lallanji. 1962. "The 'Śukranīti'—A Nineteenth-Century Text." *Bulletin of the School of Oriental and African Studies, University of London* 25 (1/3): 524–556.

Gowda, Nagappa. 2011. *The Bhagawadgita in the Nationalist Discourse*. New Delhi: Oxford University Press.

Gowen, Herbert Henry. 1929. *"The Indian Machiavelli"; or, Political Theory in India Two Thousand Years Ago . . .* New York: Academy of Political Science.

Goyal, Parikshit. 2021. "Understanding Open Prisons in India." *Economic and Political Weekly (Engage)* 56 (4). https://www.epw.in/engage/article/understanding-open-prisons-india.

Gray, Stuart. 2014. "Reexamining Kautilya and Machiavelli: Flexibility and the Problem of Legitimacy in Brahmanical and Secular Realism." *Political Theory* 42 (6): 635–657.

Gupta, Bhuvi, and Jacob Copeman. 2019. "Awakening Hindu Nationalism Through Yoga: Swami Ramdev and the Bharat Swabhiman Movement." *Contemporary South Asia* 27 (3): 313–329.

Gupta, Vijay Kumar. 2004. *Kauṭilīya Arthaśāstram: A Legal, Critical, and Analytical Study*. Rev. and enlarged ed. Delhi: Bharatiya Kala Prakashan.

Harvey, Scott L., Winfred P. Lehmann, and Jonathan Slocum. 2019. "Old Iranian Online: Lesson 4: Old Avestan." University of Texas, Austin's Linguistic Research Center. https://lrc.la.utexas.edu/eieol/aveol/40#glossed_text_gloss_21306. Accessed March 18, 2019.

Hatley, Shaman. 2007a. "The Brahmayāmalatantra and Early Śaiva Cult of Yoginīs." PhD diss., University of Pennsylvania.

Hatley, Shaman. 2007b. "Mapping the Esoteric Body in the Islamic Yoga of Bengal." *History of Religions* 46 (4): 351–368.

Hatley, Shaman. 2013. "South Asia—Dharma Pātañjala: A Śaiva Scripture from Ancient Java Studied in Light of Related Old Javanese and Sanskrit Texts." *Religious Studies Review* 39 (2): 125–126.

Hatley, Shaman. 2020. "Tantra." In *Encyclopedia of Indian Religions. Hinduism and Tribal Religions*. Edited by Arvind Sharma, 2426–2434. Dordrecht, Netherlands: Springer.

Heehs, Peter. 1993. *The Bomb in Bengal: The Rise of Revolutionary Terrorism in India, 1900–1910*. Delhi: Oxford University Press.

Heehs, Peter. 2008. *The Lives of Sri Aurobindo*. New York: Columbia University Press.

Heesterman, J. C. 1985. *The Inner Conflict of Tradition: Essays in Indian Ritual, Kingship, and Society*. Chicago: University of Chicago Press.

Heesterman, J. C. 1993. *The Broken World of Sacrifice: An Essay in Ancient Indian Ritual*. Chicago: University of Chicago Press.

Ikegame, Aya. 2013. *Princely India Re-Imagined: A Historical Anthropology of Mysore from 1799 to the Present*. London: Routledge.

Imy, Kate. 2016. "Fascist Yogis: Martial Bodies and Imperial Impotence." *Journal of British Studies* 55 (2): 320–343.

Irani, Ayesha. 2021. *The Muhammad Avatara Salvation History, Translation, and the Making of Bengali Islam*. New York: Oxford University Press.

Jaffrelot, Christophe. 2012. "The Political Guru: The Guru as éminence Grise." In *The Guru in South Asia: New Interdisciplinary Perspectives*. Edited by Jacob Copeman and Aya Ikegame. London: Routledge.

Jain, Andrea R. 2015. *Selling Yoga: From Counterculture to Pop Culture*. Oxford: Oxford University Press.

Jain, Andrea R. 2020. *Peace, Love, Yoga: The Politics of Global Spirituality*. New York: Oxford University Press.

Jamison, Stephanie W. 1991. "Natural History Notes on the Rigvedic 'Frog' Hymn." *Annals of the Bhandarkar Oriental Research Institute* 72/73 (1/4): 137–144.

Johnson, W. J. 2005. *Mahabharata. Book Three, The Forest. Volume Four*. New York: New York University Press.

Joseph, Simon. 2012. "Jesus in India? Transgressing Social and Religious Boundaries." *Journal of the American Academy of Religion* 80 (1): 161–169.

Kale, Sunila S. 2014. *Electrifying India: Regional Political Economies of Development*. Palo Alto, CA: Stanford University Press.

Kale, Sunila S. 2020. "From Company Town to Company Village: CSR and the Management of Rural Aspirations in Eastern India's Extractive Economies." *Journal of Peasant Studies* 47 (6): 1211–1232.

Kale, Sunila S., and Nimah Mazaheri. 2019. "Indigenous Politics, Tribal Homelands, and the Impact of Civil Society Organizations." In *Inside Countries: Subnational Research in Comparative Politics*. Edited by Agustina Giraudy, Eduardo Moncada, and Richard Snyder, 287–317. New York: Cambridge University Press.

Kale, Sunila S., and Christian Lee Novetzke. 2016. "Some Reflections on Yoga as Political Theology," *The Wire* (India), January 28.

Kale, Sunila S., and Christian Lee Novetzke. 2017. "Yoga and the Means and Ends of Secularism," *The Wire* (India), June 21.

Kale, Sunila S., and Christian Lee Novetzke. 2020a. "Legal Yoga." In *A History of Hindu Practice*. Edited by Gavin Flood, 404–424. Oxford: Oxford University Press.

Kale, Sunila S., and Christian Lee Novetzke. 2020b. "The Yogic Ethic and the Spirit of Development." In *Political Theologies and Development in Asia: Transcendence, Sacrifice and Aspiration*. Edited by Guiseppe Bolotta, Philip Fountain, and Michael Feener, 40–54, esp. 43–44. Manchester: Manchester University Press.

Kale, Sunila S., and Christian Lee Novetzke. 2021. "The Cultural Politics of Yoga in and Between the US and India." In *At Home and Abroad*. Edited by Elizabeth Shakman Hurd and Winnifred Fallers Sullivan, 210–227. New York: Columbia University Press.

Kamal, Kajari. 2022. "In Search of 'The India Way': Ancient Indian Statecraft and Contemporary Geopolitics." *India Quarterly* 78 (2): 381–387.

Kangle, R. P. 1965. *The Kauṭilīya Arthaśāstra: A Study*. Part III. Delhi: Motilal Banarsidass.

Kangle, R. P. 1972. *The Kauṭilīya Arthaśāstra: An English Translation with Critical and Explanatory Notes*. Part II. 2nd ed. Bombay: University of Bombay.

Kapila, Shruti. 2021. *Violent Fraternity: Indian Political Thought in the Global Age*. Princeton, NJ: Princeton University Press.

Kapila, Shruti, and Faisal Devji, eds. 2013. *Political Thought in Action: The Bhagavad Gita and Modern India*. Cambridge: Cambridge University Press.

Kersten, Holger. 1986. *Jesus Lived in India*. London: Element.

Kharge, Mallikarjun. 2022. "FM Nirmala Sitharaman Invokes Mahabharate; Mallikarjum Kharge Hits Back." *Business Standard*. https://www.business-standard.com/budget/article/fm-nirmala-sitharaman-invokes-mahabharata-mallikarjun-kharge-hits-back-122020101897_1.html.

Kiehnle, Catharina. 1998. *Jnandev Studies, Vols. I and II: Songs on Yoga: Teaching of the Maharastrian Naths*. Stuttgart: Franz Steiner Verlag.

Kirfel, Willibald. 1926. *Beiträge zur literaturwissenschaft und geistesgeschichte Indiens*. Bonn: Kommissionsverlag F. Klopp.

Krishnamacharya, Tirumalai. 2006 [1934]. *Yoga Makaranda: The Nectar of Yoga*. Translated by Lakshmi Ranganathan and Nandini Ranganathan. Chennai: Krishnamacharya Yoga Mandiram.

Kumar, Aishwary. 2015. *Radical Equality: Ambedkar, Gandhi, and the Risk of Democracy*. Redwood City, CA: Stanford University Press.

Laine, James W. 2003. *Shivaji: Hindu King in an Islamic India*. Oxford: Oxford University Press.

Lakshmi, Anusha. 2020. "Choreographing Tolerance: Narendra Modi, Hindu Nationalism, and International Yoga Day." *Race and Yoga* 5 (1).

Lee, Joel. 2021. *Deceptive Majority: Dalits, Hinduism, and Underground Religion*. Cambridge: Cambridge University Press.

List, Friedrich, George-Auguste Matile, Henri Richelot, and Stephen Colwell. 1856. *National System of Political Economy*. Translated by George-Auguste Matile and Henri Richelot. Philadelphia: J. B. Lippincott.

Lorenzen, David N. 1978. "Warrior Ascetics in Indian History." *Journal of the American Oriental Society* 98 (1): 61–75.

Lorenzen, David N., ed. 1995. *Bhakti Religion in North India: Community Identity and Political Action*. Albany: State University of New York Press.

Lubin, Timothy. 2015. "Writing and the Recognition of Customary Law in Premodern India and Java." *Journal of the American Oriental Society* 135 (2): 225–259.

Lucia, Amanda J. 2020. *White Utopias: The Religious Exoticism of Transformational Festivals*. Berkeley: University of California Press.

Mahony, William K. 1998. *The Artful Universe: An Introduction to the Vedic Religious Imagination*. Albany: State University of New York Press.

Malamoud, Charles. 2003. "Remarks on Dissuasion in Ancient India." In *Violence/Non-Violence: Some Hindu Perspectives*. Edited by Denis Vidal, Gilles Tarabout, and Eric Meyer Vidal, 209–218. New Delhi: Manohar and Centre de Sciences Humaines.

Malinar, Angelika. 2007. *The Bhagavadgītā: Doctrines and Contexts*. Cambridge: Cambridge University Press.

Mallinson, James, and Mark Singleton. 2017. *Roots of Yoga*. London: Penguin.

Manjapra, Kris. 2012. "Knowledgeable Internationalism and the Swadeshi Movement, 1903–1921." *Economic and Political Weekly* 47 (42): 53–62.

Manjapra, Kris. 2014. *Age of Entanglement: German and Indian Intellectuals Across Empire*. Cambridge, MA: Harvard University Press.

Mantena, Karuna. 2012. "Another Realism: The Politics of Gandhian Nonviolence." *American Political Science Review* 106 (2): 455–470.

Marrewa-Karwoski, Christine. 2017. "Far from Hindutva, Yogi Adityanath's Sect Comes from a Tradition That Was Neither Hindu Nor Muslim." *Scroll*. April 9.

Marwah, Inder S. 2024. "The View from the Future: Aurobindo Ghose's Anticolonial Darwinism." *American Political Science Review* 118 (2): 123–145.

Mayrhofer, Manfred. 1986. *Etymologisches Wörterbuch des Altindoarischen*. Heidelberg: C. Winter.

McCartney, Patrick. 2019. "Spiritual Bypass and Entanglement in Yogaland (योगस्तान): How Neoliberalism, Soft Hindutva and Banal Nationalism Facilitates Yoga Fundamentalism." *Politikologija Religije* 13 (1): 137–175.

McCartney, Patrick S. D. 2023. "Poles Apart? From Wrestling and *Mallkhāmb* to Pole Yoga." *Journal of Yoga Studies* 4: 215–270.

McClish, Mark. 2019. *The History of the Arthaśāstra: Sovereignty and Sacred Law in Ancient India*. Cambridge: Cambridge University Press.

McClish, Mark, and Patrick Olivelle. 2012. *The Arthaśāstra: Selections from the Classic Indian Work on Statecraft*. Indianapolis, IN: Hackett.

McLain, Karline. 2019. "Living the Bhagavad Gita at Gandhi's Ashrams." *Religions (Basel, Switzerland)* 10 (11).

Mehendale, Madhukar Anant. 1995. *Reflections on the Mahābhārata War*. Shimla: Indian Institute of Advanced Study.

Mill, James. 1826. *A History of British India Vol. 1*. 3rd ed. London: Baldwin, Cradock and Joy.

Miller, Christopher Patrick. 2020. "Soft Power and Biopower: Narendra Modi's 'Double Discourse' Concerning Yoga for Climate Change and Self-Care." *Journal of Dharma Studies* 3 (1): 93–106.

Misra, Maria. 2016. "The Indian Machiavelli: Pragmatism Versus Morality, and the Reception of the Arthasastra in India, 1905–2014." *Modern Asian Studies* 50 (1): 310–344.

Mital, Surendra Nath. 2000. *Kauṭilīya Arthaśāstra Revisited*. New Delhi: Centre for Studies in Civilizations.

Modi, P. M. 1950. "Each Adhyāya of Bhagavadgītā: A Unit by Itself." *Bhāratīya Vidyā* 11 (1&2): 85–94.

Moin, A. Azfar. 2012. *The Millennial Sovereign: Sacred Kingship and Sainthood in Islam*. New York: Columbia University Press.

Monier-Williams, Monier, Ernst Leumann, and Carl Cappeller. 1899. *A Sanskrit-English Dictionary Etymologically and Philologically Arranged with Special Reference to Cognate Indo-European Languages*. Oxford: Clarendon.

Mouffe, Chantal. 2013. *Agonistics: Thinking the World Politically*. London: Verso.

Mukherjee, Mithi. 2020. "Sedition, Law and the British Empire in India: The Trial of Tilak (1908)." *Law, Culture and the Humanities* 16 (3): 454–476.

Mulgund, Deepti. 2016. "The Museum at Aundh: Reflecting on Citizenship and the Art Museum in the Colony." In *Eurasian Encounters*, 2:25–46. Amsterdam: Amsterdam University Press.

Mulgund, Deepti. 2017. "Imaginaries of the Art Museum: Banaras and Aundh in Colonial India." In *Images of the Art Museum*, 3:215–38. Berlin: De Gruyter.

Nair, Janaki. 2011. *Mysore Modern: Rethinking the Region under Princely Rule*. Minneapolis: University of Minnesota Press.

Neelsen, J. P., ed. 1992. *Gender, Caste and Power in South Asia: Social Status and Mobility in Transitional Society*. Delhi: Manohar.

Neri, Chiara, and Tiziana Pontillo. 2019. "On the Boundary Between 'Yogakkhema' in the 'Suttapiṭaka' and 'Yogakṣema' in the 'Upaniṣads' and 'Bhagavadgītā.' " *Cracow Indological Studies* 21 (2): 139–157.

Notovitch, Nicolas. 1894. *The Unknown Life of Jesus Christ: The Original Text of Nicolas Notovitch's 1877 Discovery*. Project Gutenberg.

Novetzke, Christian. 1993. "Twice Dalit." *Journal of South Asian Literature* 28 (1): 279–296.

Novetzke, Christian Lee. 2008. *Religion and Public Memory: A Cultural History of Saint Namdev in India*. New York: Columbia University Press.

Novetzke, Christian Lee. 2011. "The Brahmin Double: The Brahminical Construction of Anti-Brahminism and Anti-Caste Sentiment in the Religious Cultures of Precolonial Maharashtra." *South Asian History and Culture* 2 (2): 232–252.

Novetzke, Christian Lee. 2016. *The Quotidian Revolution: Vernacularization, Religion, and the Premodern Public Sphere in India*. New York: Columbia University Press.

Novetzke, Christian Lee. Forthcoming in 2026. *Savitribai and Jotirao Phule*. Indian Lives Series. Delhi: HarperCollins.

Oak, Alok. 2022. *Political Ideas of B. G. Tilak: Colonialism, Self and Hindu Nationalism*. PhD diss., Leiden University.

Oguibénine, Boris. 1984. "Sur le terme yóga, le verbe yuj- et quelques-uns de leurs dérivés dans les hymnes védiques." *Indo-Iranian Journal* 27 (2): 85–101.

Oguibénine, Boris. 1998 [1984]. *Essays on Vedic and Indo-European Culture*. New Delhi: Motilal Banarsidass.

O'Hanlon, Rosalind. 2007. "Military Sports and the History of the Martial Body in India." *Journal of the Economic and Social History of the Orient* 50 (4): 490–523.

Oman, John Campbell. 1903. *The Mystics, Ascetics, and Saints of India; A Study of Sadhuism, with an Account of the Yogis, Sanyasis, Bairagis, and Other Strange Hindu Sectarians*. London: T. F. Unwin.

Pal, Bipin Chandra. 1909. "The Etiology of the Bomb in Bengal." *Swaraj*. June 16, 3–5.

Palihawadana, M. 1968. "Yoga and Kṣema: The Significance of Their Usage in the Ṛg Veda." *Vidyodaya Journal of Arts, Sciences, and Letters* 1 (2): 185–190.
Parikh, Rachel. 2015. "Yoga Under the Mughals: From Practice to Paintings." *South Asian Studies (Society for South Asian Studies)* 31 (2): 215–236.
Parpola, Asko. 1994. *Deciphering the Indus Script*. New York: Cambridge University Press.
Pathak, M. M., and Peter Schreiner. 1997. *The Critical Edition of the Viṣṇupurāṇam*. Vadodara: Oriental Institute.
Pati, Biswamoy. 2005. "Interrogating Stereotypes: Exploring the Princely States in Colonial Orissa." *South Asia Research* 25 (2): 165–182.
Patton, Laurie L. 2008. *The Bhagavad Gita*. London: Penguin.
Pillai, Sarath. 2023. "German Lessons: Comparative Constitutionalism, States' Rights, and Federalist Imaginaries in Interwar India." *Comparative Studies in Society and History* 65 (4): 801–827.
Pinch, William. 1996. "Soldier, Monks, and Militant Sadhus." In *Contesting the Nation*. Edited by David Ludden, 141–156. Philadelphia: University of Pennsylvania Press.
Pinch, William R. 2006. *Warrior Ascetics and Indian Empires*. Cambridge: Cambridge University Press.
Pinney, Christopher. 2009. "Iatrogenic Religion and Politics." In *Censorship in South Asia: Cultural Regulation from Sedition to Seduction*. Edited by Raminder Kaur and William Mazzarella, 29–62. Bloomington: Indiana University Press.
Pollock, Sheldon. 1985. "The Theory of Practice and the Practice of Theory in Indian Intellectual History." *Journal of the American Oriental Society* 105 (3): 499–519.
Potter, Karl. 1977. *Encyclopedia of Indian Philosophies*. Vol. II. Delhi: Motilal Banarsidass.
Puri, Jyoti. 2019. "Sculpting the Saffron Body: Yoga, Hindutva, and the International Marketplace." In *Majoritarian State: How Hindu Nationalism Is Changing India*. Edited by Angana P. Chatterji, Thomas Blom Hansen, and Christophe Jaffrelot, 317–334. Oxford: Oxford University Press.
Ramanujan, A. K. 1999. "Repetition in the Mahabharata." In *The Collected Essays of A. K. Ramanujan*. Edited by Vinay Dharwadker, 161–183. New Delhi: Oxford University Press.
Ramaswamy Aiyangar, K. V. 1935. *Considerations of Some Aspects of Ancient Indian Polity*. Madras: University of Madras Press.
Rangarajan, L. N. 1992. *The Arthashastra*. New Delhi: Penguin India.
Rao, Rajesh P. N., Nisha Yada, Mayank N. Vahia, Hrishikesh Jodlekar, R. Adhikari, and Iravatham Mahadevan. 2009. "A Markov Model of the Indus Script." *Proceedings of the National Academy of Science* 106 (33): 13685–13690.
Rathore, Aakash Singh, and Rimina Mohapatra. 2017. *Hegel's India: A Reinterpretation, with Texts*. New Delhi: Oxford University Press.
Renan, Ernest, and M. F. N. Giglioli. 2018 [1882]. *What Is a Nation? and Other Political Writings*. New York: Columbia University Press.
Rothermund, Indira. 1983. *The Aundh Experiment: A Gandhian Grass-Roots Democracy*. Bombay: Somaiya.
Roy, Kaushik. 2013. "Race and Recruitment in the Indian Army: 1880–1918." *Modern Asian Studies* 47 (4): 1310–1347.
Ruben, Walter. 1926. "Beiträge zur Literaturwissenschaft und Geistesgeschichte Indiens." In *Beiträge zur Literaturwissenschaft und Geistesgeschichte Indiens*. Edited by Wilibald Kirfel, 346–357. Bonn: Kommissionsverlag F. Klopp.

Rudolph, Lloyd I., and Susanne Hoeber Rudolph. 1967. *The Modernity of Tradition: Political Development in India*. Chicago: University of Chicago Press.

Rudolph, Lloyd I., and Susanne Hoeber Rudolph. 2006. *Postmodern Gandhi and Other Essays: Gandhi in the World and at Home*. Chicago: University of Chicago Press.

Sadhukhan, Ankita. 2021. "The Trial of the Colonial Legal Order: The Tilak Trial 1908 and the Colonial Fiat." *International Journal of Law Management & Humanities* 5 (3): 3025–3033.

Sagar, Rahul. 2022. *The Progressive Maharaja: Sir Madhava Rao's Hints on the Art and Science of Government*. New Delhi: HarperCollins India.

Samuel, Geoffrey. 2008. *The Origins of Yoga and Tantra: Indic Religions to the Thirteenth Century*. Cambridge: Cambridge University Press.

Sanderson, Alexis. 1988. "Śaivism and the Tantric Traditions." In *The World's Religions*. Edited by Peter Clarke, Friedhelm Hardy, Leslie Houlden, and Stewart Sutherland, 660–704. London: Routledge.

Sanderson, Alexis. 2009. "The Śaiva Age: The Rise and Dominance of Śaivism During the Early Medieval Period." In *Genesis and Development of Tantrism*. Edited by Shingo Einoo, 41–350. Tokyo: Institute of Oriental Culture Special Series.

Sarbacker, Stuart Ray. 2021. *Tracing the Path of Yoga: The History and Philosophy of Indian Mind-Body Discipline*. Albany: State University of New York Press.

Sarbacker, Stuart Ray. 2023. "Prostration or Potentiation? Hindu Ritual, Physical Culture, and the 'Sun Salutation' (Sūryanamaskār)." *Journal of Yoga Studies* 4: 303–329.

Sarkar, Sumit. 1973. *The Swadeshi Movement in Bengal, 1903–1908*. New Delhi: People's Publishing House.

Sartori, Andrew. 2013. "The Transfiguration of Duty in Aurobindo's *Essays on the Gita*." In *Political Thought in Action: The Bhagavad Gita and Modern India*. Edited by Shruti Kapila and Faisal Devji, 48–65. Cambridge: Cambridge University Press.

Scharfe, Hartmut. 1989. *The State in Indian Tradition*. Leiden: Brill.

Schmitt, Carl. 1976 [1932]. *The Concept of the Political*. New Brunswick, NJ: Rutgers University Press.

Schmitt, Carl. 2005 [1922]. *Political Theology: Four Chapters on the Concept of Sovereignty*. Chicago: University of Chicago Press.

Schmitt, Carl. 2007 [1963]. *The Theory of the Partisan*. Translated by G. L. Ulmen. New York: Telos.

Schreiner, Peter. 1999. "What Comes First (in the *Mahābhārata*): Sāṃkhya or Yoga?" *Asiatische Studien/Études Asiatiques* 53: 755–777.

Scott, J. Barton. 2016. *Spiritual Despots: Modern Hinduism and the Genealogies of Self-Rule*. Chicago: University of Chicago Press.

Senapaty, Trishna. 2023. "The Closed and the Open Prison: Contested Imaginaries and the Limits of Openness." *Legal Pluralism and Critical Social Analysis* 55 (2): 272–292.

Shamasastry, R. 1929 [1915]. *Kautilya's Arthaśāstra*. 3rd ed. Mysore: Mysore Printing and Publishing House.

Sharma, R. S. 1977. "Conflict, Distribution and Differentiation in Rg Vedic Society." *Proceedings of the Indian History Congress* 38: 177–191.

Shearer, Alistair. 2020. *The Story of Yoga: From Ancient India to the Modern West*. London: Hurst.

Sil, Narasingha Prosad. 1985. "Political Morality vs. Political Necessity: Kautilya and Machiavelli Revisited." *Journal of Asian History* 19 (2): 101–142.

Singh, Upinder. 2017. *Political Violence in Ancient India*. E-book. Cambridge, MA: Harvard University Press.

Singleton, Mark. 2010. *Yoga Body: The Origins of Modern Posture Practice*. Oxford: Oxford University Press.

Singleton, Mark. 2016. "Yoga and Physical Culture: Transnational History and Blurred Discursive Contexts." In *Routledge Handbook of Contemporary India*. Edited by Knut A. Jacobsen, 172–184. London: Routledge.

Sinha, Mishka. 2013. "The Transnational Gita." In *Political Thought in Action: The Bhagavad Gita and Modern India*. Edited by Shruti Kapila and Faisal Devji, 25–47. Cambridge: Cambridge University Press.

Skaria, Ajay. 2016. *Unconditional Equality: Gandhi's Religion of Resistance*. Minneapolis: University of Minnesota Press.

Sood, Sheena. 2018. "Cultivating a Yogic Theology of Collective Healing: A Yogini's Journey Disrupting White Supremacy, Hindu Fundamentalism, and Casteism." *Race and Yoga* 3 (1): 12–20.

Sood, Sheena. 2023. " 'Om-Washing': Why Modi's Yoga Day Pose Is Deceptive." *Al Jazeera*, June 22. https://www.aljazeera.com/opinions/2023/6/22/om-washing-modis-yoga-day-pose-of-deception.

Southard, Barbara. 1980. "The Political Strategy of Aurobindo Ghosh." *Modern Asian Studies* 14 (3): 353–376.

South Asia Scholar Activist Collective. 2023 [2021]. *Hindutva Harassment Field Manual*. https://www.hindutvaharassmentfieldmanual.org. Accessed February 21, 2024.

Spellman, John W. 1964. *Political Theory of Ancient India: A Study of Kingship from the Earliest Times to Circa A.D. 300*. Oxford: Clarendon.

Strand, Eric. 2021. "Du Bois's Dark Princess, Kautilya's Arthashastra, and the Welfare State." *Publications of the Modern Language Association of America* 136 (1): 72–87.

Sukthankar, Vishnu Sitaram. 1933. *Prologomena (to the Critical Edition of the Ādiparvan, Book 1 of the Mahābhārata)*. Poona: Bhandarkar Oriental Research Institute.

Syman, Stefanie. 2010. *The Subtle Body: The Story of Yoga in America*. New York: Farrar, Straus and Giroux.

Tambiah, Stanley Jeyaraja. 1985. *Culture, Thought, and Social Action: An Anthropological Perspective*. Cambridge, MA: Harvard University Press.

Tambwekar, W. G. 1991. *Dasbodh, an English Version, an Elixir of Human Excellence: A Treatise in Marathi of Shri Samartha Ramdas Swami, a Great Motivator Saint*. Bombay: Shri Samarth Ramdas Swami Krupa Trust.

Tietke, Mathias. 2011. *Yoga im Nationalsozialismus*. Kiel, Germany: Ludwig.

Trautmann, Thomas R. 1968. *The Structure and Composition of the Kautiliya "Arthasastra."* PhD diss., University of London.

Trautmann, Thomas R., and Gurcharan Das. 2012. *Arthashastra: The Science of Wealth*. Haryana, India: Portfolio Penguin.

Truschke, Audrey. 2016. *Culture of Encounters: Sanskrit at the Mughal Court*. New York: Columbia University Press.

Truschke, Audrey. 2020. "A Padshah Like Manu: Political Advice for Akbar in the Persian *Māhabhārata*." *Philological Encounters* 5 (2): 112–133.

Tupe, Bapurao U. 2000. *Socio-Economic Study of Aundh State (1854–1948)*. PhD diss., Shivaji University, Kolhapur.

Urban, Hugh B. 2006. *Magia Sexualis: Sex, Magic, and Liberation in Modern Western Esotericism*. Berkeley: University of California Press.

van Buitenen, J. A. B., trans. and ed. 1973. *The Mahābhārata: I. The Book of the Beginning*. Chicago: University of Chicago Press.

Varma, Vishwanath Prasad. 1976. *The Political Philosophy of Sri Aurobindo*. 2nd rev. ed. Delhi: Motilal Banarsidas.

Verdon, Noémie. 2024. *The Books Sāṅk and Pātanǧal: A Socio-Cultural History of al-Bīrūnī's Interpretations of Sāṅkhya and Yoga*. Leiden: Brill.

Vishveshvaranand, Swami, and Swami Nityanand. 1908. *Ṛgvedapadānāṃ* [A Complete Alphabetical Index of All the Words in the Rigveda]. Bombay: Nirnaya-Sagara.

Weber, Max. 2004 [1917]. *The Vocation Lectures*. Edited and translated by David S. Owen and Tracy B. Strong. Indianapolis, IN: Hackett.

Werner, Karel. 1977. "Yoga and the Ṛg Veda: An Interpretation of the Keśin Hymn (RV 10, 136)." *Religious Studies* 13 (3): 289–302.

Whitaker, Jarrod. 2011. *Strong Arms and Drinking Strength: Masculinity, Violence, and the Body in Ancient India*. New York: Oxford University Press.

White, David Gordon. 1996. *The Alchemical Body: Siddha Traditions in Medieval India*. Chicago: University of Chicago Press.

White, David Gordon. 2000. *Tantra in Practice*. Princeton, NJ: Princeton University Press.

White, David Gordon. 2003. *Kiss of the Yoginī: "Tantric Sex" in Its South Asian Contexts*. Chicago: University of Chicago Press.

White, David Gordon. 2009. *Sinister Yogis*. Chicago: University of Chicago Press.

White, David Gordon. 2011. *Yoga in Practice*. Princeton, NJ: Princeton University Press.

White, David Gordon. 2014. *The Yoga Sutra of Patanjali: A Biography*. Princeton, NJ: Princeton University Press.

Whitney, William Dwight. 1885. *The Roots, Verb-Forms, and Primary Derivatives of the Sanskrit Language*. Leipzig: Breitkipf and Härtel.

Witzel, Michael. 1995. "Rgvedic History: Poets, Chieftains, and Polities." In *The Indo-Aryans of Ancient South Asia: Language, Material Culture, and Ethnicity*. Edited by George Erdosy, 307–352. Berlin: Walter de Gruyter.

Index

Abhinav Bharat, 120
Acharya Atre. *See* Atre, P. K.
"Ages of Action," 100
"Ages of Renunciation," 100
agonism, 11–12, 24, 62, 109, 189n26, 194n24
ahiṃsā, 106, 108, 215n87
Aiyangar, K. V. Ramaswamy, 53
Akbar, Mughal king, 76
Akbarnāma, 76
Al-Biruni, 75
Alfassa, Mirra ("The Mother"), 88, 93
Alipore bomb case, 87, 94
Alter, Joseph, 108, 141, 158
amarolī mudrā, 167
Ambedkar, B. R., 19, 83, 108, 111, 216–217n118, 217n132, 217n136, 224n95; on *Bhagavad Gītā*, 110–116; on Buddha's despair, 110–116; on *karma-yoga*, 110–116
Amṛtakunda, 75
Amṛtasiddhi, 73–74, 210n8
Ānandamaṭh (Chattopadhyay), 84, 212n12
anāsakti-yoga, 102, 104
Annual Administration Report of the Aundh State for the Year 1928–1929, The, 220n32, 223n79
Annual Administration Report of the Aundh State for the Year 1935–1936, The, 223n79, 224n99
anticolonial nationalism, 81–117; and *Bhagavad Gītā*, 93–98, 110–116; and "cult of the bomb," 93–98; and *karma-yoga*, 98–116; political sphere of, 90; Rai, Lala Lajpat, 85–87; yoga as revolution in, 81–117
anti-renunciate yoga, 85–87
ānvīkṣikī, 61, 67–70, 179, 208n130
āpaddharma, 42–44, 179
ariṣaḍvarga, 68
arjuna-viṣāda-yoga, 43
Arnold, Edwin, 82, 86, 104, 212–213n22
art: esoteric, 58; martial, 12, 31, 166; meditative, 166; political, 84–85
artfulness universe, 31
artha, 51–52, 55, 64, 179
Arthaśāstra, 2, 6, 10, 15, 16, 18–19, 24, 66–70, 81, 84, 95, 101, 105, 107, 128, 171, 202n7; ascetics of, 57; modern commentators on, 53; overview, 51–52; translation into English, 54–55; yoga as political strategy in, 49–71; *yoga-kṣema*, 31, 33, 61–62, 66
Aryabhatta, 163, 228n17
Arya Samaj, 85
āsanas (body positions), 1–2, 133, 135, 148, 221–222n55, 228n12
ascetics, 56–59, 81; apostate, 204n43; female, 202n8; martial, 173; phony, 205n57; warrior, 76, 84
Ashtanga Yoga, 2
aśvamedha, 26, 193n11
atisaṁdhā, 10
Ātmacaritra, 221n44
ātman, 40, 43, 179

INDEX

Philosophy of Renunciation (*nivṛtti*), 98
Phule, Jotirao, 110
Phule, Savitribai, 110
physical education, 161, 163
political activism, 90
political art, 84–85
political theology, 13–15, 204n30; and yoga, 15–16
political theory, yoga as, 3, 10–12
Political Theory of Ancient India (Spellman), 55
Political Violence in Ancient India (Singh), 55
Pollock, Sheldon, 70
postcolonialism, 3
postmodernism, 3
poststructuralism, 3
Potter, Karl, 69
power: defined, 7; yoga as instrumentalization of, 6–7
Power Yoga, 2
prāṇāyāma (breathing techniques), 1–2, 87, 134–135, 229–230n42
Prasad, Rajendra, 230n43
premākhyān, 75
Prince, The (Machiavelli), 54
Princely States, 2, 20, 116, 119–120, 123, 133, 148–152, 218n2
psychophysical yoga, 1–2, 5–6, 9, 12, 18–20, 24, 37–41, 52, 56–57, 76, 84, 108, 122, 128, 134–136; *haṭha yoga*, 6; and mind-body problem, 9; modern systems of, 23
public education, 150, 163
public health, 166–173
Pune Pact, 108
Purāṇa literature, 88
Puruṣārth, 124, 220n24
Pūrva Mimāṃsa, 112

Qutban, 75

"radical 'Machiavellianism,'" 55
radical political action, 92
Rahasya-Vivecan arthāt Gītece Karmayogapar Nirūpaṇ, 98
Rai, Lala Lajpat, 19, 83, 85–87, 100, 104, 212n17; anti-renunciate yoga, 85–87
rājadharma, 42–44
rājarṣi, 68, 105, 182
Raja Yoga (Vivekananda), 2, 82
Rajopadhyaye, Hemant, 200n112
Rajwade, V. K., 221–222n55
Raj Yoga, 88
Ramana Maharshi, 139, 140
Ramanujan, A. K., 50
Ramdas, Samartha, 78, 120, 122, 130, 146, 148, 211n27, 219n15
Ramdev, Baba, 164
Ranade, Mahadev Govind, 149
Rangarajan, L. N., 61
Rao, P. V. Narasimha, 162, 168, 230n43
rathya ("charioteers"), 28–29
Razm-nāma, 76
Rebellion/Mutiny of 1857, 84
religion, 83; minorities, 111; and political theology, 13–14; and yoga, 15
"renunciation" (*saṃnyāsa*), 87
Ṛg Veda, 2, 14, 16, 18, 47–48, 171, 188n9, 192n4; making war, 26–31; preparing for war in, 25–26; yoga in, 24–35; *yoga-kṣema*, 31–32
Richardson, Thomas William, 96
Roots of Yoga (Mallinson and Singleton), 18, 73, 187n1
Rothermund, Indira, 139, 141, 218n5, 223n79, 227n139
Rotman, Andy, 197n60
Roy, Kaushik, 217n124
ṛta-yoga, 31, 48

sacrificial rituals, 25
ṣāḍguṇya, 63
Saiva Age, 75
śama, 55, 62–65, 183, 206n99
samādhi (transcendence), 2, 64
saṃdhi, 64
sāṃkhya, 67, 69–70, 171, 197n58, 204n34, 209n156
saṃkhya (calculation), 69
Sāṃkhya (philosophy), 37, 39, 42–43, 67–69, 76, 114, 171, 188n11, 189n16, 197n58, 198n75, 202n10, 208n133
Saṃnyāsī Rebellion, 78, 81, 84, 212n12
Sanatana Dharma, 90
Sanderson, Alexis, 72, 197n60
Sandow, Eugen, 124, 219–220n22
Sanskrit, 3–5, 9–10, 189n21; use in study of yoga, 13
śānti, 41, 43, 73, 183
Sarkar, Sumit, 93–94, 214n57
Sartori, Andrew, 214n55
sāṣṭāṅga namaskār, 122, 124, 129, 134, 219n15, 220n24
śāstra, 51, 70, 183, 202n6
Satara Conspiracy Case, 120
Satavlekar, S. D., 225n107
śatru, 65

transitive property of yoga, 28–29, 34
Trautmann, Thomas, 203n12, 203n22
trayī, 61, 68
Truschke, Audrey, 76
Trust for the Promotion of Yoga, 167
Tukaram, 100

udāsthita, 58
ud-yoga, 199n104
United Nations General Assembly, 91, 165
"Untouchables," 225n107. *See also* Dalits
Upaniṣad literature, 88
upaniṣad-yoga, 56
U.S. popular cultures, 15

vaiśya, 111
vāja, 31
Vajpayee, Atal Bihari, 163, 168
Vande Mataram ("I Praise You, Mother"), 84
vāṇija, 58
varṇa-caste typology, 111
vārttā, 61, 68
vāruṇa-yoga, 60
vedavid, 59
"Vedic Karma Yoga," 99
Vedic sacrifice, 25, 27, 30–31, 34
vegetarian ethics, 103
Verdon, Noémie, 75
vidyā, 68
vijigīṣu, 10
village democracy, 141
vinayamūla, 61
vinyāsa method, 221–222n55
Vinyasa Yoga, 2
viṣāda-yoga, 114, 116
Vishwayatan Yoga Ashram, 167
viśvāsa, 64
vṛttikāma, 58
vṛttikṣīṇa, 58
vyañjana, 58
vyāyāma (exercise), 63–65, 133, 206n99, 221–222n55

Walden Pond, 36
warrior ascetics, 76, 84
Weber, Max, 13, 54–55
Western esoteric practices, 82
Whitaker, Jarrod, 192n8
White, David Gordon, 56, 202n8
Whitman, Walt, 82, 211n6
Witzel, Michael, 192n8

yoga: as apprehension, 67–70; and *Bhagavad Gītā*, 93–98; and bomb, 93–98; bureaucratic infrastructure for education, 160–166; defined, 7; dialectical, 8–9; disciplines and fields, 13–17; on film, 125–131; infrastructure for public health, 166–173; infrastructure in bureaucracy, 159–173; intramural, 7–8; overview, 1, 3–5; philosophical, 1; as political art, 84–85; as political strategy in *Arthaśāstra*, 49–71; as political theory and practice, 3, 10–12; and power, 6–7; as revolution in anticolonial nationalism, 81–117; in *Ṛg Veda*, 24–35; as sovereignty in Princely India, 118–158; and Surya Namaskar, 121–125; three spheres of, 3; updated three spheres of, 172; transitive, 5–7; as war and peace in, 23–48
yoga-abhyās, 138
"Yoga and Its Objects, The," 95
yoga-āsana, 138
yogābhyās, 134
yoga-darśana, 56
yogād ātmavatteti, 68
Yoga Institute of Santa Cruz, 161
yoga-kṣema, 19, 31–33, 44, 47, 49–50, 107, 110, 200n110, 200n111, 201n116; *Arthaśāstra*, 31, 33; as aim of politics, 60–67; *Bhagavad Gītā*, 33, 45–46, 206n87; defined, 55, 66; ideals of, 74; *Mahābhārata*, 31, 33, 45; *Ṛg Veda*, 31–33
yoga-kṣema-sādhana, 68
Yoga Makaranda (Krishnamacharya), 125, 147–148, 220n30
yogam ātiṣṭha, 40
"Yoga of Non-Attachment, The," 102
"Yoga Pamphlets," 94
yogapuruṣa, 59, 95
yogaśāstra, 39, 40
yogaś citta-vṛtti-nirodhaḥ, 23
yogāśrama, 88, 156
Yoga Sūtras (Patanjali), 2, 23, 67–68, 75, 135, 171, 187n2
yoga-vṛtta, 60
Yog Darshan, 85
Yogendra, Shri, 161
yogeśvara, 40
Yogi Adityanath, 164
"yogic detachment," 81
yogis, 81, 84, 211n3
"Yogi Sadhana," 94
yogya vyāyām, 223n66
yoke, 4, 6, 188n9